FOREWORD BY DR. JOHN C. LOWE

RECOVERING WITH T3

My Journey from Hypothyroidism to Good Health Using the T3 Thyroid Hormone

PAUL ROBINSON

The information provided in *RECOVERING WITH T3 My Journey from Hypothyroidism to Good Health Using the T3 Thyroid Hormone* is for educational purposes only. This book is not meant to provide directions for the treatment of any individual. This book is not intended to replace the care by a qualified, licensed and competent medical professional. Care by a medical professional may be necessary to meet the unique needs of an individual patient. The author and publisher are clear that this book does not in <u>any</u> way represent the practice of medicine.

The author, publisher and others involved in the production and publication of this book do <u>not</u> recommend that readers alter their treatment that has been created for them by their own doctor or other health care professionals without individualised and clear guidance from these health care professionals.

Neither the author, publisher, nor any medical or health practitioners or researchers mentioned, nor any other parties involved in the preparation or publication of this book warrant that the information contained in this book is indicated, applicable, effective or safe in any individual case.

The author, publisher and others involved in the preparation or publication of this book disclaims any liability resulting directly or indirectly from the use of the information contained in this book. A qualified doctor should supervise in <u>all</u> matters relevant to physical or mental health.

Every effort has been made to make this book as complete and accurate as possible. However, there may be mistakes, both typographical and in content. Therefore, this book should be read as a record of the author's personal experience and <u>not</u> as a source of information on thyroid or any related health issues. Furthermore, this book contains information that is current only up to the date of publishing.

First published by Elephant in the Room Books 2011

ISBN: 978-0-9570993-0-2

To my wife Karen and my sons, Tom and Josh.

Acknowledgements

Janie A. Bowthorpe - for providing me with honest feedback on the quality of my writing in my original short essay.

Dr. C.M. Dayan - for being the most helpful and most approachable endocrinologist I have encountered, for trying to help me at times when things appeared confusing and most of all, for being committed to uncovering the truth through relevant thyroid medical research.

Dr. Barry Durrant-Peatfield - I will always be thankful for Dr. Peatfield's kindness, patience and good humour and for the lifebelt that he threw to me, in the form of T3. Dr. Peatfield rescued me and I was able to begin to work on my recovery.

Jim Harwood - for helping me clarify the correct terminology regarding thyroid laboratory reference ranges and encouraging me to eliminate any use of the highly misleading 'normal range'.

Dr. R. Kennedy - for being, without doubt, one of the kindest, most sympathetic and most encouraging family doctors I could ever have wished to have.

Dr. John C. Lowe - for writing *The Metabolic Treatment of Fibromyalgia*, which was the first book I read that had a scientific basis that was consistent with what I believed my own problems with T4 replacement therapy actually were. I was already on T3 replacement therapy and had regained my health by the time I bought and read this book. After I'd read it, for this first time in over ten years, I felt relieved that I really did understand what had gone wrong within my body. This was a massive turning point for me. I am also indebted to Dr. Lowe for reviewing this book and writing the foreword.

Lyn Mynott - for making the initial introduction on my behalf to Dr. John C. Lowe. Lyn has worked hard for many years as chairperson of Thyroid UK.

Bob Orme - for kindly providing me with information regarding the importance of magnesium to everyone and especially to thyroid patients.

Sheila Turner - for final proof reading and encouraging me when I really needed it. Sheila has dedicated many years of her life to helping thyroid patients and yet she still managed to find time to help me. Sheila works on behalf of Thyroid Patient Advocacy in the UK.

Thyroid Patients and family members - Alexandrina, Caroline, David, Dawn, Deborah, Diane, Jeannine, Laura, Lynn, Natasha, Sally and Sandra who reviewed and suggested improvements to this book at various stages in its development. You all helped to give me the confidence to see this project through.

Please note that Dr. C.M. Dayan, Dr. Barry Durrant-Peatfield and Dr. R. Kennedy have not reviewed this book prior to publication and so their inclusion in the acknowledgements does not constitute their endorsement of any of the information that is contained herein.

Contents

Foreword

Paul Robinson and I have not yet met face-to-face. Nonetheless, I feel that I know him well, and I feel a kinship with him. He and I have communicated extensively, and I have read this book, *Recovering with T₃*, cover to cover. I was delighted to read in his book the similarities of his and my experiences in recovering with T_3. Virtually all that he writes on the topic rings true when I reflect on my personal experiences with T_3 and my twenty-five years of clinical work treating patients with T_3. In addition, I respect Paul's sound problem-solving abilities and the superb discourse in his book. For all these reasons, I asked him to allow me to write this Foreword to his book.

As I indicated, in Paul's and my own route to recovery, we had similar experiences. Those experiences led us to good health and well-being. Following those routes, we first accepted the falsehood that T_4 replacement is the be-all and end-all in thyroid hormone therapy. It failed us both, however. We next tried T_4/T_3 therapy. But we found that it, too, failed us. And then, through diligent study and straight thinking, we both tried synthetic T_3 alone. This worked for both of us, and it did so safely and effectively. Paul and I are not alone in this series of experiences. I have worked with hundreds of patients who fruitlessly used every other available approach to thyroid hormone therapy, only to find in the end that only T_3 safely and fully restored their health.

In *Recovering with T₃*, Paul describes the onset of his illness and his route back to good health. In his description, it's obvious to me that he and I have something else in common. He has a skill set from a career in research and development that is similar to mine, although we differ in professional fields. That we were in different fields does not matter; effective problem solving is a matter of exercising the rules of logic, which are the steps to effective problem solving no matter what the field of endeavor. Both he and I used this skill set to find T_3 therapy as the thyroid hormone treatment that gave us good health and wellbeing. In telling his story and explaining how he has used T_3 therapy, he has applied his sound reasoning. As part of that skill, he obviously has exercised conscientious observation, good faith, and dependability in reporting the available evidence. These qualities so clearly displayed in *Recovering with T₃* make the book an exemplary learning tool for both patients and clinicians.

Clinicians, scientists, engineers, and all other problem-solving people generally disagree on certain points in their common fields of study. This, of course, is also true of Paul and me in regard to T_3 therapy. These points of differing opinions, however, can be of little or no practical consequence. Our main point of disagreement is that, from personal experience, he believes that optimal benefits from T_3 therapy come from taking the hormone in divided daily doses. For me, once per day has worked well for some twenty-five years. As I said, though, this is of little or no practical importance, as long as one effectively absorbs the daily dose of T_3 from the gastrointestinal tract into the blood.

What is of practical importance is this: Paul Robinson has written a book chock-full of information on T_3 that is *vitally* important to many people. Those people are ones who have too little thyroid hormone regulation but have failed—as he and I did—to benefit from T_4 alone and T_4/T_3 therapies. The information in the book may not only be health-recovering for many people—it may in fact be life saving.

In the late 1990s, studies by my research team at the Fibromyalgia Research Foundation (in affiliation with Baylor Medical College and the Texas Health Science Center) showed in double-blind, placebo-controlled, crossover studies how vitally important T_3 treatment is for some patients. Recently, researchers at other institutions (Stanford Medical College and the National Institute of Health) have begun to investigate T_3 therapy for what we have long called "fibromyalgia" (FMS) and "chronic fatigue syndrome" (CFS). These studies may confirm what my research team found: that T_3 alone is the *only* thyroid hormone therapy that relieves their supposed FMS or CFS, which actually turned out to be symptoms from too little thyroid hormone regulation.

Research, of course, is our most reliable way of learning what is likely to be true or false. I have learned over the years, though, that most patients trust the reported experiences of other patients over research reports. Both Paul Robinson and I have been patients; as such, we learned a fact of great importance that I intentionally repeat for emphasis: T_3 therapy is the *only* thyroid hormone therapy that works for many people.

I believe that reading *Recovering with T_3* will be a splendid experience for thousands of people, whether clinicians, patients, patient advocates, or patients' loved ones. His prose is not in the stilted style of many modern books on health; instead, it is peppered with unique figures of speech and is a truly delightful and informative read. Most important, though, I believe readers will enjoy and value Paul's book for another reason: the importance of the information he provides for those who are inquisitive about what gave him and me the gift of good health— the thyroid hormone we call "T_3."

Dr. John C. Lowe
Editor-in-Chief: *Thyroid Science*
Director of Research: Fibromyalgia Research Foundation

SECTION 1

INTRODUCTORY INFORMATION

Chapter 1

Introduction

I did not want to write this book. I am not a writer and writing was never a critical part of my working life. Neither am I a doctor, a medical researcher or a biochemist. I am simply a man who had his life derailed by thyroid disease and suffered for many years whilst on an ineffective thyroid hormone treatment. Eventually managing to recover my health through research, determination and trying other treatments, my life was forever altered in the process.

The critical part of my recovery involved the use of a currently, rarely prescribed thyroid hormone, known most often by its simplified name - T3. The correct name of this naturally produced hormone is *triiodothyronine* and its synthetic equivalent is known as *liothyronine*. It is the biologically active form of thyroid hormone, hereafter referred to as T3 - because it's a lot easier.

Had my family doctor not encouraged me to write about my twenty years of experience with thyroid disease, I would not have considered writing this book. She is retired now but she provided me with wonderful and unfaltering support whilst I was trying to develop an effective, safe and stable thyroid hormone replacement regime using T3.

Originally I thought that I would be able to produce a short article that covered my experience of thyroid disease and the important facts and techniques I required in order to use T3 successfully. However, as I began to work on this I soon came to realise how much information there was to convey and I reluctantly began to consider writing a book.

Why is it important to communicate my experience of using T3?

The majority of patients who are diagnosed with hypothyroidism are prescribed a synthetic version of the thyroid hormone thyroxine and we are led to believe that this resolves the patient's symptoms. Natural thyroxine produced by the thyroid is often known as T4, because it contains four iodine atoms. When produced as a tablet by a pharmaceutical company it may be referred to as synthetic T4, levothyroxine or a brand name. T4 replacement therapy often does succeed in alleviating the symptoms of patients. However, the assumption that T4 replacement therapy is successful for most or all patients is increasingly becoming more suspect. The doubts are arising for two reasons.

Firstly, more and more patients are coming forward and sharing their stories of the failure of synthetic T4 to resolve their symptoms. The advent of Internet forums has been very important in allowing vast numbers of disenchanted and despairing patients to come together to exchange stories and gather clues that might aid them in recovering their health. On a purely anecdotal level, I have always asked local people that use synthetic T4 what their experience has been with it. I am yet to talk to anyone who is totally satisfied that they feel as well as they did before the onset of their thyroid problems and the majority I have spoken to have some remaining symptoms of hypothyroidism.

The second source of increasing doubt about the effectiveness of synthetic T4 is that very slowly but surely, medical research is delivering findings that indicate that this treatment does not work well for some patients, that thyroid blood test results can be misleading and that some patients, who do not recover on synthetic T4, may require additional or alternative thyroid hormones prescribed in order to get well.

I have no doubt that many patients feel well on synthetic T4. It may be that the majority of patients who receive synthetic T4 feel reasonably well. The percentages do not concern me. My concern is for the large number of patients who clearly do not feel well on T4 replacement.

In my own case, T4 treatment utterly failed to resolve my symptoms and I continued to experience an extremely poor quality of life as a result. This went on for many years regardless of the dosage of synthetic T4 prescribed. For a long time I thought that mine was a rare case and this was enforced by the responses that I received from the medical profession.

I have since discovered that my experience with T4 replacement therapy is not unusual or rare at all. Because of books, Internet articles, medical research and my involvement with Internet forums, I now know that many thyroid patients all over the world have had, or are currently having, severe problems with their T4 treatment.

It was only after I received a carefully designed, full replacement dosage of T3 that my symptoms disappeared and I returned to full health.

The impact of incorrectly treated hypothyroidism

Unfortunately, by the time that I was on the right treatment, a considerable amount of what I can only describe as devastation had already been unleashed on my life. The ripples of this went well beyond me and affected other family members. I will not dwell on this aspect extensively in this book but some elements have to be mentioned, as it is important for doctors to realise that the consequences of thyroid treatment that leaves symptoms unresolved, go far beyond the individual patient.

I had been developing a successful career prior to the onset of thyroid disease but this was totally destroyed. My career was ripped away through this illness and through the T4 treatment that simply did not address my symptoms. More importantly, I had a toddler and a young baby at the time of my diagnosis. For many years on T4 treatment I felt very ill indeed. I had no patience with my children when I needed to have the greatest levels of patience. I had no time to provide two bright, demanding boys with the stimulation and attention that they needed from a father. I was irritable and often quick tempered. I was a poor father to both of them at that time. This was a direct consequence of thyroid disease and a treatment that did not resolve my symptoms but simply made my thyroid blood tests appear normal. This is no consolation to me. It removes none of the guilt from me that I will always carry. My relationship with my eldest son was damaged and I am still in the process of trying to repair this. Our relationship is a lot better now and I hope it will continue to improve. But there are memories and pain inside both of us that will always be there. I will never, ever think about thyroid disease without also thinking of the emotional damage that it can cause.

The human consequences of not resolving patients' symptoms adequately can be huge, especially with an illness like this, as it affects so many of the body's systems. Much of the damage that is done by thyroid disease may happen beyond the patient and is not visible in the doctor's consultation room. I lost what I consider to be very important years of my life. These were the years where I should have been a good father and been engaged in a satisfying and productive career.

One of my largest concerns is that progress in the treatment of thyroid disease in the past twenty years, since I was first diagnosed, appears to have been dreadfully slow. In some countries there have been some improvements in treatment options that are being offered to patients who do not recover on synthetic T4 alone. However, in many countries, including the UK, there appears to have been little change. This is an extremely sad and depressing state of affairs, especially since there are several excellent alternative treatments available.

When I consider the impact of this slow progress, I think of the human consequences. I have spent a considerable amount of time over the past several years on Internet forums dedicated to thyroid patients, listening to their often heart breaking stories. Because of this, I am now far more aware of how thyroid disease has affected the lives of many people. Some men and women find it difficult to cope with their young children and homes. In some cases relationships between patients and their partners are strained to breaking point. Many of these patients have had to reduce their working hours, or have lost their jobs and have no way of getting back to work. Some are having financial problems. Some have also been 'labelled' by their own doctor or family as having depression, psychological problems or just not being able to cope with life. This is a dreadful condition and it upsets me to see the same kinds of things happening to patients today that happened to me so many years ago.

Continuing lack of good information on T3

Let me now briefly discuss T3 itself. Many people, doctors included, think that T3 won't work properly as a long-term treatment for hypothyroidism. A lot of doctors and patients think that T3 is dangerous and can't be used safely. Some doctors think T3 causes heart attacks or heart palpitations. Many doctors think that patients need to take synthetic T4 and that it is not healthy to have little or no T4 in the body. Very few doctors consider T3 as a serious treatment option for hypothyroidism. I hope to dispel these myths and misrepresentations. Certainly, only a few enlightened doctors consider T3 as an ideal potential treatment for patients that have not responded to any form of T4 replacement therapy. Hardly anyone has considered the use of T3 as a potential treatment for other conditions that involve a low metabolic rate. These conditions include chronic fatigue syndrome, myalgic encephalopathy (ME) and fibromyalgia.

Medical training practices relating to the treatment of hypothyroidism are continuing to perpetuate two strong beliefs, which I believe are a major problem for thyroid patients today.

Firstly, there is the belief that T4 replacement therapy always works and is the only appropriate treatment for patients with low thyroid hormone levels. This is clearly flawed because I have spoken to too many patients now that have spent many years on T4 replacement therapy and who still feel ill. In a lot of cases, synthetic T4 simply does not make the patient feel well again. What is in no doubt to me and to a growing body of dissatisfied patients, is that T4 treatment is not guaranteed to eradicate the symptoms of hypothyroidism, regardless of what effect the treatment has on thyroid hormone levels in the bloodstream evident in thyroid blood test results.

Secondly, there is the belief that thyroid blood test results may be relied upon to determine whether a patient has been adequately treated or not. Doctors run thyroid blood tests to determine the levels of various thyroid hormones in the bloodstream. In the case of hypothyroidism, the patient is given T4 replacement therapy and thyroid blood test results are used to determine when the treatment is deemed to be successful. For some patients, when this point of supposedly successful treatment is arrived at, the patient may still have some, or all, of the symptoms that they first walked into the doctor's office with. However, the doctor may have correctly followed the standard procedure used to treat this illness and may be convinced that the patient's thyroid hormone levels are now normal.

In fact, many doctors are so focused on thyroid blood test results that they don't put equal effort into assessing their patient's symptoms and gauging whether there has been any significant response to T4 treatment (such was the emphasis on thyroid blood tests in their training rather than the presenting symptoms of the patient). I hear many complaints on Internet forums about doctors and endocrinologists. However, the issue really lies in the fundamental policies that drive medical training practices.

Over the past twenty to thirty years there have been a number of very important medical research papers that have been published. Issues have been highlighted with the current standard T4 replacement therapy. This research has not appeared to make any difference to the treatment protocol for hypothyroidism in all but a few countries where change does appear to be occurring very slowly. Unfortunately, the UK is not one of these countries. Of course there are a few doctors and endocrinologists across the UK who are more enlightened and I welcome this and am grateful for the work that they do. There are just too few of these doctors.

In my case, I found that I had to use T3, entirely on its own, in order to resolve my symptoms. I had to stop using T4 completely. However, once I was on the correct dosage of T3, I did regain my health and my symptoms associated with hypothyroidism disappeared. I know that if used correctly, T3 is perfectly safe and can provide a highly effective and stable long-term thyroid hormone replacement and I intend to provide information to support this view. Once some of the physiological facts about T3 are understood and some of the basic pitfalls are made clear, then using T3 for full thyroid hormone replacement is quite a practical proposition, as I hope this book will make clear.

This relatively unknown, barely used, frequently misunderstood and much maligned thyroid hormone, is critical to life itself and should be one of the treatments available to all doctors for cases of hypothyroidism that have not responded to T4 replacement therapy or combined T4/T3 treatment.

When I began to use T3 I searched extensively for knowledge and information on how to use it as a full thyroid hormone replacement therapy. I found almost no information about the practicalities of T3 use. The few examples I did find were wholly inadequate and did not prepare me for some of the difficulties I would face when using this hormone. Some of the important information that I needed to know about the use of T3 could only be acquired through actual use and through small experiments that I performed upon myself. It took me several years to fully grasp the important lessons that I needed to be aware of prior to commencing a trial with T3. Given what I know now about using T3, I could easily have determined my own T3 dosage within several months. This is not a significantly dissimilar time to arrive at a stable T4 dosage, but the process is entirely different and does require careful consideration, as it is more complex than T4 dosage management.

T3 replacement therapy should only be used after all other forms of thyroid hormone replacement have been exhausted. However, if a patient is still suffering with the symptoms associated with hypothyroidism, after all due care and attention has been given to other forms of thyroid hormone replacement, then I have no doubt that working under the supervision of a family doctor or endocrinologist that it is possible to use T3 safely, effectively and in an organised manner.

Someone said to me recently that no thyroid treatment is a silver bullet. Over the past several years I have been fortunate to witness many people make a complete recovery using T3, after years, or decades in some cases, of ill health on other forms of thyroid replacement. I believe that T3 is the closest treatment we actually have to a silver bullet. Unfortunately, hardly anyone is aware of this, because in most cases when T3 is prescribed it is not used optimally and alongside appropriate nutritional support. Therefore, the power of this wonderful thyroid hormone is never realised.

Although there are plenty of excellent books on hypothyroidism, T4 and T4/T3 thyroid hormone replacement, there aren't any that have their main focus on the practical use of T3 in the treatment of hypothyroidism. There are also some excellent Internet websites that contain key pieces of information regarding the use of T3 but even these are not comprehensive.

Technical Content

Some parts of *Recovering with T3* are quite complicated. This is because the nature of what is being written about is inherently complex. I have done my best to explain everything as clearly as possible but I have chosen to communicate virtually all my accumulated knowledge and wisdom in the hope that it can benefit others. I could have made the book less detailed but then its usefulness would also have diminished. *Recovering with T3* should become a resource that readers continue to come back to month after month and year after year, such is the level of information contained within it.

Some hopes looking forward

The above should explain my motivation for documenting my experience of using T3. In truth, despite my initial reluctance, I simply had to write this book. I have been compelled to write it, even though I would rather have spent my time in other ways. The information demands to be communicated.

There are many topics that are relevant to the effectiveness of thyroid hormone that I am either not going to cover at all, or will barely touch the surface of. This is because there are already excellent sources of information on these. My focus will be on the practical aspects of how I used T3 as a long-term thyroid hormone replacement and on insights and experience relating to the safe and systematic use of the T3 thyroid hormone. I am going to relate the story of how I became ill and how I recovered through the use of T3 and I will share the information and practical lessons that I have learnt over the years. My hope is that open minded doctors, who have patients who are desperate to get well but have failed to do so using T4 replacement therapy, may find this book of some value.

T3 is a potent thyroid hormone that needs to be used cautiously and in an organised manner. In order to do this most effectively, I believe that T3 replacement therapy should be prescribed and managed by family doctors and endocrinologists. I am no great fan of self-medication. My view is that, in the interests of patients, the medical profession need to embrace T3 replacement therapy and T4/T3 based treatment and provide trials of these to those patients that have not regained their health with synthetic T4. I believe that this is by far the best way to provide the improvement in thyroid treatment that patients so desperately require. So, I hope that some doctors do take the time to read this.

At the present time, it is often only those patients who are determined, resourceful and financially able that can eventually find an appropriate thyroid treatment other than synthetic T4. This is not how it should be. Effective thyroid treatment should be available to all thyroid patients. To achieve this, change must come from within the medical profession. I am hoping that my personal experience of using T3 will allay fears and encourage more doctors to conduct trials of T3 with those patients that have failed to recover with any other form of thyroid treatment. However, there does appear to be a great deal of reluctance to make any changes in the methods used in the diagnosis and treatment of thyroid disease.

Increasing numbers of doctors and patients are finding success with a variety of thyroid hormone replacement therapies other than synthetic T4. However, there is still strong resistance to these treatments from many in the medical profession. Whether that is down to lack of information, poor communication of relevant research, resistance to change or the strong belief that only synthetic T4 is required, I do not know. I also have the rather cynical view that many pharmaceutical companies, whose balance sheets depend upon the sales of synthetic T4, may be partly responsible for some of this resistance.

There are many examples from history where changes in areas of science or medicine were slow to occur due to the inertia of the day. A classic example of this is when Galileo Galilei, the famous astronomer, proved conclusively that the Earth was not at the centre of the known universe. Many scholars understood immediately that he was right but it took over a hundred years for Galileo's view to gain wide acceptance, such was the resistance from the Catholic Church at the time. In reality, it took the death and retirement from public life of the 'old guard' before Galileo's work was accepted. Thyroid patients who remain unwell on T4 treatment cannot wait for history to repeat itself.

If any doctors read this book, then I beg them to read the entire book before forming any conclusions. If the plight of thyroid patients, who do not regain their health on synthetic T4, is to be improved, then it is critical that more doctors are prepared to offer trials of alternative thyroid hormone treatments including T3. It is very important that this is acted upon soon, in order to reduce the number of women and men who are condemned to the cold embrace of low thyroid symptoms for the rest of their lives.

My background and a few words of caution

My background is in science. I initially began studying physics but part way through my university degree I realised that I was far more interested in the burgeoning computer industry. Consequently, I changed my degree course and studied computer science. My working life was focused on the development and management of a variety of large computer software projects and computer sub-systems. I eventually managed research and development areas, which included software and electronics design. I also spent several years in applied research investigating new technology. It is clear from this that I am **not** a doctor and have had no medical training. What I do have is logical deduction, systematic problem solving and an ability to understand technical information.

I do use the word 'patient' extensively throughout the book. When I use this term I always mean that this is a 'thyroid patient' just as I have been a thyroid patient. I never mean that this is a patient of mine - because I have none.

This book was written in order to document my own experience in the hope that the medical profession will take some of this on board. I do not believe that this book can in any way replace the relationship between a patient and their doctor. I also do not recommend that any patient changes any of their current treatment based on reading this book. Any changes to a patient's medications or supplements should only be done under the supervision of the patient's own doctor, with their doctor's support for any changes and with proper medical supervision thereafter.

I am not proposing that anyone applies any of the information, methods or suggestions contained within this book. A qualified doctor should supervise any course of treatment involving thyroid hormones, other hormones, prescription medicines, vitamins, minerals, or food supplements. If someone attempts to apply any of the information described in this book then I can take no responsibility for any consequences of this. My intention is to document my own experience of thyroid disease and how the T3 thyroid hormone helped me to regain my health. I am hoping that the medical profession will begin to consider the use of T3 as more mainstream and valuable thyroid medication than it appears to do at the present time.

Chapter 2

The Thyroid Gland and Hypothyroidism

The thyroid gland is one of several glands that are collectively referred to as the endocrine system. The thyroid gland is located at the front of the neck just below the Adam's apple. It has two lobes and the gland is butterfly shaped. The thyroid gland controls the metabolic rate of all the tissues of the body.

Metabolic rate means the rate at which the cells produce and consume energy and therefore, the thyroid gland is in charge of energy regulation in every cell of our body. This encompasses almost every physiological process in the body, including growth and development, metabolism, body temperature, and heart rate.

Throughout this book I use the terms 'tissues' and 'cells' quite frequently. These terms are equivalent and I use both just for variety.

Thyroid hormone production is controlled by the pituitary gland, which in turn is controlled by the hypothalamus. The pituitary gland is an endocrine gland about the size of a pea in humans that is a protrusion from the bottom of the hypothalamus at the base of the brain. The hypothalamus is a portion of the brain that is located just above the brain stem and is about the size of an almond in humans.

The pituitary gland produces thyroid-stimulating hormone (also known as TSH). TSH then stimulates the thyroid gland in order for it to secrete thyroxine (abbreviated to T4) and a very small amount of triiodothyronine (also known as T3). Thyroxine and triiodothyronine are the natural forms of the T4 and T3 thyroid hormones produced by the thyroid gland, which circulate in the bloodstream.

A significant amount of the circulating T4 is converted into T3 by the cells in the liver and kidneys. The remaining T4 is converted in the gut and in other peripheral tissues throughout the body. The T3 converted from T4, as well as the relatively small amount of T3 produced by the thyroid gland itself, increases the level of circulating T3 in the bloodstream. Although the thyroid gland does produce some T3, it is thought that around 80% of the circulating T3 is derived from conversion from T4, primarily by the liver and kidneys.

It is essential to understand that it is only the T3 thyroid hormone that is the biologically active thyroid hormone within our cells. T3 can only achieve this biological action, once it is inside the cells. T3 does nothing of any use when it remains in the bloodstream.

Thyroid hormones are similar to fuel in a car. Without enough fuel, a car's engine cannot generate the energy required to move the car. Cells cannot function properly if they are deprived of the right amount of T3 that acts as their fuel. It should be evident from this, just how critical thyroid hormones are in optimising our metabolism, so that we can stay alive and feel well.

Let us briefly look again at the control mechanism for the thyroid gland. The level of production of TSH by the pituitary gland is controlled by a thyrotropin-releasing hormone (TRH), which is produced in the hypothalamus. The TRH reaches the pituitary gland, which triggers increased TSH production and its release. Somatostatin, which is also produced by the hypothalamus, has the opposite effect on the production of TSH, decreasing the rate of its release.

In addition, the levels of T4 and T3 in the bloodstream have an added effect on the release of TSH by the pituitary. When the levels of T4 and T3 in the bloodstream are low, the production of TSH is increased. Equally, when levels of T4 and T3 are high then TSH production is decreased. This effect creates a regulatory negative feedback loop as the TSH signals to the thyroid that lower levels of T4 and T3 are required.

The thyroid gland also produces a hormone called calcitonin, which plays a significant role in calcium homeostasis.

So, the above is all fine and dandy when everything is working correctly. Let us now begin to consider a situation where things have gone wrong.

HYPOTHYROIDISM

The most concise definition of hypothyroidism is that the body does not have enough T4 and T3. Some of the main symptoms associated with hypothyroidism include:

- Feeling cold.
- Low body temperature.
- Reduced sweating.
- Myxoedema (swollen skin especially on the face, eyelids, upper arms and hands).
- Weak muscles.
- Muscular cramps or pain.
- Joint pain.
- Fatigue/tiredness.
- Slow movement.
- Constipation.
- Depression.
- Thin, brittle, cracked fingernails.

- Coarse hair.
- Hair loss.
- Dry, coarse, itchy skin.
- Acne and skin infections.
- Pale skin.
- Weight gain.
- Water retention.
- Low heart rate (lower than sixty beats per minute).
- Heart palpitations.
- Changes in voice (slower, rougher).
- Swollen tongue.
- Abnormal or painful menstrual cycles.
- Poor memory.
- Impaired thinking ability (brain fog).
- Lack of concentration.
- Headaches.
- Sluggish reflexes.
- Anaemia.
- Swallowing problems.
- Loss of appetite.
- Shortness of breath, laboured breathing.
- Need for more sleep than normal.
- Decreased libido.
- Irritability, mood swings.

Myxoedema is common in severely hypothyroid patients and it is caused by mucin, which is a glue-like substance that fills parts of the skin. If myxoedema is present then it is often difficult to slightly lift up areas of the skin, using the thumb and forefinger. The presence of this particular clinical feature, combined with a low body temperature and any of the other more common symptoms listed above, used to be the main method of diagnosing hypothyroidism prior to the advent of thyroid blood tests.

Primary hypothyroidism, where the thyroid gland fails to produce enough T4 and T3, is the most common type of hypothyroidism and the patient is therefore said to have an under-active thyroid.

Secondary hypothyroidism is less common and occurs if the pituitary gland itself fails to produce enough TSH. This condition is called secondary hypothyroidism.

Tertiary hypothyroidism is due to a fault within the hypothalamus gland.

Secondary and tertiary hypothyroidism may be collectively referred to as *central hypothyroidism*.

Diagnosis of hypothyroidism

Primary hypothyroidism is usually detected when numerous symptoms begin to appear, which prompt the patient to seek medical advice. As the thyroid gland is no longer able to adequately respond to the demand of TSH, this usually results in lower than normal levels of T4 and T3 appearing in thyroid blood test results. In addition, TSH levels are often higher than normal. This is because the pituitary gland is attempting to stimulate more thyroid hormone production by releasing more TSH. One of the most common causes of primary hypothyroidism is an autoimmune disease known as Hashimoto's thyroiditis or Hashimoto's disease. This is when the immune system attacks the thyroid gland with autoantibodies and gradually destroys it.

Treatment for hypothyroidism

When the patient seeks medical advice it is common for a blood test to be performed to measure the level of the patient's TSH. Some well-informed doctors will run a more comprehensive blood test that includes TSH, thyroid hormones as well as thyroid autoantibodies. Any thyroid patient who has not had the full range of thyroid blood tests performed would be well advised to do so, because the results from these will provide a far more complete picture of their thyroid condition than is possible from the TSH alone.

The most common treatment available for primary hypothyroidism is to provide a once daily amount of synthetic T4 medication in tablet form. Synthetic T4 is sometimes referred to as levothyroxine or L-thyroxine. It's actual chemical name is 3,5,3',5'-tetraiodo-L-thyronine but I prefer to call it synthetic T4. It is called T4 because its molecular structure has four iodine atoms within it, unlike T3, which has only three iodine atoms. Common brand names for T4 include L-thyroxine, Eltroxin and Thyrax in Europe, Eutirox, Tirosint, Levoxyl, Unithroid and Synthroid in North America. There are also numerous generic versions and some of these are referred to as levothyroxine.

The standard protocol for thyroid hormone replacement is to slowly increase the dosage of synthetic T4 until the TSH level decreases back into the laboratory reference range as determined by a thyroid blood test. The patient will usually require T4 replacement therapy for life. Other available forms of thyroid hormone replacement will be discussed later.

To avoid any ambiguity with naturally produced T4, the term *synthetic T4* will be used from now on when the replacement medication is referred to, rather than referring to any particular brand of tablet. When *T4 replacement*, *T4 replacement therapy*, *T4 treatment*, or *T4 dosage* are used within the book, this implicitly means the use of synthetic T4, unless otherwise stated.

There is no naturally produced T3 that exists as a medication containing only T3. Therefore, any reference to T3 medication implicitly means synthetic T3.

When referring to T4 or T3 within the bloodstream or cells, it is not possible, or necessary, to identify whether the hormones came from medication or from a thyroid gland, so in this context only *T4* or *T3* will be used.

Alternative treatments and focus of this book

As already mentioned, there are growing numbers of patients who are extremely dissatisfied with T4 treatment, because they have found that their symptoms have not been adequately addressed by it. I intend to discuss the false belief that synthetic T4 is always successful and should always be used.

I will spend very little time discussing the merits of the alternative protocols that typically use either natural desiccated thyroid preparations or synthetic T4 combined with T3. Despite having had some experience of being treated with natural thyroid and with a combination of synthetic T4 and T3, I do not consider my knowledge to be great enough in the use of natural thyroid or T4/T3 combinations to attempt to cover these properly. In any case, there are many excellent books that discuss all of these other treatments.[1, 2] Natural thyroid and T4/T3 combinations all have their place. They can be excellent therapies and are often far more successful than the use of synthetic T4 on its own, for some patients.

My primary concern is to communicate to doctors and patients the incredible value that the T3 thyroid hormone can have in those severe cases that have not responded to any form of T4 replacement therapy. I also want to communicate just how I went about using T3 in order to recover my own health.

THYROID BLOOD TESTS

The levels of TSH, T4 and T3 circulating in the bloodstream can all be measured by routine thyroid blood tests. Once hypothyroidism has been diagnosed, adults will usually be given a daily T4 replacement dosage of between 50 and 200 micrograms.

TSH blood tests are usually performed every few weeks at the start of treatment and the T4 dosage is adjusted according to the result. It typically takes six to eight weeks for an increase of synthetic T4 to stabilise in the body, so the blood tests are usually spaced six to eight weeks apart, to allow sufficient time for the new T4 dosage to take full effect. Once the TSH falls to a level that is within the laboratory reference range, it is assumed that the correct amount of synthetic T4 is being prescribed. It is then common practice to check the TSH blood level approximately once a year. However, this standard protocol does not always succeed in resolving patients' symptoms.

Total T4 and free T4 are two separate tests that can help a doctor evaluate thyroid hormone levels in the blood in more detail. The results of the total T4 test are affected by the amount of protein available in the blood to bind to the hormone. The free T4 test is a more recent test that measures the unbound portion of T4, i.e. the T4 that is unaffected by protein levels. Since free T4 is the active form of thyroxine, it is considered to be a more accurate reflection of thyroid hormone function. Free T4 may be written as FT4.

T3 circulates in the blood, with almost all of the T3 bound to carrier proteins. The main transport protein is thyroxine-binding globulin (TBG). Only the free (unbound) portion of T3 is believed to be biologically active. Therefore, it is free T3 that is commonly measured, as it provides a more accurate reflection of the patient's clinical status than the total T3 level. Free T3 may be written as FT3. It is the FT4 and FT3 that enters the cells of the pituitary gland and are used to determine TSH. The hypothalamus controls the pituitary and this too uses FT4 and FT3 to determine its actions.

Typical blood test laboratory reference ranges

A typical TSH reference range for UK laboratories is 0.4–4.5 mU/L.[3] For FT4 the range is 9.0–25 pmol/L.[4] For FT3 the range is 3.5–7.8 nmol/L.[3] However, it is important to note that for a number of reasons, reference ranges may vary in different laboratories. One cause of this is that the reference population studied by each laboratory is likely to have been different.

It is very important to be aware that laboratory reference ranges are simply reference intervals derived statistically and at best they only represent 95% of the population - not the entire population. Therefore, these ranges are actually statistical concepts that cannot be used as absolute cast-in-stone diagnostic or therapeutic ranges. I will discuss this further in Chapter 8.

Many patient groups and some doctors in the USA are convinced that it makes more sense to manage a patient's T4 replacement dosage based on their FT4 and FT3 levels combined with close monitoring of the remaining symptoms.

The concern that many of these patients and doctors have is that TSH is simply a pituitary hormone and, as such, is only very useful in assessing the state of the pituitary. They believe that using the TSH to determine a patient's thyroid hormone replacement level, in preference to the actual levels of FT4 and FT3 and the presenting symptoms of the patient, is a flawed approach.

Thyroid autoantibodies

It is also common practice to test for thyroid autoantibodies. The three most common autoantibody tests are for:

- *Thyroid peroxidase antibody (TPOAb).* Thyroid peroxidase is an enzyme produced in the thyroid that causes iodine to become available during the process of T4 and T3 production within the thyroid gland. These autoantibodies are often extremely high in Hashimoto's thyroiditis. The TPOAb autoantibodies are thought to be cytotoxic to the thyroid cells and high levels of these often precede thyroid gland destruction.

- *Thyroglobulin antibody (TgAb)*. Thyroglobulin is a protein produced and used entirely within the thyroid gland during the production of T4 and T3. These autoantibodies are often raised in Hashimoto's thyroiditis.

- *Thyroid stimulating hormone receptor antibody (TRAb)*. This refers to the receptors in the thyroid gland that respond to the stimulus of TSH from the pituitary gland. These autoantibodies may be raised in Hashimoto's thyroiditis and also in another type of autoimmune thyroid problem that causes high levels of thyroid hormones to be produced (Graves' disease).

Usually a patient's family doctor will determine which of the autoantibodies to test for and how frequently to do the tests, based on the medical history of the patient. It is sensible to test for the presence of autoantibodies when the patient is initially suspected of having thyroid disease.

Unless a patient knows whether they have TPO and/or Tg autoantibodies they won't know if they have Hashimoto's thyroiditis and therefore, they won't know if they should expect further deterioration of their thyroid gland over time. It is highly advantageous for a thyroid patient, who is taking any form of thyroid medication, to understand whether they are likely to require more medication over time.

Any thyroid patient, who does not already know if they have thyroid autoantibodies, may want to insist upon having the TPO and Tg autoantibody tests. The results will help both patient and doctor to understand the nature of their thyroid problem and how it may develop in the future. If Hashimoto's thyroiditis is detected, through raised autoantibodies, then this result will provide the motivation to take measures aimed at calming the immune system and slowing the destruction of the thyroid. I will discuss the possibility of calming the immune system later.

THYROID URINE TESTS

Thyroid urine tests are currently not available on the NHS in the UK. I am not going to make many comments on their usefulness yet, because many health organisations in different countries are still in the process of evaluating thyroid hormone urine tests. Some doctors in the USA believe that thyroid urine tests, which involve a twenty-four hour urine collection, are more sensitive at detecting low levels of thyroid hormones than blood tests. If this proves to be true then thyroid urine tests may be very valuable in detecting previously undiagnosed hypothyroidism.

I will very briefly return to the topic of thyroid urine tests later in the book after more information has been presented.

METABOLISM AND ACTION OF THYROID HORMONES

In order to understand what can go wrong with thyroid hormone metabolism within the body, I need to become a little more technical.

I will continue to use many of the terms mentioned here, as they are useful when describing what may have gone wrong with my health and why the thyroid hormone T3 was so important to me. The information I am about to discuss is quite challenging and contains answers to many of the questions that I asked for a long time. If any reader does not immediately grasp every single aspect of this, please don't worry, pick up what you can and then come back and re-read it at another time.

To help me make this a little clearer, let me provide a very simple block diagram of a typical human cell.

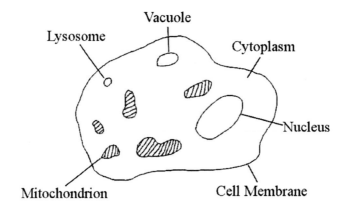

In this simplified cell block-diagram, the cell is completely enclosed by a cell membrane. Inside are the cytoplasm, the nucleus and various other entities that human biologists refer to as organelles.

It is primarily the T3 thyroid hormone that is the biologically active thyroid hormone within our cells. Thyroid hormones have to be within our cells to achieve any effect. Circulating levels of thyroid hormones in the bloodstream are not actively affecting our bodies.

Free T4 and free T3 thyroid hormones pass into the cells through the cell membrane. High-affinity binding proteins in the blood restrict the entrance of T4 into the cells, much more than they do T3. This is because T3 is bound less strongly to these proteins. When discussing T4 and T3 within the cells, I implicitly mean FT4 and FT3, because only *unbound* thyroid hormones may enter cells.

It used to be thought that this movement of thyroid hormones occurred by passive diffusion through the cell membrane. However, during the past twenty or thirty years, it has become clear that thyroid hormones are transported into cells by specific transporter proteins. There is now a growing body of medical research showing that diffusion probably plays a minor role, if any. Several thyroid hormone transporter proteins have recently been identified and some problems have even been identified that can cause issues with thyroid hormone uptake into cells.

Incidentally, cortisol is not directly involved in the process of movement of thyroid hormone into the cells. There is no published medical research that supports the idea that cortisol is directly involved in thyroid hormone transport into cells (sometimes referred to as thyroid hormone take up by cells). Unfortunately, it is all too easy to browse the Internet or Internet forums and come across the myth that cortisol is actively involved in the process of transporting thyroid hormone into our cells. I suspect that as a result of this, more people are taking adrenal hormones than really need to because of the mistaken believe that any thyroid hormone they take won't be able to access their cells unless they raise their cortisol level.

Dr. John C. Lowe specifically suggested that I make this clarification of the role of cortisol regarding thyroid hormone metabolism, as he recognised that some people have been assuming that cortisol has a far more direct role with thyroid hormones than it actually does.

Of course it is possible to view cortisol as being important to thyroid hormone take up into our cells because cortisol is involved in glucose metabolism. Glucose is used by the mitochondria to produce cellular energy. Consequently, with chronically low cortisol levels the mitochondria will not be able to sustain our metabolic rate. However, this argument also applies to many other co-factors that the mitochondria require, e.g. vitamin B1. However, it is important to be very clear that low cortisol levels do not automatically bring down a barrier between thyroid hormone and our cells because cortisol is not directly involved in the process of transporting thyroid hormone into our cells or to the thyroid hormone receptors. The link between cortisol and the effectiveness of thyroid hormone, via the supply of cellular glucose, is further explored in Chapters 3 and 5.

What would be needed to show any closer connection between thyroid hormone uptake and cortisol would be scientific research resulting in experimental evidence that proved the biochemical interaction between thyroid hormone, cortisol and any other necessary agents at the cell membrane (where thyroid hormones enter the cells via transporter proteins) and in the cell nucleus where thyroid hormone binds to its receptors. Right now all that exists is a plethora of publications that assume that this research exists or make inferences based on observations of hormone levels and other measures, which cannot be used to conclude any specific chemical interaction or dependence between thyroid hormone and cortisol at either the cell membrane or nuclear thyroid receptors. This research of course might one day be done and it may be found to be true but for the moment this is not the case.

T4 needs to be converted to T3 to be of use

Once inside the cells, some T4 may be converted into biologically active T3. T4 may be converted to T3 only in those tissues that have high levels of the right type of enzymes present. The enzymes that are involved in the conversion of thyroid hormones to their simpler forms are called collectively the deiodinases. It is through the action of two of these enzymes (D1 and D2 deiodinase) that T4 may be converted to T3. This conversion only occurs in those cells that have the ability to create the necessary deiodinase enzymes.

T4 to T3 conversion mainly occurs within the cells of the liver, kidneys and thyroid, through the action of the D1 deiodinase enzyme, where much of the converted T3 is returned through the cell membranes to circulate in the bloodstream (some bound by carrier protein and some free T3). It is thought that a special type of structure (a type of organelle called an endoplasmic reticulum) is present within liver cells that is specialised and manufactures and contains the D1 deiodinase. Some of this physiology is still subject to research.

The liver also controls how much of the T4 and T3 are bound to protein and how much exists as free T4 and free T3 in the bloodstream.

Around a fifth of the conversion from T4 to T3 occurs within the gastrointestinal tract, but this only happens if the gut is healthy and has the right level of friendly gut bacteria. Some conversion also occurs within the cells of the brain, pituitary, bones, and muscles, through the action of the D2 deiodinase enzyme, where the T3 is used locally and does not re-enter the circulation. T4 to T3 conversion requires adequate amounts of the right deiodinase enzymes and, since these enzymes are heavily dependent on selenium in their construction, it is very important to have adequate levels of selenium in the diet or through supplementation.

The activity of the D1 deiodinase enzyme involved in T4 to T3 conversion within the liver does not occur at a fixed rate. The conversion rate is regulated. There are a variety of studies that indicate that the conversion rate of T4 to T3 is affected by the level of TSH that is present in the bloodstream.[4, 5, 6] A higher level of TSH appears to have a tendency to increase the conversion rate of T4 to T3 and a lower level of TSH appears to do the reverse. We also know that conversion rate is reduced by starvation, extreme stress and severe illness, especially liver diseases.

What is clear is that the conversion rate of T4 to T3 is variable and is certainly affected by TSH and probably by other factors. Some people believe that this may be a natural defence mechanism that helps to maintain the health of the individual for as long as possible when they have a slowly deteriorating thyroid gland.

As an important aside, the above information goes a long way to explaining why some people experience a worsening of symptoms, or no improvement in symptoms, if a little T3 medication is added alongside their synthetic T4 medication.

T3 has to reach its targets for us to feel healthy

The T3 that is present in our cells has either entered directly, or through conversion from T4 that has entered these cells.

Once inside each cell, T3 needs to reach **two main targets:**

- One target is the thyroid hormone receptors on the mitochondrion that is responsible for generating the energy that the cell requires.

- The second target is the thyroid hormone receptors on the genes within the cell nucleus.

I will refer to these targets collectively as the *intra-cellular targets of T3* because they are the two ultimate targets that enough T3 must reach, in order for us to feel healthy.

The mitochondrion is the energy-producing factory within each cell. The mitochondrion is responsible for producing each cell's supply of adenosine triphospate (ATP), which is used as a source of chemical energy. As well as being the cellular power plant, the mitochondrion is involved in a range of other processes. Along with various co-factors, like vitamin B1, Glucose is a critical chemical required by the mitochondria in order for ATP to be produced; therefore, having normal blood sugar metabolism is very important. Various natural chemicals have a significant effect on blood sugar metabolism including insulin and cortisol. This is why it is so important to have good blood sugar regulation and adequate cortisol levels, because without these even adequate levels of thyroid hormones will not make us feel well.

The nucleus contains the genes of the individual. Genes are made up of a chemical called DNA that most of us have heard of these days. DNA is a nucleic acid that contains the genetic instructions used in our development - what we look like on the outside and also how we work on the inside. DNA is often compared to a set of blueprints, since it contains the instructions needed to construct other components of cells, such as proteins. It is the genes that contain the information our bodies need to make proteins, which form the structure of our bodies and play an important role in the processes that keep us alive. Specifically, a gene is a length of DNA that codes for a specific protein.

When T3 binds to the thyroid hormone receptors on the genes within the cell nucleus, it causes certain genes to be activated and others to be inhibited. This effect on the genes is known as gene transcription. This process, which is reliant on T3, enables the cells of the body to perform the necessary function of making proteins, which is essential for good health. The binding of T3 to the thyroid hormone receptors within the cell nuclei and the resultant action on the genes is sometimes referred to as the *genomic action of T3* and it is through this action that the regulation of cell function occurs.

It is absolutely essential that an adequate amount of T3 is available and binds to the intra-cellular targets of T3 (nuclear and mitochondrial thyroid hormone receptors) in order to ensure that all of our tissues function as they are supposed to and we remain healthy.

This genomic action of T3 is the most significant way in which thyroid hormone affects the tissues. The clinical effects may take hours, days or weeks to fully occur.

T3 absolutely has to reach its targets!

This is such an important point that I will allow myself to repeat it in a different way. If you or I do not have enough of the T3 thyroid hormone within our cells, or the T3 is not being utilised correctly once it is there, then we will not feel well and we may have some or all of the symptoms of hypothyroidism, regardless of how much T4 and T3 is circulating in our bloodstream.

The problems that arise from insufficient T3 reaching its intra-cellular targets and correctly regulating cell function are at the heart of this book.

T4 is a pro-hormone and having enough T4 is no guarantee of good health

T4 is also capable of binding to the nuclear thyroid receptors but T3 has an affinity for the nuclear thyroid receptors of ten to fifteen times the affinity of T4, i.e. T3 is significantly more likely to bind to the thyroid hormone receptors in the cell nuclei. Even if T4 does manage to bind with some of the nuclear thyroid receptors, researchers believe that the effect of T3 on the cell nucleus is at least ten times more powerful than that of T4. For these reasons, T4, in isolation, is believed to have no biological action of any significance.

T4 therefore acts as a 'pro-hormone' as it can be converted into the biologically active hormone, T3. T4 is sometimes referred to as a storage hormone because, if working correctly, it should provide a reservoir of thyroid hormone for future use within the body. Many biochemical problems can occur that prevent T4 from enabling sufficient T3 reaching its intra-cellular targets.

It should be clear from all the above that many things have to work correctly for us to continue to feel well.

REVERSE T3 THYROID HORMONE

I am now going to discuss a thyroid hormone that I have not yet alluded to.

T4 is a metabolically inactive hormone. It only becomes useful to the body after an enzyme called 5'-deiodinase converts it into the active hormone, T3. A different enzyme, 5-deiodinase, is able to convert some of the T4 into reverse T3. From now on I will use the terms rT3 or RT3 instead of reverse T3.

The conversion process of T4 to rT3 occurs on an on-going basis within the cells, in order to clear excess levels of T4 from the body or to lower metabolic rate in certain circumstances. RT3 is eventually broken down by other enzymes and converted into T2, which in turn is converted into T1. T2 and T1 are simpler molecules with fewer iodine atoms. The body then eliminates these molecules within roughly twenty-four hours.

The proper name of rT3 is 3,3',5'-Triiodothyronine. RT3 is an isomer of T3, which means that it has the same molecular formula as T3 but the atoms form a slightly different internal structure. RT3 is very similar to T3 but it is not biologically active.

Like T3, rT3 may reach the same intra-cellular targets but it is unable to trigger any metabolic effects. If too much rT3 is produced then it may have a negative effect on metabolic rate and the regulation of cellular function.

RT3 is thought to exist in order to provide a dynamic mechanism to match the amount of available T3 to the body's actual needs. Some studies show that most people convert over 50% of their FT4 to rT3 and therefore, they convert less than 50% of FT4 to the metabolically active hormone FT3. The levels of rT3 fluctuate up and down through the day. Therefore, it is impossible to set an ideal level for rT3 or any ideal ratio of FT3 to rT3.

RT3 also provides a mechanism for slowing down the metabolism in the event of starvation, serious illness or high stress and in these circumstances the conversion rate of T4 to T3 decreases and more rT3 is made. The reduced T3 level that occurs during illness, fasting, or stress slows the metabolism of many tissues. Because of the slowed metabolism, the body does not eliminate rT3 as rapidly as usual. The slowed elimination from the body allows the rT3 level in the blood to increase considerably.

During stressful experiences such as surgery and combat, the amount of the stress hormone cortisol increases. The increase in this stress hormone is thought to inhibit the conversion of T4 to T3 and to increase the conversion of T4 to rT3. The same inhibition occurs when a patient has Cushing's syndrome, a disease in which the adrenal glands produce too much cortisol.

There is medical research that suggests that the inhibition of T4 to T3 conversion due to elevated stress hormone is temporary, even if the stress and cortisol continues to be high. Some studies have documented that the inhibition is temporary.[7, 8, 9]

However, there is still considerable anecdotal evidence from thyroid patients that suggests that elevated cortisol levels do in fact impede thyroid hormone effectiveness. It is quite common to hear of patients who have elevated cortisol levels for only certain parts of the day. I have wondered whether in such cases the body may never adjust to the elevated cortisol because it is not permanently elevated and if this might be one reason why some thyroid patients with elevated cortisol might continue to experience thyroid hormone problems.

One study of a group of patients who ultimately required the provision of T3 to enable them to recover their health, spent some time initially assessing these patients for any evidence of impaired T4 to T3 conversion and elevated rT3.[10] No laboratory evidence was present to suggest any impairment in T4 to T3 conversion or increased level of rT3 in any of these patients. So, it appears that not everyone who requires T3 hormone replacement therapy has elevated reverse T3.

The dynamic nature of rT3 can make it hard to know if an individual has an rT3 issue or not, unless multiple blood tests are taken during a 24-hour period because the rT3 level in the bloodstream can vary so much from hour to hour. There are conditions that are thought to upset the balance of FT3 and rT3. These include: low iron levels, low cortisol levels, insulin and blood sugar problems, excess T3 medication with T4, poor conversion of T4 due to lack of important nutrients like selenium, infections, tumours, damage to the heart muscle, aging, chronic alcohol abuse, diabetes, liver disease, kidney disease, severe illness, stress, surgery, some drugs, genetic defects affecting the deiodinase enzymes.

My personal view is that rT3 is useful in a lot of cases but that in some patients its value may be irrelevant to the real problem that the patient has or it may appear normal and yet the patient still may have problems with the T4 thyroid hormone.

THYROID HORMONE SYNTHESIS AND SECRETION

I have included this small explanation in order to make it clear how complex the processes are that lead up to the production and release of thyroid hormones and to explain the importance of the thyroid cells that the TPOAb and TgAb autoantibodies disrupt or destroy.

The thyroid is largely composed of a collection of spherical structures known as follicles. Specialised follicular cells called epithelial cells surround each follicle. Within each follicle is a colloid (a semi-liquid gelatinous substance). The follicular space and the colloid that it contains serve as a reservoir for all the materials required for producing thyroid hormones. It is within each of these thyroid follicles that much of the activity leading to the production of thyroid hormones occurs.

The thyroid gland uses the element iodine in its production of thyroid hormones. Iodine in the diet usually comes in the form of a compound such as sodium iodide or potassium iodide (iodised salt often contains these forms of inorganic iodide).

The epithelial cells surrounding each follicle collect circulating inorganic iodide and through a series of steps this form of iodine is used to create the two thyroid hormones T4 and T3. The steps are essentially:

1. Transporting the iodide into the thyroid epithelial cells. The rate of follicular transport of iodide appears to speed up with higher levels of TSH.

2. A protein called thyroglobulin (Tg) is produced within the thyroid epithelial cells. Thyroglobulin is a large complex protein, which is used to hold the majority of the iodine concentrated in the thyroid. Thyroglobulin is made from an amino acid residue called tyrosyl, which is made using the amino acid tyrosine.

3. The thyroglobulin protein is released by the epithelial cells, which surround each thyroid follicle into the colloid within each follicle. It is within this colloid that a lot of the action occurs.

4. An enzyme called thyroid peroxidase (TPO) is also made with the thyroid epithelial cells and this enzyme is also released into the colloid within each follicle.

5. Within the colloidal substance iodotyrosine molecules within each thyroglobulin protein are joined with the help of the enzyme thyroid peroxidase (TPO). An iodine atom is added with tyrosine to make mono-iodotyrosine (T1). Two iodine atoms are also combined with tyrosine to make di-iodotyrosine (T2). T1 and T2 are combined with the help of TPO to make T4 and T3 (the two iodothyronines).

6. The thyroglobulin protein is therefore altered through these processes. The thyroglobulin protein now holds the T1, T2, T3 and T4 inert within its structure.

7. Thyroglobulin contained within a little of the colloid has to move back from the main body of the colloid within the follicle and into the thyroid follicle epithelial cells.

8. Once within the epithelial cells, the free iodotyrosines (T1 and T2) and iodothyronines (T3 and T4) may be released from the complex thyroglobulin protein that they are still a part of. Specialised enzymes break down the thyroglobulin and release the separate T1, T2, T3, and T4 from the thyroglobulin protein.

9. The thyroid hormones remain as part of the thyroglobulin (Tg) protein until the thyroid is ready to secrete them, via the stimulation of TSH.

10. When the thyroid is asked to produce thyroid hormones through the stimulation of TSH several things happen:

11. Enzymes break some of the T1 and T2 down and the iodide is reused and released back into the colloid as new thyroglobulin.

12. T4 and T3 diffuse with some T1 and T2 through the epithelial cells of the thyroid and into the bloodstream.

It can be seen from the above that the thyroid follicles act as a factory and a warehouse for thyroid hormones.

It is a fairly complex process and it is a wonder that it works at all!

Chapter 3

The Adrenal Glands and Hypothyroidism

Whole books have been written on the topic of the adrenal glands and the importance of maintaining their health, particularly during the treatment of hypothyroidism. I can't complete this book without at least discussing some basic information regarding the relationship of healthy adrenals to thyroid replacement therapy.

There are two adrenal glands. Each small adrenal gland, which is the size of a walnut, sits on top of each kidney. The hormones that the adrenals produce are absolutely critical for life and I will now briefly touch on some of these. However, it is important to note that the adrenal glands produce many steroids that I will not be discussing at all. Dozens of steroid hormones are made by the adrenal glands. Consequently, maintaining the health of the adrenal glands and allowing them to work as optimally as possible is very important to our health

Let's start with adrenaline, which is known as epinephrine in the USA. Adrenaline is the hormone that is produced in the 'fight or flight' response. It is the hormone that enables you to immediately cope with stress, anger and fear.

The adrenals also produce a less well-known but incredibly important hormone called aldosterone that controls the balance between sodium and potassium in the body. Aldosterone is also involved in regulating blood pressure.

Hormones called dehydroepiandrosterone (DHEA) and androstendione are made by the adrenals glands to help the body repair itself. Sex hormones are also produced to a certain extent in the adrenal glands but not in the volumes secreted by the testes or the ovaries.

CORTISOL

The main hormone that I want to discuss is cortisol, which is produced in high volume by the adrenal glands. Cortisol is part of a family of adrenal hormones known as glucocorticoids. Cortisol has several functions in the body. One of the main functions of cortisol is to raise the level of blood sugar by affecting glucose metabolism. It can also raise blood pressure. Cortisol has a suppressive effect on the immune system and prevents the release of substances that cause inflammation. Cortisol is also important in fat, protein and carbohydrate metabolism. Cortisol may be viewed as having the opposite effect to insulin. Insulin's role is to make our cells more receptive to the glucose that they need and to facilitate the storage of excess blood glucose within the liver, muscles and fat tissues. Cortisol tends to conserve glucose in the bloodstream thus raising blood sugar levels. The adrenal glands produce more cortisol in times of intense stress, in order to protect us from the effects of this stress.

The adrenal glands produce cortisol throughout the day and night. The largest amount of cortisol is produced in the last four hours of sleep and when we first wake up, typically between the hours of 4:00 am and 8:00 am for most people. Thus the time when we wake up and get out of bed is usually when cortisol levels reach their peak and from then on, less and less cortisol is produced during the day. Typically the level of cortisol within our bloodstream drops precipitously as the day progresses. By the evening our cortisol level may have dropped to around 10% of what its peak level was, early in the morning. This is the normal daily pattern of cortisol. If someone has a very different pattern of sleeping and being awake, then the timing of cortisol release will be different.

Cortisol production is also affected by the quality of sleep that we get. Deep sleep tends to reduce cortisol secretion and light, or disturbed, sleep patterns tend to increase cortisol secretion.

There are conditions of extremely low levels of cortisol (Addison's disease) and very high levels of cortisol (Cushing's disease) that are both very serious and would need to be diagnosed and treated by an endocrinologist or qualified physician.

Addison's disease would produce symptoms that would almost certainly take a patient to their doctor quite promptly. These symptoms might include:

- Severe lethargy.
- Loss of appetite and weight loss.
- Nausea.
- Aches and pains.
- Low blood sugar.
- Darkening of the skin.
- Dizziness or fainting episodes.
- Low blood pressure.
- Emotional changes possibly including irritability or depression.
- Feeling cold due to the lowering of the metabolic rate.

These symptoms typically worsen when even a mild illness like a cold occurs. Severe low cortisol needs to be dealt with urgently, by a specialist, as it may be life threatening. Extremely serious low cortisol levels may also be produced by hypopituitarism, which is caused by diseases of the pituitary gland leading to an inability of the pituitary to make the necessary demand of the adrenals.

This chapter is concerned with the milder levels of adrenal insufficiency, which many thyroid patients experience after prolonged periods of hypothyroidism, or sustained periods of high stress. Some patients and doctors refer to milder forms of adrenal insufficiency as 'adrenal fatigue' or 'low adrenal reserve'. However, the medically documented and recognised terms for these milder cases are 'partial adrenal insufficiency' or 'mild adrenal insufficiency'. Hereafter, I will simply use 'adrenal insufficiency' to refer to this condition. Adrenal insufficiency exists on a continuum, as most diseases do, and the condition ranges from mild to severe.

Low cortisol is important to thyroid patients

There are several reasons why anyone with thyroid disease should be interested in the adrenal glands and cortisol in particular:

- Firstly, some of the symptoms of hypothyroidism may be confused with some of the symptoms of low levels of cortisol, since both can lower the metabolic rate.

- Secondly, low levels of cortisol may interfere with the conversion of T4 to T3. This may result in elevated reverse T3 levels.

- Thirdly, without sufficient cortisol the processes that lead to the generation of cellular energy will not work well. These processes that ultimately enable cellular energy (ATP) to be produced by the mitochondria require that our blood sugar metabolism is functioning normally, as glucose is one of the main chemicals that the mitochondria require in the production of ATP. Having healthy blood sugar metabolism is therefore a critical requirement if thyroid hormone treatment is to be successful. Natural chemicals like insulin and cortisol and a healthy diet all have a part to play in regulating blood sugar.

- Finally, a patient may cope quite well most of the time but at periods of real stress they may find that their adrenal glands are simply not up to the job of manufacturing enough cortisol and they become symptomatic, because they cannot adapt to the new stress level.

If someone with a susceptibility to low adrenal function has been experiencing high levels of emotional or physical stress for a long time, their adrenal glands may begin to malfunction and produce less cortisol. This may also be true for the person who has been hypothyroid for several years before diagnosis and treatment. Adrenal insufficiency may also result from exposure to environmental toxins, dietary sensitivities and allergens, as well as life events.

Not only can the total daily amount of cortisol decline but also, when a stressful event occurs, the adrenals may simply not be able to respond by producing the additional cortisol required. When this happens adrenal insufficiency is the end result.

Milder forms of adrenal insufficiency are far more common than the severe adrenal insufficiency of Addison's disease.

ADRENAL INSUFFICIENCY

Low adrenal hormone levels can be very bad news for any thyroid patient hoping for an immediate recovery from hypothyroidism. These symptoms may be due to cortisol insufficiency or aldosterone insufficiency.

There are some clues when cortisol insufficiency is present:

- Low blood sugar, which may cause dizziness, feeling unwell or more frequent hunger.
- Severe fatigue/tiredness.
- Aches and pains.
- Dizziness (even when sitting down).
- Clumsiness.
- Poor response to thyroid hormone replacement therapy.
- Anxiousness or inability to cope with stress.
- Irritability or anger or panic feelings.
- Feeling cold/low body temperature.
- Fluctuating body temperature. Some doctors in the USA ask their thyroid patients to take body temperature readings three hours after waking, three hours later and a further three hours after that. These are averaged for the day to form the daily average body temperature (DAT). If a thyroid patient's DAT varies more than 0.2 degrees Fahrenheit then this may suggest cortisol insufficiency when combined with other evidence.
- Possibly having dark rings under the eyes.
- Pale and 'washed out' skin colour or even a slight darkening of the skin.
- Skin appears thinner.
- Digestive upsets, which may including diarrhoea.
- Worsening allergies.
- Symptoms similar to a flu virus.
- Nausea.
- Trembling, shakiness or a jittery/hyper feeling.
- Rapid heartbeat or pounding.
- Difficulty sleeping.
- Low blood pressure as a result of the impact on the action of thyroid hormones.
- Low back pain - where the adrenal glands are located.
- Worsening symptoms in the presence of stress of any kind, including minor infections.

There are some clues when aldosterone insufficiency is present:

✓• Low blood pressure, which is even lower if the blood pressure is taken immediately after the patient stands up (postural hypotension).
✓• Craving for salty foods.
• Thirst.
• Dizziness when standing up, which may include fainting.
• More frequent need to urinate or frequent urination during the night.
✓• Excessive sweating.
• A slightly higher body temperature than usual.
• High heart rate.

Low levels of thyroid hormone can also cause several of the above symptoms. This can obviously make recognising adrenal insufficiency a bit of a challenge. If someone has been hypothyroid for a considerable time before diagnosis and treatment, then it is possible that there will be adrenal insufficiency present. Therefore, adrenal insufficiency is something that a family doctor or endocrinologist should either check for, or at the very least, be on the lookout for.

Other causes of adrenal insufficiency may be:

• Autoimmune attack on the adrenal glands (which may be tested).
• Environmental toxins that are interfering with cortisol production.
• Low adrenal or thyroid hormones after a woman gives birth.
• Hypothyroidism.
• A severe nutritional deficiency.
• If someone has been on adrenal hormones for a prolonged period of time, the adrenal glands can atrophy and take months to recover as the adrenal medication is withdrawn.
• A pituitary or hypothalamic disorder (like hypopituitarism).

Adrenal insufficiency may be exposed during thyroid hormone treatment

Quite often the result of prolonged hypothyroidism is not to have immediately obvious low cortisol levels, because the general slow down of the metabolism may also have slowed down the rate at which cortisol is used up and cleared by the body. In this case, it is more likely that any adrenal insufficiency will be exposed, once thyroid hormone replacement commences. Consequently, a doctor *must* be on the lookout for this and be ready to test for adrenal issues and cortisol in particular, if the thyroid treatment does not progress as expected.

As previously mentioned, thyroid hormones can only enable the body to work correctly if the processes that generate cellular energy are also working well. This requires correct blood sugar metabolism and adequate glucose reaching the interior of our cells. Cortisol plays an important role in maintaining blood glucose levels and therefore, cellular glucose levels. If there is a significant adrenal insufficiency issue then this will reduce the effectiveness of thyroid hormone, enabling the continuation of many of the symptoms associated with hypothyroidism.

For a patient with low cortisol levels, when thyroid hormone is given and gradually increased a variety of reactions can occur.

It is possible that the thyroid hormone replacement does not appear to correct the symptoms that the patient first brought to the attention of the doctor. The patient may continue to feel cold and tired, for instance. Continuing to feel cold as thyroid hormone replacement is gradually increased is probably one of the most common clues during thyroid treatment that the patient's cortisol level may be low. In addition to this a patient may find that their body temperature does not remain stable during the day but fluctuates up and down. Worse still, more unpleasant reactions can occur if cellular glucose levels fall and the generation of cellular energy is not high enough. These reactions may differ from patient to patient but might include a very rapid heart rate and intense anxiety.

However, it is important to note that in many cases when the right form of thyroid treatment is provided and it is managed carefully then the adrenal glands will begin to function well once more.

Adrenal insufficiency can be confusing

If adrenal insufficiency is present and the patient has been given increasing amounts of thyroid hormone, then it is possible that their blood test results will appear normal but they may still feel dreadfully ill. Consequently, if undetected adrenal insufficiency is present and a doctor is using only thyroid blood tests to determine whether treatment is successful or not, then the patient may never fully recover.

As soon as adrenal insufficiency is suspected the patient should seek the advice of a medical practitioner who has experience of dealing with thyroid hormone replacement in the presence of adrenal insufficiency. However, some people with adrenal insufficiency may recover quite swiftly once the correct level of appropriate thyroid hormone replacement is in place. The adrenal insufficiency may simply have been due to the inadequate level of thyroid hormone available to the adrenal glands themselves. The response of an individual will depend on the severity of the adrenal insufficiency and any other factors that might be present. Severe adrenal insufficiency may well need some form of intervention with medication. However, even with T3 replacement therapy the patient's doctor will need to be vigilant and some form of adrenal support may still be needed in severe cases.

TREATMENT OPTIONS IF ADRENAL INSUFFICIENCY IS SUSPECTED

Hopefully, by working in cooperation with a competent and knowledgeable doctor, it will be clear from the clinical picture and from the events leading to the diagnosis of hypothyroidism, whether adrenal insufficiency is likely to be an issue or not. If adrenal insufficiency is likely, then there are several schools of thought on how to proceed.

The approach that is probably the most common is to do nothing, which can occasionally result in problems during thyroid hormone replacement. However, very frequently when the correct thyroid hormones are provided at the right levels then the adrenals quickly recover. This option might be the best solution for someone who is about to be offered T3 replacement therapy by their doctor, because with T3 there is the possibility to use it to drive the adrenal glands more fully than with T4 replacement (this will be discussed at length later in the book).

Another approach used by some doctors prior to commencing thyroid hormone treatment, is to do appropriate tests for adrenal insufficiency, keeping in mind that optimal levels of cortisol are essential for proper functioning of the body. If the test results indicate a sufficiently low cortisol level then some form of treatment might be administered, prior to prescribing thyroid hormone replacement. I have also heard of doctors who tend to prescribe physiological levels of adrenal support treatment based only on the patients presenting symptoms. Physiological doses of any naturally occurring hormone are doses that are small and only raise the level of hormone in the body to the normal level and no higher. I'm obviously not a doctor but, given what I now know, I wouldn't take any adrenal hormones without test results that confirmed that I required them.

An alternative approach is to commence thyroid hormone replacement therapy and watch carefully, to see if any of the tell tale signs of adrenal insufficiency exist. If there is evidence of adrenal insufficiency during thyroid hormone replacement, then laboratory tests for cortisol levels may be done at that time. The doctor can then assess if there is any need to use any form of treatment for adrenal insufficiency.

If a doctor concludes that a patient may be suffering from adrenal insufficiency that is severe enough to prevent the success of thyroid hormone replacement, then it is possible that the patient may be offered a trial of adrenal support. This may involve the use of very small, physiological doses of hydrocortisone, which are designed to only correct a patient's cortisol to normal levels and not above this. In this case, because of the short-lived nature of hydrocortisone in the body, several small doses may be given during the day. Alternatively, a more natural form of adrenal support may be used, which is likely to contain some level of ground up adrenal glandular. Adrenal glandular products are thought by some doctors to be safer and cause less risk of suppression of the adrenal glands.[1] However, other doctors feel that these product are only effective for mild cases of adrenal insufficiency.

In the case where some form of adrenal support has been provided, once the correct dosage of thyroid hormone replacement has been established, then any form of adrenal support may usually be reduced gradually and then stopped.

The purpose of adrenal support is to ensure that the body is able to regulate blood sugar and generate sufficient cellular energy in order that the prescribed thyroid hormone can be seen to be performing correctly, until an adequate dosage for the patient has been found. At that point, the thyroid hormones themselves should ensure that the adrenals are able to function normally once again unless they are suffering damage through autoimmune attack or other disease or hypopituitarism exists.

If adrenal hormone medication that is being provided for adrenal insufficiency is not slowly reduced and discontinued when it no longer required, then there is a danger that it will have a suppressive effect on the adrenal glands and may even cause long term damage.[1, 2] The intent should therefore be to only use physiological doses of adrenal hormones for a matter of a few weeks or months at the most before gradually withdrawing them. In rare cases the individual may require adrenal hormone medication indefinitely in order to remain healthy. This is also why it is essential to get comprehensive cortisol testing performed before cortisol is supplemented. This testing should include a Synacthen test or possibly an insulin tolerance test. Saliva testing only paints a picture of what the adrenals are producing during the day and does not show how much the adrenal glands are *capable* of producing.

A new approach to the treatment of adrenal insufficiency in thyroid patients called the *Circadian T3 Method* will be discussed in Chapters 16 and 25. I discovered the Circadian T3 Method (CT3M) many years ago and have now described it in this book. The CT3M is being found to be highly effective in correcting adrenal function in many thyroid patients and requires no use of any adrenal medication. Provided that the thyroid patient has no Addison's disease or hypopituitarism then the CT3M may well be an excellent treatment for adrenal insufficiency by thyroid patients and their doctors.

For more details on this subject there are many excellent books available, written by both doctors and patients.[1, 3, 4, 5]

LABORATORY TESTS FOR ADRENAL INSUFFICIENCY

There are several laboratory tests that may be employed if it is suspected that the adrenal glands are not producing enough cortisol:

- *The ACTH stimulation test* is a test that a patient typically has done as an outpatient in a hospital. It is also known as a Synacthen test (and sometimes a cosyntropin test or tetracosactide test). There are two types of this test - a long Synacthen test or a short Synacthen test. There is some controversy over which of these is better.

This test involved a series of blood samples. It is usually done early in the morning when the patient's cortisol levels will be close to the highest for the day. One blood sample is taken at the beginning of the test. Then a chemical is injected into the patient, which is either ACTH (the pituitary hormone that stimulates the production of cortisol) or a very similar chemical. Further blood samples are taken every half an hour thereafter. Typically three blood samples are taken following the injection of ACTH.

The doctor interpreting the results can then use the initial baseline level of cortisol and the level of response to the injection, to assess the health of the adrenal glands and determine if there is a potentially serious adrenal issue. If the ACTH Stimulation test is done properly and interpreted correctly then it can be extremely useful in determining adrenal insufficiency.

- *The twenty-four hour urinary cortisol test* measures the amount of cortisol produced by the body over a twenty-four hour period. The patient is given a large collection container and told to collect all the urine they produce over an exactly timed twenty-four hour period. This is not an accurate test if the patient has renal failure. It is important for the doctor who is requesting this test to explicitly request a '24 hour urinary cortisol' because if '24 hour urinary adrenal' is requested then an adrenaline assay may be performed.

The test produces a result that estimates the total cortisol production over twenty-four hours as well as an assessment of the free (unbound) cortisol level. This test is typically used in the cases where high levels of cortisol are suspected or the patient has severe adrenal insufficiency and has been placed on some corticosteroid treatment. However, it may also be used as a general assessment of cortisol levels. Some doctors have stated that if the total and free cortisol levels that are measured by this test are in the lower third of the laboratory reference range then it is still possible that adrenal insufficiency might still be present. In this case, adrenal insufficiency should be excluded using other methods of testing.

I believe that this test provides a relatively simple, reliable and general check on adrenal cortisol production. I have used this test many times and found the results to be very helpful and always reasonably consistent with how I have actually felt.

- *The twenty-four hour adrenal saliva test* is a relatively new test compared to the previous two tests. It is only available privately through specialist companies within the UK and is not currently available via the NHS. This test is in much wider use within the USA and is considered by many to be the most useful of all the tests for cortisol insufficiency.

This test involves providing four separate saliva samples during the day, from morning to late evening, which are then sent off by mail to the specialist company. Results show the four distinct measures of salivary cortisol at each point in the day. Typically, the private laboratory will provide a chart that illustrates how the patient's cortisol level appeared to fluctuate during the day, including any time periods when the cortisol was unusually high or low. The test result may also include an estimate of the total daily cortisol production.

This type of testing, which provides an insight into how a patient's cortisol level fluctuates over a day, is sometimes referred to as dynamic testing. Some form of dynamic testing of cortisol, made available through the NHS, would be a very positive step forward.

The experience of thyroid patients and doctors who regularly use adrenal saliva testing is that healthy adrenal function will typically exhibit the following pattern: an early morning result with free cortisol at the top of the reference range; a late morning/lunchtime result with free cortisol in the upper quartile; a tea-time (approx. 5:00 pm) result with free cortisol around mid-range; and a late evening free cortisol at the bottom of the reference range.

- Sometimes a *single serum cortisol test*, usually early in the morning, may be done. This provides a quick and easy insight into the state of the adrenal glands. It should only be used to see if a gross problem exists, as it only provides a snapshot at one time of the cortisol level. It is probably the least useful of all the other tests described.

- Occasionally an endocrinologist may arrange an *insulin tolerance test* that measures the adrenal glands' response to hypoglycaemia (low blood sugar/glucose levels). Normally, the adrenals release extra cortisol when blood sugar falls below a certain level. This cortisol release raises the blood sugar back up to a healthy level. However, weak adrenals are not as efficient at doing this. So this test aims to measure adrenal function by inducing a hypoglycaemic state. The test itself involves taking a baseline cortisol level and then injecting the patient with insulin so that they become hypoglycaemic. Cortisol blood samples are then taken every 15 minutes throughout the test and during the hypoglycaemia. Once hypoglycaemia (blood glucose level of 2.2/40mg/dl) has been achieved, the patient is injected with dextrose to bring the glucose levels up as quickly as possible.

A nurse or doctor is present at all times throughout this test and they will take note of hypoglycaemic symptoms, as well as ensuring that the patiently is rapidly given dextrose if they become unconscious. The insulin tolerance test also measures growth hormone and insulin. It is considered the gold standard for diagnosing hypopituitarism and detecting hypothalamic-pituitary-adrenal axis problems. The insulin tolerance test is extremely effective at detecting more subtle cases of adrenal insufficiency (and secondary adrenal insufficiency in particular); however it does carry real risks. Therefore, many endocrinologists are reluctant to run this test.

I have had all of the above tests done apart from the insulin tolerance test, at some point in the past. If there is any serious concern over low cortisol levels, then it does make sense to have an ACTH stimulation test at least once - just to be able to be certain that no Addison's disease is present.

PUPIL DILATION TEST FOR ADRENAL INSUFFICIENCY

There is a simple test that observes the response of the pupils of the eyes that may be done easily at home with no equipment other than a mirror and a small torch. This test may provide additional evidence that adrenal insufficiency is present.

Adrenal insufficiency usually results in more than one adrenal hormone that is low. If cortisol is low then it is likely that the adrenal glands are struggling and so it is likely that **aldosterone will also be affected**. Aldosterone helps to maintain the balance of sodium and potassium in the body. With low aldosterone there is usually an increase in potassium and a reduction in sodium. This imbalance can cause the muscles of the eye to be weaker than they ought to be, which can result in a dilation (enlargement) of the pupil of the eye in response to light. There is a simple test for this.

This test is perhaps best done in the evening when adrenal hormones are at their lowest ebb and the light is fading. The test requires the subject to be in a dark room and close enough to a mirror so that they are clearly able to observe the pupils of their eyes. This may be easier to achieve in the evening and this timing may provide a more realistic result because the adrenal hormones may be lower in the latter part of the day.

The light from a bright torch is shone from the **side** of the head towards one eye (not directly at the eyes from in front). The light is held steady for about a minute, so it is ideal that the subject is sitting down in front of a fixed mirror so there is less movement. Care should be taken that the light that illuminates the pupil (sometimes torches have darker areas in the middle of the beam). It is ideal if another person can hold the torch and direct the beam carefully from the side of the head onto the pupil.

The subject's pupil should narrow and stay that way during the whole test. If the pupil narrows but then dilates again or begins to fluctuate noticeably between one state and another then this may indicate adrenal insufficiency. The longer the period of time that the pupil remains dilated for before contracting again then the more likely that adrenal insufficiency is present. This is a very simple test and may be used to add additional evidence to the laboratory test results and other symptoms and signs of adrenal insufficiency.

LABORATORY TESTS AND ADRENAL SUPPORT

If a patient is already on some form of adrenal medication then the patient's doctor may advise them to discontinue it for a period of time prior to any adrenal laboratory test. Whenever adrenal medication is stopped it must always be done slowly. This weaning process allows the adrenal glands time to respond and avoids severe problems. The patient's doctor must advise on whether this should be done and how it should be done.

Discussion on both twenty-four hour tests

I have used the twenty-four hour urinary cortisol test on numerous occasions and I have found that the test results have always been consistent with how I have felt at the time the test was taken. It has been a very useful test for me, even though using it to assess any adrenal insufficiency issue is not really what it was originally intended for.

Currently, dynamic testing of cortisol, via blood or adrenal saliva testing, is not available through the NHS in the UK but it may be done privately.

When I first released the 'Recovering with T3' book I had very little exposure to the twenty-four hour adrenal saliva test. Since that time many thyroid patients have told me how useful this test has been and how consistent with their symptoms it has been. Because of this increased experience I would now choose to do a twenty-four adrenal saliva test in preference to the twenty-four hour urinary cortisol test, although doing both may have advantages for a patient who was trying to obtain a full picture of their cortisol status.

ADRENAL TREATMENT REQUIRES CAUTION

If some form of treatment is required to improve adrenal hormone levels then this needs to be done carefully. As mentioned already one of the roles of cortisol is to raise blood levels of glucose by causing tissues that have stored sugar in various forms to release glucose into the bloodstream. If glucose levels have been low due to adrenal insufficiency then cellular levels of glucose may be low. If someone has been placed on thyroid hormone treatment already then this may have created more demand that reduces cellular glucose levels, which may cause symptoms that appear to look like hyperthyroidism. This cellular glucose deficit is often accompanied by rising adrenaline levels, which might induce raised blood pressure, a high heart rate and flushing of the skin (often on the face) and other symptoms. The adrenaline may make the detection of the underlying low cortisol quite difficult.

Once some form of adrenal treatment is given then the cellular levels of glucose may rise and the ATP generation may return to normal. However, this can result in a sudden rise in the apparent effectiveness of thyroid hormone as the cells begin to work more correctly. Some patients sometimes refer to this as a 'hyper dump' and it can appear like severe hyperthyroidism. It should be clear that it is very important that any form of adrenal treatment is provided slowly and the response is monitored as it may be necessary to reduce thyroid hormone levels.

EXCESS ADRENAL HORMONES

I have been asked by thyroid patients to include a brief description of some of the symptoms and signs of high cortisol or high aldosterone. <u>Sometimes when a thyroid patient has experienced stress for a long time then cortisol or aldosterone may become high rather than low.</u> It is quite common for cortisol to be high at certain times of the day but not at others.

The 'Recovering with T3' book does not focus on the treatment of all types of adrenal problems, so thyroid patients should work with their own medical professionals on dealing with high or low cortisol, aldosterone or other adrenal hormones. Many patients in the USA in particular are having success in treating high cortisol using herbs known collectively as *adrenal adaptogens* or with zinc, which appears to depress cortisol levels. It is important for thyroid patients to work with their own personal physician on the diagnosis and treatment of elevated adrenal hormones and to rule out any serious underlying condition, e.g. Cushing's disease.

There are some clues when high cortisol is present:

- High blood pressure.
- Bruising easily.
- Fluid retention.
- Obesity and/or Moon-shaped face, increased belly fat, fat on back of the neck.
- Fatigue.
- Weak muscles and muscle loss

There are some clues when high aldosterone is present:

- High blood pressure.
- Low potassium - which can cause weakness or muscle spasms.
- Numbness or tingling in the extremities.
- Frequent urination.

ADRENAL AUTOANTIBODY TESTS

If low cortisol levels are found through laboratory testing, then depending on the severity of the result, the doctor may request referral to an endocrinologist and further investigation. This investigation may involve testing for adrenal autoantibodies.

The most commonly tested adrenal autoantibodies are: adrenocortical autoantibodies (ACA), 21-hydroxy autoantibodies and the 21-OH autoantibodies. Two other autoantibodies that are associated with the adrenal glands but are less frequently tested for are: 17-alpha-hydroxylase autoantibodies and P450scc autoantibodies.

A competent endocrinologist will be able to investigate the patient's adrenal glands and any possible disease or autoimmunity thoroughly.

Chapter 4

Vitamins, Minerals and Hypothyroidism

Vitamins and minerals may have a huge effect on the success or failure of thyroid hormone replacement therapy. Some nutrients may have such an impact on thyroid hormone treatment that it makes sense to have laboratory tests to determine their levels prior to taking thyroid treatment, and during treatment, if the patient does not respond well.

There are several nutrients that may be beneficial to supplement, because of their critical role in the biochemical pathways involved in the creation or use of thyroid and adrenal hormones.

Someone who has a well balanced diet, high in organically grown, unprocessed foods should have a reduced need for supplementation. However, for many of us, our modern diets do not provide enough of the important nutrients we need. This may be especially true for thyroid patients, who may have impaired absorption of nutrients due to hypothyroidism.

Let me briefly review some of the nutrient information that thyroid patients need to be aware of.

HOW TO TAKE VITAMINS AND MINERALS

Vitamins are divided into two types:

- *The fat-soluble vitamins.* These are the A, D, E and K vitamins. It is possible to take these vitamins once a day, because after they have been ingested the body uses them as and when necessary. However, even these vitamins are absorbed better if they are taken in divided doses with food. The two fat-soluble vitamins, A and D, are the only ones in this group that can be toxic if taken in too high a dose.

- *The water-soluble vitamins.* These are the B vitamins and vitamin C. These are ingested and absorbed into the blood stream and the cells but any excess will be quickly excreted. It is therefore better to take these vitamins in small doses throughout the day. They may be taken with meals for convenience and better absorption, although I often taken vitamin C on its own. There is almost no risk of overdose with either vitamins B or C, although too many grams of vitamin C may cause loose bowel movements. In order to suffer from an overdose of vitamin B6, a patient would need to take over 2000 mg per day but it is unlikely that anyone would be recommended to take more than 100 mg of B6 per day.

Minerals need to be taken with food. Ideally the minerals would be taken in divided doses and taken with each meal as the body can only absorb what it needs. This may be inconvenient if a single multi-mineral is the simplest way to purchase the minerals. I take most of my minerals with one meal. This is not perfect but we do what we can and have to compromise sometimes.

It is important to look carefully at the labels on bottles containing minerals, to check the exact amounts of elemental minerals present, in order to ensure that the correct quantity of the actual element is being taken.

If a patient's doctor has found a specific deficiency of a vitamin or mineral, the doctor will usually recommend a suitable dosage of the particular nutrient.

I will now discuss some specific vitamins and minerals in turn, starting with the most important ones that may require testing, to ensure that they are not low prior to commencing thyroid hormone replacement therapy.

IRON

Iron is a trace mineral that is used to make haemoglobin and is involved in the processes that move oxygen and carbon dioxide in and out of our cells. Iron forms part of numerous enzymes and it is critical for energy production in the body.

Low levels of iron in the body are often associated with hypothyroidism, perhaps because hypothyroidism reduces the efficiency of absorption of nutrients in the gastrointestinal tract (GI tract). Therefore, hypothyroidism can lead to depleted iron levels, which in turn can result in iron deficiency anaemia.

The symptoms of anaemia may include:

- General malaise.
- Tiredness.
- Drowsiness.
- Dizziness.
- Fainting.
- Heart palpitations including a faster heart rate (very common).
- Shortness of breath.
- Chest pain (angina).
- Headaches.
- Ringing in the ears.
- Brain fog/difficulty thinking clearly.
- Irritability.
- Depression.
- Anxiety or panic attacks
- Pale skin.

52

- Brittle hair or nails.
- Pale nail beds.
- Food cravings.
- Low sex drive.
- Burning sensations in tongue.
- Dryness in mouth/throat.
- Difficulty swallowing.
- Altered sense of touch.

These symptoms can easily be misinterpreted as hypothyroidism and as a result the low iron level may be missed.

Low iron levels may also be caused by low stomach acidity that is often present in a patient with hypothyroidism, or from a prolonged period of having a low body temperature, which in turn can lead to a reduction in the number of red blood cells being produced. Iron is absorbed in the duodenum. Consequently, any condition that disrupts the health of the small intestine may have an impact on iron levels.

Thyroid patients and iron

Iron forms a component of a vast number of enzymes that are involved in energy generation within the cells. Therefore, without enough iron, the metabolic activity within the cells that is driven by T3 will grind to a halt. Iron is also used by the thyroid in its production of thyroid hormones and in the biochemical processes leading to the use of thyroid hormones within our cells. In particular, it appears that iron has a role in the conversion of T4 to T3.[1, 2]

If low iron levels have not been addressed first, the symptoms associated with hypothyroidism may continue, even when thyroid replacement therapy has started. If low iron is an issue, it is also possible to experience symptoms similar to hyperthyroidism when thyroid replacement is started, because the body may then fail to process the thyroid hormone properly. Therefore thyroid hormone replacement therapy cannot succeed without an adequate level of iron. Because of this it is very important for thyroid patients to have the most thorough range of laboratory tests for iron in order to detect any potential iron issues.

Iron should be measured by the following comprehensive laboratory tests:

- *Complete Blood Count (CBC)*. This is the first test that is used to diagnose anaemia. It measures the haemoglobin and haemocrit levels. Haemoglobin is an iron-rich protein in red blood cells that carries oxygen to the body. Haemocrit is a measure of how much space red blood cells take up in the blood. If either the haemoglobin or haemocrit are low then this may be a sign of anaemia. The blood count also checks the number of red and white blood cells and platelets in the bloodstream, which a doctor can use to diagnose a variety of conditions.

- *Serum Iron.* This test measures the amount of iron in the bloodstream that is bound to transferrin. However, because this can be normal, even though the iron stores in the body are low, other tests must also be done. Typical laboratory reference ranges for serum iron are 65-176 ug/dL for men and 50-170 ug/dL for women. Serum iron is sometimes measured in umol/L, e.g. the reference range for women would then be 10-30 umol/L rather than 50-170 ug/dL. I have heard reports from other patients and Internet forums that suggest that thyroid patients feel better if their **serum iron over 90 ug/dL and ideally close to 100-110 ug/dL** but still remaining within the laboratory reference range.

- *Total Iron Binding Capacity (TIBC).* Transferrin is a protein that carries iron in the blood. TIBC measures the ability of the blood to bind iron to transferrin. Total iron-binding capacity (TIBC) is most frequently used along with a serum iron test to evaluate people suspected of having either iron deficiency or iron overload. These two tests are used to calculate the transferrin saturation %, a more useful indicator of iron status than just iron or TIBC alone. In iron deficiency, the serum iron level is often low, but the TIBC is increased. In states of excess iron the serum iron level will be high and the TIBC will be low or normal.

If TIBC is high then there is likely to be a low amount of transferrin not carrying iron, i.e. the ability to carry additional iron is good. If TIBC is low then the transferrin has limited capacity to bind further iron, i.e. the capacity of the blood to bind additional iron is poor.

If someone is identified as having a low iron level via one of the other tests and a **low** level of TIBC is present then the patient's doctor must take care when iron supplementation is started to avoid a build up of iron in the blood. Iron supplementation must be far lower than is normally used for iron deficiency and the building up of iron stores will take a lot longer to accomplish, e.g. less than 20 mg of elemental iron per day may be required initially until the TIBC becomes higher. In practice thyroid patients have found that they appear to **handle iron supplementation reasonably well if their TIBC is at or above the lower quartile of the reference range**. The patient's doctor should be able to provide excellent advice on iron supplementation.

The typical reference range for TIBC is 240-450 ug/dL. Sometimes an alternative test called the UIBC is performed. This is the unsaturated iron binding capacity and this determines the reserve capacity of transferrin, i.e. the portion of transferrin that has not yet been saturated with iron. If serum iron and UIBC are known then TIBC may be calculated as TIBC = UIBC + serum iron. The typical reference range for UIBC is 150-375 ug/dL.

- *Transferrin Saturation %*. This is a calculation that is expressed as a percentage. TIBC is divided by serum iron to calculate the transferrin saturation %. The transferrin saturation % tells a doctor how much of the free iron is being carried by transferrin. This is a far more useful indicator of iron status than just serum iron or TIBC alone. Transferrin saturation % is sometimes referred to as the transferrin saturation index. For instance a transferrin saturation % of 15% means that only 15% of the free iron is bound to transferrin.

  Typically the transferrin saturation % will be low if there is iron deficiency because serum iron will be low and TIBC will be high. The typical reference range for transferrin saturation % is 15-50% for men and 12-45% for women.

  The feedback from experienced thyroid patients that I have received is that thyroid patients should aim to maintain their transferrin saturation % in the 25% - 45% range. However, recently I have read about some doctors in the USA who have found that thyroid treatment proceeds more smoothly once the patient's **transferrin saturation % is in the 35% - 45% range, with serum iron ideally at least 90 ug/dL**. In this situation, TIBC or UIBC may be low in their reference ranges but still not below the lower end of the reference ranges. Transferrin saturation % should not exceed 45% though.

- *Serum Ferritin*. Ferritin is a protein that is used to store iron within the tissues and it enables the steady release of iron that our cells require. The serum ferritin blood test measures how much storage iron is available.

  Typical laboratory reference ranges for serum ferritin are 22-320 ng/mL for men/post menopausal women and 10-290 ng/mL for pre menopausal women. However, many female thyroid patients report that their **serum ferritin needs to be at least in the 70 - 90 ng/mL range**, which is considerably higher than the lower reference range of most laboratories. Male thyroid patients do well with similar results or even a little higher.

  However, with conditions like hypothyroidism serum ferritin may be misleading, e.g. in the presence of inflammation, infection or cancer. In the case of prolonged hypothyroidism serum ferritin may be falsely elevated, or even sometimes low or normal, in the presence of both high and low iron levels because of the inflammation caused by the condition. Consequently, in the first instance it is important to have the broad range of tests for iron as outlined here. In particular, the combination of serum iron, serum ferritin and transferrin saturation % may be more valuable in order to gain a more accurate appreciation of iron status. If low ferritin is present with high serum iron and high transferrin saturation % then the patient's doctor must carefully assess whether this is simply a case that the ferritin level has not yet been given adequate time to improve with iron supplementation or whether some other process is at work.

The above laboratory reference ranges are only typical and may vary depending on the laboratory performing the test.

Ensuring iron levels are healthy is important for thyroid patients

Any type of thyroid hormone replacement therapy that a patient is having may be severely compromised if iron is a problem. It is critical to establish healthy levels of iron within the body prior to commencing thyroid hormone replacement therapy. However, it is dangerous to supplement with more than a few milligrams of elemental iron unless laboratory testing has suggested that irons levels ought to be higher. Therefore, the comprehensive range of iron tests should be performed prior to commencing any thyroid hormone treatment.

The comprehensive laboratory tests of CBC, serum iron, serum ferritin, TIBC and transferrin saturation % will provide insight into whether there is any iron deficiency anaemia. **It is extremely important to have the full iron panel of serum iron, serum ferritin and transferrin saturation % to get a full picture of iron levels in the body.** Thyroid treatment can be complex and confusing at times and iron is often an issue, which goes undetected, sometimes for many years. Having a comprehensive exploration of iron levels to begin with is highly desirable.

If for any reason thyroid treatment appears to stop working, or if no benefit is felt from further dosage increases, it may be advisable to re-test iron levels because an increase in metabolic rate as a result of thyroid hormone replacement therapy may reveal a previously undetected issue with storage iron.

Work with a doctor

Anyone considering iron supplementation needs to be very aware that excessive levels of iron are highly **toxic** to the body. If excess iron is present then this can cause joint pain, fatigue, abdominal pain, decreased sex drive, lack of energy and heart problems. Consequently, it is very important to take iron supplementation only if it is required and then at an appropriate level. Therefore, the decision over whether iron supplementation is required and what level it should be taken at should be done with full involvement of a patient's own family doctor.

Iron supplementation must be taken with vitamin C in order to aid the absorption of the iron. It is best to have a doctor prescribe iron in the form of ferrous gluconate or ferrous fumerate as both of these are milder on the stomach than ferrous sulphate. The amount of elemental iron in these preparations is usually quoted in milligrams and is not the same as the number of milligrams of the supplement. For instance there may only be 55 mg of elemental iron in a 325 mg ferrous sulphate tablet.

A patient's doctor will advise on how much iron to take but the experience of thyroid patients suggest that during the correction phase of raising iron levels 150-200 mg daily of elemental iron is often required and this will need to be taken in two or three divided doses. If total iron binding capacity is high then this level of iron supplementation will need to be significantly lower and the patient's doctor should be able to advise on an appropriate level.

Once supplementation of iron has begun it can take many months for the iron storage to rectify. Once iron stores are healthy once again then it is likely that some far lower level of long-term iron supplementation will be required combined with intermittent blood tests.

Practical aspects of iron supplementation

One of the side effects of iron supplements may be constipation and so an appropriate level of magnesium in the diet may be required to alleviate this. A family doctor should be able to give advice on an appropriate level of magnesium to take, if this is a problem. It is advisable to take calcium supplements away from iron, because calcium may reduce the absorption of iron.

It is also important to avoid taking iron supplements for several days prior to any laboratory tests for iron as this may compromise the test results. Recent findings suggest that vitamin C should also be suspended for a few days prior to the iron test, as vitamin C use can also artificially inflate iron results.

Patients taking thyroid hormone and iron supplements need to be aware of the possible interactions between these. Iron can bind to some of the thyroid hormone medication, making it ineffective. The advice is usually to take any thyroid hormone medication at least one hour prior to any iron supplement. Alternatively, if the iron supplement has already been taken, then it is sensible to wait for four hours before taking the thyroid medication. This should enable the maximum absorption of the thyroid hormone.

Pulse Oximeters

A portable pulse oximeter is a device that clips onto your finger and reads your heart rate as well as the percentage of oxygen in your blood. The oximeter was originally developed to detect hypoxia, which is a condition caused by insufficient oxygen. Haemoglobin in the blood bonds to oxygen and carries it to the tissues. A pulse oximeter works by emitting an infrared light that shines through your body's tissues to a photo sensor on the other side. The infrared light is able to detect the amount of haemoglobin that is saturated with (or carrying) oxygen. The pulse oximeter will display a number that indicates the percentage of haemoglobin that is saturated with oxygen. A pulse oximeter reading (denoted by SpO2) in the 97 - 99 range is typical for a healthy person. SpO2 is the shorthand that doctors use to be clear that the reading is arterial oxyhaemoglobin saturation measured non-invasively by pulse oximetry - it is a clear and unambiguous term that avoids confusing the result with another measurement.

Reading a pulse oximeter is quite simple. The pulse oximeter must be clipped onto a part of your body where light can shine through the blood flowing through your arteries. The finger is usually the best place to attach the oximeter. Alternatively, the toe, earlobe or bridge of your nose may also be used. Because pulse oximeters are most frequently used on the finger, these devices are also commonly called a finger pulse oximeter. Ensure the pulse oximeter is giving you an accurate reading. A good way to do this is to compare the pulse rate on the pulse oximeter to the heart rate you get by taking your pulse manually or through a blood pressure monitor. If they do not correspond, then the pulse oximeter is not being used correctly. The muscles in the arm and the hand of the finger that is being used need to be completely relaxed when testing. Lying down to do the test is ideal. The person undergoing the test must be breathing room air rather than using any form of oxygen or breathing apparatus and ideally in a location that is at or close to sea level (altitude may affect the readings). The finger that the oximeter is placed on needs to be clean, completely still and fingernail polish or false nails should not be present. Finally, any readings should not be done in bright ambient light.

A normal reading of SpO2 is in the high 90s, with 97 - 99 being typical. A reading of 95 or less could indicate some underlying issue and should be investigated. A reading of 90 or less indicates significant hypoxia and requires immediate action.

Iron deficiency will cause a lower oxygen level in the blood, which should result in a low oximeter reading (low percentage of oxygen). Increasing iron to a healthy level will normally raise the oxygen level in the blood. A low oxygen level can have other causes apart from iron-deficiency anaemia, such as poor fitness levels, carbon monoxide poisoning, asthma, allergies, smoking, respiratory infections, sickle cell anaemia, thalassemia and various heart conditions (where the blood is not being circulated normally).

The use of oximeters by thyroid patients who have concerns that they may be deficient in iron or are already taking iron supplementation is a fairly recent occurrence. Thyroid patients and doctors are just beginning to understand how useful these cheap and helpful devices may be. Consequently, the information contained here is as accurate as I could make it at the time of writing. However, as the use of these devices by thyroid patients increases, then hopefully we will see more information on oximeter use becoming available on the Internet.

Different models of oximeters may provide slightly different readings and care should be taken to read all the information that comes with any oximeter purchased. It's hard to be confident that an oximeter will detect the existence of low iron levels because the body makes adjustments to compensate for loss of iron. When the oxygen level falls below 90%, hospitals usually use an oxygen machine to maintain a normal oxygen level, however this level is too low for determining whether someone has an iron deficiency or not. Some thyroid patients have found that oxygen levels of 92% – 95% may be indicative of an iron deficiency and may prompt them to request a thorough panel of iron tests from their doctor.

For a patient already taking iron supplementation then no matter how much iron supplementation is taken, the highest possible oximeter reading is 99 - 100. A measurement of 99 can mean there is a healthy 99% oxygen level and an optimal level of iron supplementation is being taken. However, a reading of 99 can also mean a 99% oxygen level as a result of taking too much iron. If a patient's oximeter is constantly reading at 99 for several days then it is possible that they are taking too much iron supplementation and they should consult their doctor and ensure that their iron levels are tested.

In light of the information above, it should be clear that these devices might only act as a guide to possible iron levels. Oximeter readings may provide an indication to suggest that iron levels are low which will hopefully encourage patients to prompt their doctor to carry out a thorough set of iron blood tests. For those thyroid patients already taking iron supplementation oximeters may provide additional information that may help them to see how well the supplementation is working.

VITAMIN B12

Vitamin B12 is one of the B complex vitamins. It is used in the production of red blood cells and proteins. It helps the blood transport oxygen and therefore is vital for energy. Vitamin B12 is also used in making DNA and it plays an important role in the nervous system.

Thyroid patients and vitamin B12

Someone with hypothyroidism may not be absorbing B12 properly, possibly because of low stomach acid levels. A further and more serious reason for B12 deficiency may be due to an autoimmune issue, that reduces the level of intrinsic factor in the stomach. In this latter case, the B12 deficiency may be so serious that it leads to pernicious anaemia.

There is some evidence that B12 may also be involved in the conversion of T4 to T3, since tissue deficiencies of B12 have been seen to be associated with a reduced deiodinase activity in animal livers and in T3 levels in serum.[3]

The symptoms of B12 deficiency include:

- Tiredness.
- Weakness.
- Breathlessness after activity.
- Heart palpitations.
- Headaches.
- Mental confusion/brain fog.
- Balance issues.
- Dizziness.
- Reduced appetite.

- Easy bruising.
- Sore mouth and tongue.

If the deficiency is very severe then nerve related symptoms such as pins and needles (neuropathy) may develop.

Vitamin B12 laboratory test (cobalamin test)

The important thing to note is that many of the symptoms of B12 deficiency may overlap the symptoms of hypothyroidism and make the thyroid hormone replacement appear as though it's not working. For this reason it is very important to have a blood test for B12 performed, prior to the commencement of treatment with any thyroid hormone replacement. The typical laboratory reference range for a B12 test result is 200 - 900 pg/mL but thyroid patients usually feel better with results near the top of the reference range. Since B12 is not toxic it is advisable to supplement to achieve a very healthy level of B12, rather than have a level near the bottom of the laboratory reference range. Supplementing B12 at 500 ug or 1000 ug may be done safely in addition to any B complex. If there is a clear deficiency of B12 then a family doctor will probably prescribe a specific treatment for this. Methylcobalamin is the supplement of choice rather than cyanocobalamin (methylcobalamin is more directly usable and contains no cyanide molecule which the body needs to remove).

B12 works synergistically with folic acid, so it is important to also have a folate test done at the same time as the B12 blood test. Folic acid is usually included in any B complex supplementation. Please be aware that if someone has low B12 and they are taking folic acid supplementation then this can mask any B12 deficiency being detected through a B12 laboratory test.

New Active Vitamin B12 laboratory test (holotranscobalamin test)

The majority (up to 80%) of serum vitamin B12 is not bio-available. Current laboratory tests measure total vitamin B12. There is a poor correlation between circulatory total B12 and B12 at the tissue level. Consequently, it is possible that some vitamin B12 deficient patients might not be detected by the standard vitamin B12 laboratory test. Conversely, some patients can inappropriately be classified as being B12 deficient. The new active vitamin B12 test is only a recent development and might not yet be readily available except through private laboratories. However, it is likely that over time this new test will become readily available and might even become the de-facto vitamin B12 laboratory test.

VITAMIN D

Vitamin D is made in the skin. Under normal circumstances the body creates sufficient amounts of vitamin D simply due to being outside in sunlight. Vitamin D is also present in a small number of foods, some of which have been fortified with the vitamin during the processing of the food.

Vitamin D helps the absorption of calcium and so it is vital in the building and maintenance of strong and healthy bones. Vitamin D also modulates neuromuscular function, reduces inflammation and influences the action of many genes. Vitamin D deficiency may be implicated in osteoporosis, poor hair follicle growth, some vascular diseases, arrhythmia (abnormal heartbeats), strokes, certain cancers (breast, prostate), multiple sclerosis, rheumatoid arthritis, diabetes, Parkinson's and Alzheimer's diseases, depression, muscle weakness, chronic fatigue and seasonal affective disorder (SAD).[4]

Thyroid patients and vitamin D

Research carried out as far back as twenty years ago began to mention links between low levels of vitamin D and thyroid disease. This may be due to poor absorption of vitamin D in the GI tract as a result of a slower metabolism. More research is becoming available on the effects of vitamin D deficiency and the links with hypothyroidism and autoimmune diseases. Much more work is required but the evidence is accumulating, that suggests that vitamin D is actually extremely important.

In particular, it appears that people with autoimmune thyroid disease are more prone to low levels of vitamin D and this may even be due to a gene defect.[5] Studies show that a high percentage of people with autoimmune thyroid disease have gene defects that affect their ability to process vitamin D within cells. The defect appears to reside in the vitamin D receptors within the cells. Unfortunately, this defect is not detectable via a blood test of vitamin D, which may appear normal. So, some doctors are making recommendations that patients with Hashimoto's thyroiditis should use much higher levels of vitamin D3 supplementation to provide a greater possibility of adequate vitamin use within the tissues.[6]

Low levels of vitamin D that are accompanied by high calcium levels may be indicative of secondary hyperparathyroidism and this should be investigated by a qualified medical professional and may necessitate vitamin D supplementation.

Vitamin D is increasingly being talked about as having a calming influence on the autoimmune response in Hashimoto's thyroiditis patients.[7] To compensate for this, some doctors recommend that their patients, who have autoimmune thyroid disease, take supplemental doses of vitamin D3. However, prior testing may be safer before supplementation.

Vitamin D supplementation

Vitamin D is usually supplemented in the form of cholecalciferol or Vitamin D3, in the range of 4000-5000 IUs per day (Vitamin D Council recommendation).[8] In healthy adults, sustained intake of 50,000 IUs can produce toxicity after several months. Pregnant or breastfeeding women should consult a doctor before taking a vitamin D supplement, as should patients that have <u>known kidney problems.</u> The Institute of Medicine as of 30 November 2010, has increased the tolerable upper limit to 2500 IU per day for ages 1–3 years, 3000 IU per day for ages 4–8 years and <u>4000 IU per day for ages 9–71+</u> years (including pregnant or lactating women).[8]

Vitamin D overdose causes hypercalcaemia and the main symptoms of this are: anorexia, nausea, and vomiting can occur, frequently followed by polyuria, polydipsia, weakness, nervousness, pruritus, and, ultimately, renal failure. <u>Stopping any vitamin D3 supplementation and restricting calcium intake, is the treatment for vitamin D toxicity, although any kidney damage may be irreversible.</u> Therefore, care must be taken to ensure that if vitamin D supplementation is used then excessive amounts are not taken.

I do use vitamin D3 but prefer to be ultra cautious and only use 2500 IUs in the darker months of the year.

Working with a family doctor, or nutritionist, to ensure the safe use of vitamin D3 supplementation is very important.

Vitamin D laboratory test

Vitamin D may be tested via a 25-hydroxy vitamin D blood test. This is another test that it is important for a patient's family doctor to do in order to assess the patient's vitamin D level prior to thyroid hormone replacement, so that any deficiency may be corrected. The typical laboratory reference range for the 25-hydroxy vitamin D test is 30 - 74 ng/mL but many <u>thyroid patients appear to feel better once their results are in the 50 - 70 ng/mL range.</u>

VITAMIN B COMPLEX

B complex contains the following vitamins:

- B1 (thiamine).
- B2 (riboflavin).
- B3 (niacinamide).
- B5 (pantothenic acid).
- B6 (pyridoxine).
- B7 (biotin).
- B9 (folic acid).
- B12 (cobalamin)

The B vitamins play important roles in the metabolic processes that are regulated by thyroid hormones. These vitamins are involved in energy production, brain function, digestion, protein digestion, protein synthesis and usage, skin/hair/nerve health, the acid/alkaline balance, sugar and cholesterol management processes, inflammatory processes and the balancing of other hormones. The B complex vitamins are **hugely important**. They help us to deal with stress, which presumably is due to their positive effect on the adrenal glands.

Thyroid patients and vitamin B complex

Enzymes are critical in the metabolic pathways involving thyroid hormones. Enzymes are proteins that either have vitamins or minerals attached to them. All patients who use thyroid hormone replacement will benefit from supplementation with B complex vitamins. Sufficient levels of these micronutrients must be available at the cellular level for correct thyroid hormone operation. Vitamin B1 is extremely important since it is one of the co-factors used by the mitochondria in the generation of cellular energy (ATP). Vitamins B2, B6 and B12 are thought to be important in the conversion of T4 to T3. In addition, once thyroid hormone replacement therapy has begun, more of these important vitamins will inevitably be used up as the body starts to function properly again, which may result in nutrient deficiencies if they are not supplemented.

It is worth being aware of the effects of vitamin B1 deficiency. If a patient with a vitamin B1 deficiency begins taking thyroid hormone replacement, severe symptoms similar to hyperthyroidism, or thyrotoxicosis, may develop.[9] A severe vitamin B1 deficiency may lead to a heart disorder once thyroid hormone replacement begins. Therefore, supplementing with a strong B complex prior to thyroid treatment is a wise idea. For those people who have symptoms of fibromyalgia, a deficiency of vitamin B1 can also cause more widespread pain.

All the B vitamins are critical. Recently, I spoke to a thyroid patient whose adrenal hormone levels improved dramatically after vitamin B3 (niacin) supplementation. Ensuring that excellent levels of B vitamins are available to the body is extremely important.

Vitamin B complex supplementation

Supplementing with a high potency vitamin B complex, twice per day with meals, prior to commencing any thyroid hormone replacement is highly desirable. A high potency vitamin B complex will typically have around 50 mg of each of the vitamins B1, B2, B3, B5 and B6. This level of supplementation will support the thyroid and adrenal metabolic pathways and potentially reduce the number of confusing issues that can occur during thyroid hormone replacement. There should be no need to test deficiencies of all the B vitamins, as there is no risk of overdosing, even with the use of high potency B complex products.

Folic acid, folate testing and relevance to vitamin B12

Folic acid is one of the B vitamins. It is important to be aware that a folic acid deficiency can compromise the effectiveness of B12, which is important in thyroid hormone metabolism. A folic acid deficiency, also known as a folate deficiency, can lead to anaemia as it affects the function of B12. A deficiency of folic acid can also cause: loss of appetite, diarrhoea, stomach pains, weakness, lack of energy, prematurely greying hair, sore tongue, mouth ulcers, cracked lips, headaches, heart palpitations, shortness of breath, poor memory, mental confusion and irritability. Folic acid and B12 also play a role in depression as they are both used in the production of neurotransmitters. Low levels of folic acid and B12 may lead to a build up of homocysteine, which ultimately may cause cerebral dysfunction and depression. Relatively recent research has identified low levels of the B vitamins, B12, folic acid and elevated homocysteine levels as increasing the risk of cognitive decline such as that occurring in Alzheimer's disease.[10,11]

For all the above reasons it is highly desirable to have a folate test done at the same time as having a B12 test, because folic acid and B12 work synergistically together. The typical laboratory reference range for folate test results is 2.7 - 17.0 ng/mL. It is sensible to use diet or supplementation to ensure that folate levels are at least in the middle of this reference range.

VITAMIN C

Vitamin C helps the immune system and helps to fight infections. It is used to make collagen and helps to maintain bones, skin and joint health. It is also a powerful antioxidant that removes toxins and helps to protect us from disease. Vitamin C is also critical for the production of adrenal hormones and the adrenal glands have the highest concentration of vitamin C of all the organs of the body. Vitamin C is also used in the conversion of food into energy.

Humans used to make vitamin C naturally - lots of it!

There is now widely accepted scientific evidence that suggests that human beings experienced a genetic mutation about 5000 years ago, causing us to lose the ability to manufacture ascorbic acid (vitamin C). The most likely reason for this genetic mutation was that food was very scarce at that point in time. Producing high levels of vitamin C in the body would have consumed a lot of energy and so losing this ability would have offered the mutated human an advantage in times of food shortages. Many mammals, including cats, dogs and rats, can still manufacture vitamin C within their bodies and they do this in very large quantities. If we take account of the difference in body weight between some of these animals and humans, it would suggest that humans would have produced many grams of vitamin C per day prior to the genetic mutation. These mammals produce even more of their own vitamin C, sometimes a factor of 100 times their normal rate, in times of stress and illness.

Based on the above, it is very easy to believe that we humans were meant to have much higher levels of vitamin C circulating in our blood, than the rather low current RDA would have us believe.

I have read two books that very clearly and with extensive reference to experimental data, set out a solid scientific case that indicates that the rationale behind the current RDA for vitamin C is flawed.[12, 13]

Vitamin C Supplementation

Hickey and Roberts develop what they refer to as a 'Dynamic Flow theory' that explains the factors affecting blood and cellular levels of vitamin C. One of the main conclusions of their book is that it is far better to take many smaller doses of vitamin C per day than a single large dose. The Hickey/Roberts Dynamic Flow findings indicate that the half-life of vitamin C in the blood stream is around 30 minutes and that doses of 500-1000 mg every few hours ensures a high concentration of vitamin C all day long. This might translate into a supplementation regime of four to six 500-1000 mg vitamin C tablets each day.

It is only by maintaining high levels of vitamin C in the tissues that the benefits of this vitamin can truly be felt. Animals that can produce vitamin C themselves are able to achieve this high concentration naturally.

Vitamin C is also a good general antioxidant and can help to protect against toxicity induced by heavy metals like cadmium. I try to use the Hickey/Roberts Dynamic Flow method but I have a sensitive GI tract. Some people with sensitive systems may find that vitamin C causes loose bowels. I am careful to take 500 mg of vitamin C in buffered form (sodium ascorbate), rather than in the pure ascorbic acid form and I do this six times per day.

There is no risk of toxicity from vitamin C and taking as much vitamin C, as is easily tolerated, is sensible. The only cautionary note is that for those that already have some form of PH imbalance in the body then high doses of vitamin C can make things worse and the patient should consult with their doctor prior to supplementing with vitamin C.

MAGNESIUM

Magnesium plays a key role in many metabolic functions: it promotes muscle and nerve action, it is essential for normal heart beat, health of the blood vessels, bone and teeth formation and generally for the growth and repair of body cells. It is involved in energy production and regulates body temperature. It ensures the right distribution of phosphorus, sodium, potassium and calcium across cell membranes as well as the proper absorption of B-complex vitamins, vitamin C and E. It is also necessary in the production of testosterone and progesterone.

Low magnesium levels can cause various heart related issues including:

- Arrhythmias (irregular beats), tachycardia (rapid heart rate) due to poor cellular potassium regulation.
- Abnormal electrical activity shown on ECGs.
- Arteriosclerosis (stiffening of blood vessels).
- Narrowing of arteries.
- High blood pressure.
- Angina.

- Heart attacks due to low oxygen reaching the heart (because of too much calcium and not enough magnesium reaching the heart).
- Blood clots, which might lead to a heart attack or stroke.
- Heart valve problems.

People with rapid/slow or irregular heart rhythm or any other cardiovascular issue should consider low magnesium as a possible factor.[14]

Magnesium deficiency is also associated with migraine headaches, insomnia, depression, irritability, fatigue and a number of other neurological, muscular metabolic and cardiovascular problems. It is also works as a co-factor with many enzymes. Low magnesium also can lead to bone loss, as the body will strip out magnesium and calcium from the bones to compensate for low available magnesium levels.

It is important to take magnesium if you are using calcium supplements as too much calcium in the diet in the absence of magnesium can cause excess calcium to enter the cells and a state of hyperactivity can occur, which may include cardiovascular effects.[15] Having both a healthy amount of magnesium in the diet and through supplementation combined with healthy amounts of calcium is the ideal situation. I recommend the book I have just referenced as it contains a wealth of information on this topic.

Hypothyroidism tends to lead to our cells dumping magnesium (and potassium) in order to reduce overall energy output. This magnesium is then excreted from the body. The combination of hypothyroidism and magnesium deficiency can put such a strain on the heart that in rare cases this can result in sudden cardiac failure with absolutely no warning. Consequently, eating enough fruit and vegetables and supplementing with magnesium is very sensible indeed.

Once there is sufficient magnesium in our cells this activates the sodium/potassium 'pump' that swaps sodium and potassium across the cell membrane. Consequently, by supplementing with magnesium and eating enough fresh fruit and vegetables we can ensure that we have enough of both magnesium and potassium in our cells, without the need to supplement with potassium. So, people with apparently low potassium levels may be advised to supplement with magnesium to raise both magnesium and potassium levels.

It is common for people to have far too little magnesium in their diets. However, in the unusual circumstance of having too much magnesium in the diet, this can lead to kidney problems and digestive upsets.

I have been told that we need roughly a little less than half the amount of magnesium in our diet as calcium. Therefore, some doctors suggest taking 500-1000mg per day of magnesium supplementation. People who have very sensitive GI tracts find that they cannot tolerate the above levels of magnesium without experiencing some digestive upsets.

The chelated form of magnesium is significantly gentler on the digestive system. I have found that adding 200 mg chelated magnesium twice a day to my own supplementation regime has dramatically improved my recovery rate after intense cardiovascular exercise, which I can only conclude means that I did have some level of magnesium deficiency.

In order to reduce any confusing symptoms that may occur during thyroid hormone replacement it is advisable to supplement with enough magnesium. It can sometimes be difficult to understand why issues arise during thyroid hormone replacement. Removing as many of the possible nutrient deficiencies that can create confusing symptoms during thyroid hormone replacement is critical if a straightforward and quick treatment process is desired.

SELENIUM

Selenium is one of the trace minerals and it is extremely important in thyroid hormone metabolism. Selenium is of special interest because it forms a key component of the deiodinase enzymes. In animal experiments, deficiencies of selenium were associated with reduced T3 levels, as a result of impaired deiodinase activity.[16, 17] It is because selenium is an important component of the deiodinase enzymes that low selenium levels are thought to have the potential to adversely affect the conversion of T4 to T3. Selenium is also an antioxidant and it protects us from free radicals, reduces inflammation and helps the immune system. It also helps the heart, as it works synergistically with vitamin E. Some research that suggests that selenium may help to reduce thyroid autoantibodies.[18]

Selenium supplementation

Many soils have become depleted in selenium over the years. Consequently, ensuring there is enough selenium in the diet, or via a supplement, is very important for a thyroid patient. Selenium is easy to supplement and has no known toxicity below 750 micrograms. It is often recommended that thyroid patients supplement with 200 micrograms of selenium each day.

CALCIUM

Calcium is good for the heart, blood, nerves, muscle activation, skin, bones and teeth. Calcium helps muscles recover from use and it plays an important role in maintaining our acid/alkaline balance.

Endocrinologists and doctors often advise thyroid patients to take a 500 mg calcium supplement once or twice a day, as well as some vitamin D3 to aid the absorption of the calcium. The idea behind this is that those people who use any form of thyroid hormone replacement may be slightly more at risk of suffering from osteoporosis later in life. Some form of regular weight bearing exercise needs to be combined with the calcium intake for the maximum benefit to be obtained in the maintenance of healthy bones. Calcium in the diet is important in order to maintain bone density but it is also vital in other areas of the body, including the muscles and the nervous system. Taking some vitamin D3 with the calcium is essential in order to ensure that the calcium will actually be used to build new bone.

It is very important to be aware that taking calcium supplements without sufficient magnesium may create an unhealthy calcium-magnesium balance, as too much calcium entering our cells is dangerous. Consequently, taking magnesium supplements also may be advisable. As mentioned in the earlier information regarding magnesium too much calcium or calcium in the presence of inadequate magnesium may be over-stimulatory.

Some endocrinologists also advise thyroid patients to have a bone density scan (Dexa scan), every two or three years, to monitor the health of the bones.

It is advisable to take any thyroid medication at least one hour before any calcium supplement, or alternatively, wait four hours after the calcium has been taken, before taking any thyroid hormone medication.

ZINC

Zinc is a component of hundreds of enzymes as well as being used in DNA. It is essential for growth, healing, and hormone control. Zinc helps us to cope with stress and aids the brain and nervous system. It is also important for the health of the teeth, bones and hair.

Zinc is also necessary for normal thyroid function and to maintain normal energy levels. Low levels of zinc are associated with decreased levels of total and free T3 and increased rT3, so it appears that zinc has some role to play in the conversion of T4 to T3. Zinc is also thought to be necessary in the binding of T3 to the nuclear thyroid receptors.[19] Zinc helps to protect us against heavy metal toxicity. The symptoms of zinc deficiency can overlap those of hypothyroidism because of its role in many enzymes. Zinc is often supplemented at 15 mg per day. However, it is important to be aware that zinc supplementation is thought to lower cortisol levels and patients with low cortisol may be advised by their doctor not to supplement with zinc.[20] In fact, zinc is often used by thyroid patients to suppress elevated cortisol levels that can occur at certain times of the day, along with adrenal adaptogens.

VITAMIN E

Vitamin E is a powerful antioxidant, which protects cells from damage and helps the body utilise oxygen. It is also very good for the heart as it helps to reduce blood clots, thrombosis and long-term damage to the cardiovascular system. It improves healing and the skin. Vitamin E is thought by many to reduce the risk of heart disease and is useful in reducing heavy metal toxicity. A typical supplementation level is 400 IUs of vitamin E.

CHROMIUM

Chromium is one of the trace minerals. It is critical in the maintenance of blood sugar balance and in protecting DNA from damage. It is also important in heart function. Chromium is a part of a metal-protein complex known as glucose tolerance factor (GTF) because it appears to help insulin work more efficiently. When supplemented, 200 micrograms is typical. Chromium is also thought by some to lower cortisol levels and a patient's doctor may advise them not to supplement with chromium.[21]

OTHER TRACE ELEMENTS

Trace elements include boron, copper, chromium, iodine, manganese, molybdenum, selenium and iron. I have already discussed those that are of special interest for thyroid patients (chromium, iron and selenium).

Manganese is important in the formation of bones, cartilage, tissues and nerves. It is also important in the activation of many enzymes and helps with blood sugar balance and brain function. Manganese also helps to maintain healthy DNA and is essential for the creation of red blood cells and insulin. It is therefore useful to have manganese in the diet, or in some form of supplement.

Iodine is reported to benefit some thyroid patients. I do not have any personal experience of using it, other than in the tiny quantities found in salt, or in my multi-mineral supplement. There are mixed reports on the benefits of iodine. Some thyroid patients believe it plays a critical part in achieving optimal thyroid or adrenal function and others say that it has made their autoimmune condition worse. I have no specific recommendations on iodine but it is important to be aware of the mixed opinions on its usage. My advice to any thyroid patient is to do your own research and talk to your own doctor about the value that iodine supplementation may or may not offer you.

Copper is also thought to have a role in thyroid hormone metabolism and is used by the body within many enzymes, often in conjunction with zinc. Copper deficiency or a zinc-copper imbalance can cause: irregular heartbeats; lack of response to iron in cases of anaemia; skin problems and nor-adrenaline production issues.

Supplementing with a good multi-mineral

Using a general-purpose multi-mineral that contains a sprinkling of these trace elements may provide some protection against any deficiencies caused by processed foods, or our modern diets. I consider the use of a good chelated multi-mineral to be of great value in eliminating another potential source of issues during thyroid hormone replacement. If one of the minerals is deficient then this may undermine thyroid hormone treatment and give rise to confusing symptoms that may be difficult to understand and may cause significant delays in achieving a return to good health.

OMEGA-3 FATTY ACIDS

The Omega-3 fatty acids contain EPA (eicosapentaenoic acid) and DHA (docosahexaenoic acid), which are important in heart and brain function. EPA and DHA are involved in vision, learning ability, coordination, and mood. They also reduce the stickiness of blood and help to control cholesterol and fat levels. Omega-3s help to improve immune function, metabolism and reduce inflammation.

Although they are not directly implicated in thyroid hormone processing, our modern diets are often quite low in Omega-3 fatty acids and so these are usually well worth supplementing.

NUTRIENT SUPPLEMENTATION AND LABORATORY TESTING

Thyroid patients who wish to use supplementation, to ensure that they have the broad range of nutrients available, should consult their own doctor, or a qualified nutritionist, for advice on which supplements to use and safe levels to take. Laboratory testing may also be available, which can provide evidence of nutrients that are low and may be safely supplemented. There are also some excellent books that cover a range of useful information including safe levels of supplementation.[22]

Anyone who continues to have problems when they using an appropriate thyroid hormone replacement therapy should consider having a wide range of tests that include iron, B12, folate, vitamin D and all the macro and trace minerals. It is extremely easy for someone to overlook a nutrient issue and continue to have symptomatic issues interfere with a perfectly good thyroid replacement regime.

Laboratory testing of nutrients should only be done if any supplementation containing the nutrients is stopped for a period of time prior to the test. It is sensible to stop the relevant nutrients for at least several days before the test, although I usually allow one week without the nutrient in order to be confident in the test result. This should be discussed with the patient's own doctor to confirm this approach and how long that any supplementation should be ceased prior to laboratory testing.

MY OWN SUPPLEMENTATION REGIME

My personal supplementation regime is summarised in a table. It is **not** in any way intended to be a recommendation for anyone. I have simply included the supplements I use so that any reader can see how I have implemented some of the information above.

I began taking most of these supplements when I started thyroid hormone replacement but I have modified the regime over time to reflect my own personal needs and any new findings about thyroid or adrenal hormone metabolism.

Ideally, I would take a little more vitamin C but I develop digestive problems at higher levels. I also use chelated magnesium to avoid digestive issues.

If I had a specific nutritional deficiency, such as low levels of iron, B12, folate or vitamin D3, then I may have had to use a higher level of supplementation, recommended by my family doctor, to fully correct the deficiency.

I use vitamin C, L-methionine and anti-histamines as part of an on-going programme to control my histamine levels as a result of internal urticaria, which I have previously alluded to.

I have been on T3 for around fifteen years and I am obviously getting older now. However, my health is now the best it has been since I first developed thyroid problems. I attribute most of this improvement in my health in the past few years entirely to the use of appropriate supplements of vitamins and minerals.

I consider the use of the supplements of important vitamins and minerals as a critical part of my recovery. The use of vitamins and minerals should **not** be viewed as a short-term measure designed to kick start the metabolism. They are a lifetime commitment to good health and a working thyroid hormone metabolism.

My daily nutritional regime is as follows:

Supplement	Amount	Taken	Comment
Protein drink		Breakfast	Slow release energy
Vitamin C	500 mg	Breakfast	Sodium ascorbate.
Vitamin C	500 mg	Morning	To reduce histamine levels.
Vitamin B Complex:		Lunch	
B1 (thiamine)	50 mg		
B2 (riboflavin)	50 mg		
B3 (niacin)	50 mg		
B5 (pantothenic acid)	50 mg		
B6 (pyridoxine)	50 mg		
B12	50 ug		
Folic acid	400 ug		
Biotin	50 ug		
Choline Bitartrate	50 mg		
Inositol	50 mg		
PABA	50 mg		
Vitamin C	500 mg	Lunch	
Vitamin B12	500 ug	Lunch	Ideally in the methylcobalamin form
Vitamin D3	2400 IUs	Lunch	October-March **only.**
Vitamin E	400 IUs	Lunch	
Calcium+200 IUs D3	250 mg	Lunch	
L-Methionine	500mg	Lunch	To reduce histamine levels.
Multi-Mineral:		Lunch	
Calcium	250 mg		
Iodine	75 ug		
Iron	5 mg		
Magnesium	125 mg		
Phosphorus	100 mg		
Zinc	5 mg		
Boron	1 mg		
Copper	0.125 mg		
Chromium	10 ug		
Manganese	5 mg		
Potassium	33 mg		
Selenium	13 ug		
Chelated Magnesium	200 mg	Lunch	Additional to mineral (only form I can tolerate)
Selenium	200 ug	Lunch	Additional to mineral.
Omega-3 Fish Oil	1000 mg	Lunch	(180 mg EPA, 120 mg DHA)
Vitamin C	500 mg	Mid Afternoon	
Vitamin B Complex	As above	Dinner	
Vitamin C	500 mg	Dinner	
Calcium+200 IUs D3	250 mg	Dinner	
Chelated Magnesium	200 mg	Dinner	
L-Methionine	500 mg	Dinner	
Cod Liver Oil	1000 mg	3 days/week	(2600 IUs Vitamin A, 200 IUs Vit. D, 110 mg EPA, 100 mg DHA)
Vitamin C	500 mg	Late Evening	

Chapter 5

Other Factors and Hypothyroidism

Before I begin to tell my own story of how I recovered from hypothyroidism, I need to outline some other factors that may affect thyroid hormone metabolism.

ENVIRONMENTAL TOXINS

There are many chemicals that we unfortunately come into contact with all too often. Some of these may be avoided with a little knowledge, whereas others are actually increasingly more difficult to avoid, as they are in our food, water and the air that we breathe.

Pesticides are used in the production of our food. Livestock are given antibiotics and are treated with pesticides. The foods that livestock are fed have been treated at some stage with pesticides. Our foods are processed and treated to aid their presentation, storage and shelf-life.[1] Many of the 'treatments' used throughout the lifecycle of the foods that we consume are known to have adverse effects on our bodies and, especially in this context, our thyroid hormones.

The list of toxins that we find in our modern life appears to be growing. Here are just a few:

* *Mercury*. This is highly toxic and is found in amalgam based dental fillings. It is also used in the composition of some vaccines. Mercury stays in the body for a long time and can affect the biochemical pathways associated with thyroid hormones. I have had all my amalgam fillings removed and replaced with white mercury-free fillings, which look better and are healthier. If mercury fillings are removed, then this needs to be done by a professional, who can perform the procedure without releasing mercury into the body. My dentist used a rubber dam at the back of my mouth, to prevent any mercury from being ingested.

* *Heavy Metals*. Lead, cadmium and mercury (already singled out) are produced by industry and contaminate the food chain (fish especially). They are all capable of blocking the uptake of selenium, crucial in the processing of thyroid hormones. Cadmium is known to induce a lowering of TSH. The use of nutrients like zinc, vitamin E and vitamin C, may be beneficial to protect against heavy metal toxicity.

* *Dioxins and PCBs (polychlorinated biphenols)*. If ingested then these remain in fatty tissues in our bodies for many years. Dioxins interfere with the uptake of iodine and how it is processed

into thyroid hormones. PCBs are used in many electrical products, in plastic manufacture, paints, adhesives, flame-retardants and inks. There has been a phasing out of their use but the contamination of the environment and food chain has already occurred, according to some. Dioxins and PCBs are toxic and can damage our immune systems, liver and the processing of thyroid hormones. PCBs can also prevent enough thyroid hormone from binding to a protein called transthyretin, which is the protein responsible for carrying thyroid hormone to the brain.[2] PCBs and other chemical contaminants can directly reduce thyroid hormone production of T4 and T3 and speed up thyroid hormones clearance.

- *Fluorine*. Fluorides are compounds containing fluorine and they are all toxic to the body to some extent. A common exposure to fluoride is from toothpaste, although we have the option to buy toothpaste without fluoride. Fluorides are present in many other applications, including numerous drugs, like antibiotics and anaesthetics. Fluoride is also added to the water supplies in some areas, to reduce tooth decay. Unfortunately, fluoride tends to destroy and disrupt enzymes and can have a disastrous effect on the processing of thyroid hormones.[3] We should all oppose the fluoridation of our water supplies in my opinion.

- *Silica, beryllium, aluminium and fluorine*. These are all capable of increasing the level of a protein (Gq/11), which can reduce the action of the T3 thyroid hormone within our cells.[4] The Gq/11 protein also desensitizes the thyroid to the stimulation of TSH, which in turn will lower the production of T4 and T3 from the thyroid.

- *Lithium*. This is not really a toxin but a component of some drugs for anxiety and depression. This will interfere significantly with thyroid hormone release, as will drugs containing bromine (used in some sedatives).

Having researched some of this, I was left with the question - well, what do we do about it? I think the answer has to be that we need to do our own research and, based on our own diet and lifestyle, we need to make our own choices and when possible we should eat freshly grown, organically produced foods.

INTERACTION WITH SEX HORMONES

Sex hormone imbalances may occur in both men and women at any age. This is nothing to be ashamed of and paying attention to these hormones can be very important, as it is possible that an imbalance in sex hormones can cause some symptoms that may be confused with symptoms of hypothyroidism, which can make any treatment for hypothyroidism appear as though it is not working ideally.

If there is a genuine issue with one or more sex hormones as well as hypothyroidism then this can cause confusion for the patient and the doctor involved. For example treatment of hypothyroidism in women that has improved symptoms but has not eradicated them may be due to a sex hormone imbalance that might cause: fatigue, headaches, menstrual issues, low libido, weight gain or a feeling of coldness.[5] Since these symptoms are nearly identical to those experienced with hypothyroidism, additional testing of the sex hormones can provide invaluable information that may lead to a complete solution to unresolved problems.

Sex hormone imbalances in women can have many causes including: the menopause; exogenous estrogen exposure from environmental factors (e.g. foods, pesticides); birth control pills; stress and adrenal insufficiency; pregnancy; obesity; luteal phase defects causing low progesterone; hypothyroidism; anorexia; high sex hormone binding globulin (SHBG) due to past/current usage of birth control pills or oral estrogen supplementation - to name but a few.

If a sex hormone issue is suspected, then in the case of women, it may be sensible to find a doctor who is knowledgeable in diagnosing and treating common oestrogen, progesterone and testosterone imbalances. Various laboratory tests exist to provide help in diagnosing these types of issues. Progesterone and oestrogen should be tested. Oestrogen is a class of hormones, including estriol, estradiol and estrone, which should ideally be present in the correct ratios, although it is common for only estradiol to be tested of the three along with progesterone. It is also common for testosterone and SHBG to be tested.

Dehydroepiandrosterone sulphate (DHEAS) may also be tested along with the other hormones whenever excess or deficient androgen production is suspected or when a doctor wants to evaluate a patient's adrenal gland function. Dehydroepiandrosterone (DHEA) is produced by the adrenal glands primarily in the early morning. Around 90% of the DHEA in the bloodstream exists in the form of DHEAS (which is converted from DHEA by adding an extra sulphate molecule. Orally ingested DHEA is converted to DHEA when passing through the intestines and liver). DHEA peaks in the early morning, whereas DHEAS levels appear to remain far more stable showing no clear circadian rhythm and consequently, it is usually DHEAS that is tested.

DHEAS, testosterone, SHBG and possibly other androgens may be tested as part of a sex hormone evaluation or to evaluate a patient's adrenal gland function. Concentrations of DHEAS are often measured along with other hormones such as FSH, LH, prolactin, oestrogen and testosterone to help diagnose polycystic ovarian syndrome (PCOS) and to rule out other causes of infertility, amenorrhea and hirsutism. An increased level of DHEAS is not diagnostic of any specific condition but if sufficiently high it may suggest the need for further more specific tests to find the source of any hormonal imbalance.

Sex hormone testing for women who are still ovulating and having a menstrual cycle is usually done on a fixed day of a woman's monthly cycle, often between days 19 and 23 of a 28-day menstrual cycle. This ensures that ovulation has passed and the woman is well into the luteal phase of her cycle with progesterone levels that are reaching a peak level for the month.

The post-ovulation luteal phase is typically about 14 days and so testing of sex hormones between days 19 and 23 is the most reliable approach.

A woman who is postmenopausal may have the testing done on any day of the month.

Men too can have their own problems. Men may have various symptoms, some of which may overlap with hypothyroidism, making a potential sex hormone problem less obvious. Men may have low total testosterone, low free testosterone, or a high ratio of oestrogen to testosterone. Sex hormone imbalances in men can be related to such things as high estrogen levels due to obesity; a diet that includes exposure to exogenous hormones from milk or meat from animals that had been given hormones; elevated levels of aromatase (an enzyme that converts androgens into oestrogens); and hypothyroidism.

If a man suspects that he may have a sex hormone imbalance then a competent doctor could investigate these potential hormone imbalances, often by testing for total testosterone, free testosterone, SHBG (the main protein that binds most of the testosterone) and estradiol. Low testosterone may impact the conversion of T4 to T3.

A variety of options are available for both men and women for the correction of any imbalances. These range from simple herbs and natural substances to natural bio-identical hormone replacement, which is often delivered by applying creams or gels to the skin (transdermal replacement).[5, 6] Transdermal hormone replacement using bio-identical hormones is increasingly common these days and most doctors continue to use blood testing to determine the patient's response while under treatment for sex hormone imbalances. Saliva testing has proven to be a very accurate measure of free cortisol but it is not clear whether all hormones move passively and equally into the saliva. In addition, once a patient begins using transdermal sex hormone replacement then the levels in the saliva are thought to become quite high and may misrepresent the effective levels of the sex hormones in the blood and tissues. Consequently, blood tests are thought by many doctors to be a better tool to use to monitor sex hormone replacement levels, although it can take several weeks for bloodstream levels of sex hormones to rise when transdermal hormone replacement is being used. The counter argument to this is that more sex hormone tests are becoming available via saliva testing, e.g. it is possible to get the oestrogens estradiol, estriol and estrone tested via saliva testing and imbalances in the ratios of these may be corrected as a result. Consequently, some doctors do use saliva testing and over time the relative merits of the two types of testing may become clearer.

Some patients and their doctors find that they need to balance sex hormones, before they can achieve adequate FT3 levels.

GASTROINTESTINAL ISSUES

If a patient's thyroid hormone replacement therapy has arrived at a point, where the correct medication is being provided at the ideal level and problems still persist, then one or more of the following issues might provide some ideas for further things to investigate:

• *Coeliac disease.* Coeliac disease is an autoimmune disease that affects the small hairs, or villi, that line the small intestine. It is caused by a reaction to gliadin, which is a gluten protein found in wheat, barley, oats and rye. The resultant inflammation interferes with the ability of the villi of the small intestine to absorb nutrients. It is also known as celiac sprue and gluten intolerance. As well as reducing the ability of the gut to absorb nutrients, it is also thought to weaken the walls of the intestines and make them more permeable, allowing some proteins and chemicals to leak through the walls of the gut into the bloodstream.

Severe coeliac disease leads to diarrhoea, with loose, pale stools, weight loss, abdominal pain/cramping, bloating with abdominal distension and fatigue. Many findings are used to form a diagnosis of coeliac disease, including several key antibody tests but the final confirmation is often done via an endoscopic biopsy, to look at the damaged villi.

The only known treatment is to avoid the protein responsible for the condition and adopt a gluten-free diet for life. The poor absorption, as a result of coeliac disease, can cause poor absorption of iron, B12, calcium and vitamin D. Anaemia can be one result. Low blood sugar can be another. All of this can cause a related problem with thyroid hormone metabolism. Coeliac disease is an autoimmune disease and it often goes hand in hand with other autoimmune conditions like Hashimoto's thyroiditis. This may be partly due to any permeability of the gut that allows undesirable proteins into the blood, which then cause more stress on the immune system.

Because of the similarity to the symptoms of irritable bowel syndrome, some patients may initially be informed that they have irritable bowel syndrome, rather than coeliac disease.

• *Irritable bowel syndrome (IBS).* IBS is defined as a functional bowel disorder in the absence of any detectable organic cause. Typical symptoms include: chronic abdominal pain, discomfort, diarrhoea or constipation, bloating and alteration of bowel habits and fatigue as a result of the other symptoms. Some patients with coeliac disease were initially diagnosed with IBS. Consequently, doctors should consider testing for coeliac disease if there is any possibility that this could be the underlying cause.

There is no cure for IBS but various treatments, including pain relief, are used to relieve the symptoms. The exact cause of IBS is unknown. Some foods may appear to trigger the symptoms. There is some research that suggests that IBS may be caused by an as-yet undiscovered infection, as one recent study found that an antibiotic (Rifaximin) provided relief for IBS patients. Some doctors have suggested that IBS may have links to a bacterial overgrowth in the intestines (small intestinal bacterial overgrowth - SIBO).

Several medical conditions often occur in patients diagnosed with IBS. These include: headaches, fibromyalgia, chronic fatigue syndrome and depression.

The reason that I wanted to include IBS is that there are a number of interesting links to hypothyroidism. In hypothyroidism, the patient may have a number of digestive symptoms, which may overlap with those of IBS. In fact, many thyroid patients complain of having IBS as a part of their condition. Fibromyalgia is thought in many cases to be linked to low levels of thyroid hormone. IBS is often associated with a number of food sensitivities. Recent research has suggested links between histamine production from mast cells and IBS.[7] In addition to this, we also know that low thyroid conditions are associated with an increase in release of chemicals, like histamine, from mast cells.[8]

I have experienced severe problems with excess stomach acidity and depression, which were being caused by excess histamine production. Using a combination of anti-histamines and vitamin C resolved my symptoms. An immunologist told me that there are genetic links between autoimmune thyroid disease and urticaria and that this may have been responsible for my excess mast cell release of histamine.

My own conclusion is that where there are low thyroid conditions, do not be surprised to see IBS and where there is IBS, consider whether low thyroid levels might also be an issue.

• *Gut dysbiosis.* The gut contains many of the immune system tissues of the body. This is known as the gut-associated lymphoid tissue (GALT). The GALT helps to fight against disease. If the gut becomes compromised for any reason, then these immune system tissues are also compromised. Dysbiosis of the gut occurs when bad bacteria and other flora or fauna, like candida or parasites, take residence. The balance of good bacteria in the gut can change and this can be extremely bad for the GALT aspects of the gut. Often, diet has a part to play, with too much red meat, too little fibre and too many simple carbohydrates and sugar in our foods. In addition, there may be gluten intolerance issues, infections, low stomach acidity or even an initial infection that can start the problems.

Why should I include anything about gut dysbiosis here? A severe imbalance in the gut may allow proteins, that should remain contained there, to 'leak' through the normally well-protected gut walls and behave as antigens in our bloodstream. A 'leaky gut' may cause the immune system to go into overdrive and this is one route, according to some doctors, that can see the development of autoimmune diseases like Hashimoto's thyroiditis.

There are many other connections between gut health and thyroid hormones. The gut is involved in a certain amount of conversion of T4 to T3. Consequently, inflammation or disease in the gut could potentially reduce the levels of T3 hormone converted from T4. Low stomach acid often results from hypothyroidism and is associated with gut dysbiosis.

Therefore, patients with hypothyroidism may also have to address any digestive system issues, as well as treating the thyroid problem, if they are to achieve a full and swift recovery. Diet may have a part to play in this. In my own case, I developed many digestive system issues, which did not respond to any form of treatment until I eventually was prescribed T3 and at this point all of my digestive problems rapidly disappeared.

- *Immune system dysregulation*. I recently read a book, which really improved my understanding of some of the factors that can cause stress on the immune system and may set the scene for the development of diseases like Hashimoto's thyroiditis.[9] In this book, the author makes the case for addressing the stressors of the immune system, as a major part of treating any hypothyroidism.

These stressors include: stress at work or home, gluten intolerance, oestrogen surges, insulin resistance, polycystic ovary syndrome, vitamin D deficiency, toxicity issues, infections and inflammatory conditions.

The author's approach is focused on calming the immune system with dietary changes and appropriate nutrients. He is particularly insistent on removing gluten completely from the diet and possibly dairy products. The author goes as far as to say that simply treating the low thyroid hormones won't necessarily fix the symptoms and he argues that many of these symptoms can persist unless the immune system itself is calmed.

BLOOD SUGAR BALANCE

I mentioned in Chapters 2 and 3 that even with adequate thyroid hormones we won't feel well unless we have enough cellular energy (ATP) being generated by the mitochondria. The mitochondria require glucose as a critical input chemical. For sufficient glucose to reach the mitochondria our blood sugar metabolism needs to be in good working order. Consequently, healthy levels of chemicals such as insulin and cortisol play are very important.

One of the functions of cortisol is to raise blood sugar levels through a process called gluconeogenesis. Insulin's role is to facilitate the entry of glucose into our cells and to enable excess blood sugar to be stored for future use. If cortisol is low or insulin is low then the result can be that our cells do not receive the glucose levels that they need. Both cortisol from the adrenal glands and insulin from the pancreas need to be in balance in order for our cells to maintain healthy glucose levels. If our cells have sufficient glucose then the mitochondria can generate enough cellular energy. As mentioned earlier in this chapter our digestion and dietary intake can also have a bearing on all of this.

It naturally follows that if there is a problem with blood sugar metabolism then any pre-existing hypothyroid symptoms may be made significantly worse. Perhaps more importantly than the worsening of symptoms is the potential for any form of thyroid hormone treatment to fail to work as expected. It should not be surprising that severe problems with blood sugar metabolism might prevent a rise in overall metabolic rate.

If a patient has any suspicions that their blood sugar levels may be high, low or fluctuating, they should consult their own doctor or a suitable specialist. A patient's doctor may arrange for one or more tests to be performed, which may include a glucose tolerance test (GTT). A GTT typically requires the patient to fast from the previous night and then a series of blood sugar measurements are taken, prior to and after, the ingestion of a measured amount of glucose. In a healthy response, the blood sugar should rise and then, within a few hours, the blood sugar will steadily fall back to normal. In a patient with blood sugar metabolism issues, this pattern will not be followed and periods of both high and low blood sugar may exist. A knowledgeable doctor will be able to interpret the results of a GTT and identify potential problems. A GTT may be combined with the measurement of insulin levels in order to more clearly diagnose any potential pre-diabetes or insulin resistance or other issues.

Diet may be a factor, as too often, many of us eat too many refined carbohydrates. Over time, this may cause a blood sugar imbalance involving a large rise and subsequent steep fall in blood sugar levels, before the blood sugar level normalises. If this is allowed to continue, prolonged periods of low blood sugar, known as hypoglycaemia, can develop, resulting in a confusing set of symptoms including: fatigue, trembling or shaking, sleeplessness, confusion, anxiety, mood swings, feeling faint, headaches, depression, heart palpitations, hunger, cold hands/feet, clammy skin, sweating, dizziness and allergies. If someone finds that they 'crash' after meals and have feelings of fatigue, then blood sugar metabolism may be part of the picture as well as hypothyroidism.

If a patient has a diet that is rich in high amounts of simple carbohydrates then this may be an issue. In many cases, dietary changes may be all that are required to slowly re-establish a normal blood sugar balance. Often these changes may require the exclusion of high sugar foods and the introduction of more complex carbohydrates, protein and some good quality fat into the diet, to ensure a more steady release of glucose from food over time.

More seriously, other chemicals such as insulin and cortisol may be involved.

Insulin is produced by the pancreas and is central to regulating carbohydrate and fat metabolism in the body. Insulin causes cells in the liver, muscles and fat tissues to accept glucose and store it for future use, as glycogen in the liver and muscles. Insulin also stimulates our cell membranes to more readily receive glucose into the cells. Some tissues do not require insulin in order to accept glucose from the blood, e.g. the brain and liver.

If insulin levels are too low then the bulk of the cells in our body become unable to take up glucose. This will result in the inability of the mitochondria to produce enough cellular energy. In this case, it is highly likely that any thyroid treatment will be undermined and may appear not to be working. In the worst case, the thyroid treatment may use up the remaining glucose in the cells so rapidly that the patient may become severely low in cellular levels of glucose. Diabetes is one well-known disease that can result in low levels of insulin and high levels of blood sugar. This can leave blood sugar levels high but the cellular levels of glucose may be desperately low because the insulin is not available to enable the entry of glucose into the cells.

If any blood sugar metabolism issue is suspected, then a full investigation by a competent doctor or specialist is important and they may well do a GTT as well as other investigations.

I have already discussed the issues that low levels of cortisol can cause in Chapter 3. The relevant point to repeat here is that cortisol is important in blood sugar metabolism as it causes blood sugar to be maintained at healthy levels. In the presence of low cortisol levels, people tend to develop low blood sugar or hypoglycaemia. So, if blood sugar metabolism issues are suspected then adrenal insufficiency should also be considered, as this too can result in inadequate cellular energy being generated by the mitochondria. Again, a GTT may be required, as well as investigation of the adrenal glands and cortisol levels.

Regardless of what causes the low availability of glucose to the cells, if thyroid treatment proceeds and does not correct the cause of the low glucose level then serious symptoms can result. As the thyroid hormone is increased then this may cause the cells to use up the available glucose as they attempt to produce the required amount of ATP. The consequence can be a severe depletion of glucose levels within the cells and a lowering of available ATP. This may result in a variety of unpleasant effects including a very rapid heart rate, raised blood pressure, shaking, fainting and other symptoms associated with severe hypoglycaemia.

Some of these symptoms may be caused by the increase in adrenaline levels that can occur in response to the low cellular glucose and low ATP production. These symptoms may often get confused with those arising from excess thyroid hormones or even excess cortisol levels in the case of high blood pressure, whereas they may in fact be caused by the large increase in adrenaline in response to this cellular glucose deficit. It is also important to remember that it is cellular glucose that is the issue because in the cases of pre-diabetes, diabetes or insulin resistance the glucose level in the blood may be normal or even high.

In many cases the provision of the right form and dosage of thyroid hormone will simply correct the issue but in some cases treatment may be needed for the underlying problem.

For all the above reasons it is essential to have any suspicions of blood sugar metabolism issues investigated further by an appropriate medical professional.

EXERCISE AND RE-BUILDING MUSCLE MASS

For the hypothyroid patient who may have been ill for a long time, it is likely they will have lost muscle mass. Muscle tissue creates a higher metabolic demand than any other tissue type in the body.

One of the main ways of recovering during thyroid hormone replacement therapy is to do regular exercise but not so much as to make you feel exhausted. Cardiovascular exercise is important, as is exercise designed to tone and rebuild muscle mass. By improving fitness levels and building, or toning, muscles, the metabolism is asked to work harder. This creates the demand for more thyroid hormone and allows the thyroid hormone replacement to be utilised correctly within the body. This is a critical part of the recovery from hypothyroidism.

OTHER MEDICATIONS

Some prescription drugs have a long list of side effects. Most of the time we just assume that we are not going to suffer any of these. Many of us do not even read the information on the leaflet that comes with the medication. The leaflet provided with the medication is one source of information and the Internet offers the opportunity to find out more about how medications work and what the potential side effects and drug interactions are.

Why should anyone be interested in this type of information? Sometimes, medication side effects can be significant and may be confused with one of more symptoms of a thyroid or adrenal disorder. There may also be interactions with the thyroid treatment being used. I have seen situations where months of confusion occurred only to discover that someone was taken a medication that was causing a range of serious side effects that were assumed to be part of the failure of thyroid treatment. This is an area not to be overlooked.

CONCLUSIONS

The above represent some of the conditions and factors that may need to be considered, before and during the treatment of a patient's hypothyroidism. Some of the above health issues may correct automatically, once the correct treatment for hypothyroidism is in place, whilst others may not and will take intervention by the patient's doctor or another specialist. The biggest challenge may be recognising that one or more of these other factors are present, because of the overlap with the symptoms of hypothyroidism.

SECTION 2

MY STORY

Chapter 6

Realising I Was Sick

I am fifty-two years of age now and am battle-scarred by the consequences of the thyroid problems that changed my life over the past twenty years.

It was on a particular day in the spring of 1992 that I began to realise I was really quite unwell. I was in my early thirties at the time. This was the day that my second child was born and it should have been a good day. My wife was due to have given birth nearly two weeks earlier and on this day I had taken her into hospital to have her labour induced. I stayed with her during the early part of the day but, because it was clear that the birth was not going to happen immediately, I left in the afternoon and picked up my son from school. All I had to do then was wait for a signal from the maternity hospital that my wife had started labour. The call came in the early hours of the morning. I hurriedly dropped my son off with a friend and drove to the hospital.

Probably because he was our second child he arrived quite quickly. I only just made it to the delivery room in time. Fortunately, the birth was straightforward and my wife and I found we had a noisy and lively baby boy. As we were waiting in the delivery suite for the staff to move my wife to a different room, I quite by chance and purely for fun, decided to put my wife's heart rate monitor on. My heart rate was fractionally over forty beats per minute!

Now, if I was a marathon runner with an elite athlete's level of fitness this might not have alarmed me. However, I wasn't an athlete and even when I was younger my heart rate rarely dropped below seventy-five beats per minute. If this measurement was right then I knew I was in some kind of trouble. I repeated the test with the heart rate monitor a few times until I was satisfied that it was correct. Yes, it was really very low. Something was wrong. My heart rate was so far below my normal level that both my wife and I were immediately concerned.

I had not been feeling well for about a year. I was responsible for a large electronics project at work and I was under a lot of pressure and stress to ensure it completed on time. I had not stopped and assessed my health. I already had a young son at home and, like so many people, I was just too busy at home and at work to take notice of any of the indicators that pointed to a health issue. The indicators were actually lit up in neon and flashing on and off in front of me. It took one of these flashing health lights to catch me being still for a moment, in that delivery suite, in order for me to notice it.

Over a period of about a year I had put on about 35 pounds in weight. I was permanently tired and exhausted at the end of each day. During the past winter I had been complaining about feeling the cold far more than usual. I had also begun to develop digestive problems that included constipation, bloating and discomfort in my abdomen. After eating a meal, I would feel nausea. One of the strange things I had not even realised was happening, was that my memory had deteriorated and my thinking ability had slowed. I had been struggling with remembering the names of people I worked with, as well as family members. I was even starting to have trouble arranging my own thoughts and plans at work. My face was not only fatter than it used to be but it also looked like it was puffy and swollen. For any reader that knows anything about thyroid disease this last item should be a clincher.

I was just over thirty years of age and my career was developing nicely. I was in a job I loved and my family was growing. Who considers being ill at an age when everything appears to be going well? I had also never even heard of thyroid disease and I wouldn't have recognised the symptoms if someone had written them on a frying pan and hit me over the head with it.

The symptoms of thyroid disease are manifold because the thyroid affects every system of the body. I don't think I stood a chance at that time in my life of recognising that all of my different symptoms were linked.

At the time of my son's birth I was working for one of the largest computer companies in the world. I was a senior manager with a large department of elite software and electronics designers. I loved my job. I was extremely lucky because as I have got older it is clear how few people can actually say that they enjoy their job. In those days I couldn't get into my car fast enough in the morning to get to work. Life was good! That was soon to stop, completely and utterly. The previous few years at work had been enormously stressful. I was involved in the development of several new products and the pressure on me personally was intense. The stress must have wreaked havoc with my body and particularly my thyroid, adrenal glands and immune system.

Prior to this point in my life my health had been very good. Apart from the usual childhood illnesses, I have only had a few medical conditions that might be worth mentioning.

Firstly, I had continual bouts of tonsillitis as a child. Now, this should surely fall into the category of 'usual childhood illnesses' shouldn't it? Some endocrinologists now think that even this minor illness may have a bearing on the future health of the thyroid gland. It is suspected that the inflammation that accompanies tonsillitis may cause the blood supply to the thyroid gland to be restricted and may lead to future problems with the thyroid.

Secondly, I had a skin condition known as urticaria (hives) that developed when I was eleven years of age. Urticaria causes redness, thick swelling and itchiness of the skin. When I had an urticaria episode it would sometimes cover my entire body, even inside my mouth and throat. I was close to hospitalisation on a couple of occasions because my throat closed so much that I could barely breathe. I was prescribed antihistamines for about six years and then for some reason the urticaria just stopped as quickly as it had begun. I developed hay fever immediately after this but that wasn't a problem by comparison. I mention the urticaria because I will refer to it again later as there are links between urticaria and thyroid disease.

The third issue worth noting is that I had glandular fever when I was about twenty years of age. Glandular fever is also known as mononucleosis or Epstein Barr virus. I had this nasty little virus during my last year at university and it was so virulent that when the nurse in the university medical centre drew a blood sample, it was more pink than red. My blood was so full of white cells that not only had my blood become paler but according to the doctor, who diagnosed me with glandular fever, I should not have been conscious at all at the time the blood was drawn. I highlight this because there is a possible link between the virus involved in glandular fever and thyroid disease.

Anyway, back to my story. Once my wife had been moved to a different hospital room and we had agreed that I had to visit our family doctor, I went and picked my son up and returned home. However, before I went to sleep, I began to make a list of any other changes in my health that I thought had happened over the past year.

During the coming days my wife and I refined this list. The main symptoms included:

- Permanent fatigue.
- Lower level of enthusiasm.
- Slow movement.
- Feeling cold.
- Cold skin.
- Digestive problems.
- Weight gain.
- Puffy skin on my face.
- Dry hair.
- Dry skin.
- Cracked nails.
- Low body temperature.
- Low heart rate.
- Poor memory.
- Difficulty in thinking clearly.
- Irritability.
- Decreased libido.
- Needing far more sleep than I ever had in my life.

When we looked at the list it was hard to believe that neither of us had spotted that I had clearly developed a health problem. I booked an appointment with my family doctor.

Chapter 7

The Diagnosis and T4 Treatment

Clutching my list of symptoms in my cold, dry-skinned hand, I went to see my family doctor.

The doctor listened to the whole story as I described the long list of problems that my wife and I thought might be important. She took my blood pressure and listened to my heart and agreed that my heart rate was unusually slow. Taking a syringe and needle from a drawer she took a blood sample, saying that she was going to run a wide range of tests and making it quite clear that she did not necessarily expect to find anything wrong. It seemed clear that the most likely result would be that the tests would be negative and that stress at work was largely responsible. However, my doctor did tell me that on no account was I to go into work until she knew what was going on. Fortunately, I had already planned to take a few days of holiday, to be at home with my wife and the new baby.

Four or five days later my family doctor paid a routine visit to see my wife and our new son. She informed us both that my blood tests had come back from the laboratory and that she now knew exactly what was wrong with me.

It was explained that my thyroid gland was not producing enough thyroid hormones. She briefly described what the thyroid did and then she told us that in my case the problem was due to my body attacking my own thyroid with autoantibodies. I was told that once this process had started that it was likely to continue to do more damage to my thyroid over time. She gave me the blood test results, which I wrote down but didn't fully grasp at the time. My TSH was extremely elevated at nearly 50 mU/L compared with the laboratory reference range of 0.4 - 4.5 mU/L. Both my FT4 and FT3 levels were desperately low. My TPO autoantibodies were over 750 IUs/ml and my Tg autoantibodies were also elevated.

I had Hashimoto's thyroiditis, the most common cause of hypothyroidism. The diagnosis was clear-cut according to my doctor and it fitted the symptoms that I had been experiencing completely. It was an extremely good decision by my family doctor not only to ask for laboratory tests of TSH, FT4 and FT3 but also to request a test for thyroid autoantibodies.

I was completely surprised. This diagnosis was not something I had considered. Even my family doctor was surprised. She said that she had asked for quite a large number of conditions to be checked for, including hypothyroidism but she had not really expected this to be the problem. She made the point that it was much more unusual for a man to have hypothyroidism than a woman and that it usually occurs in older people than me; her comment that most of her patients with this condition were old ladies made my wife laugh.

However, the good news, according to my doctor, was that by taking some thyroid hormone replacement medication once a day, I should be back to normal in no time at all. I was naive and optimistic in those days and I thought that I would feel completely healthy once I was taking the medication.

T4 TREATMENT BEGINS

I was prescribed synthetic T4 immediately and was assured that I would feel well once my thyroid replacement dosage was at the correct level. My doctor had the pills with her already and I popped the first into my mouth there and then. I was also warned that I would have to remain on T4 treatment for the rest of my life. The synthetic T4 that I was prescribed during this period was sometimes Eltroxin and at others it was a generic levothyroxine.

This was the point in time when I began to learn the basics about low thyroid hormone levels and autoimmune thyroid disease.

The first few weeks of taking synthetic T4 were probably the best weeks that I ever experienced on it. There were some immediate improvements in heart rate and I did feel slightly warmer. My energy level improved a little during those first few weeks, even though I was only taking 25 micrograms of synthetic T4. I went back to work and tried to perform as well as I was able to. I continued to find doing my job and dealing with home life extremely difficult. However, I had been assured that this would improve as my thyroid hormone levels returned to normal.

Over many months my doctor slowly increased my daily dosage of synthetic T4. The normal treatment process is to increase the daily dosage, perhaps by 25 micrograms, then to wait for around six or eight weeks for the increased T4 levels in the body to stabilise. After that time another TSH test is done and if the TSH has still not lowered into the laboratory reference range then a further increase of synthetic T4 is made. Typically, this process is repeated over time until the TSH blood test result indicates that adequate levels of thyroid hormones are present in the bloodstream and at that point the patient should be feeling well.

Of course complete stability rarely occurs with any form of hypothyroidism but autoimmune hypothyroidism is often less stable because the thyroid gland may deteriorate further, which over time may require the addition of more thyroid hormone medication to compensate. This process of deterioration and modification of medication can go on for years unless the autoimmune response halts or the thyroid gland is totally destroyed.

So, as my synthetic T4 was increased, I waited for my health to improve. However, after the initial improvement that occurred during the first couple weeks of treatment, my health did not continue to get better and in fact my energy level and feeling of warmth deteriorated again.

The myxoedema that was visible on my face did go away completely and my heart rate did rise back to a more normal level. However, the rest of the symptoms remained similar to how they were before my treatment began. My doctor seemed encouraged that my blood tests were beginning to appear to be more normal. However, I did not feel well. This feeling grew over the coming months.

I WAS TOLD I WAS NOW 'CURED'

Eventually, when I was taking 150 micrograms per day of synthetic T4, my family doctor pronounced me cured, or words to that effect. I was told that my TSH was normal, which meant that my pituitary gland thought I had enough thyroid hormone. My TSH had dropped from being nearly 50 mU/L to begin with, to around 2 or 3 mU/L now. My FT4 and FT3 were now both normal and this apparently showed that I had adequate levels of T4 and T3 in my bloodstream.

There was a big problem though. Even though my blood test results were indicating loud and clear that my thyroid levels were now normal, I continued to feel unwell. I still had a long list of symptoms. I now knew, from all the reading that I had done, that these symptoms were typical of someone who has hypothyroidism.

My energy level was still poor and my muscles still felt weak. I was still extremely tired all of the time. I had succeeded in losing some of the excess weight I had gained and my skin condition improved a little but it was still abnormally dry. My memory and brain function improved slightly, however they were still significantly impaired. My digestive and abdominal problems were probably worse than they had been. I was still very tired all of the time.

I was lifeless. I found I could not be enthusiastic about work any more and I was no longer able to do my job with the energy that it required. Playing and looking after my children was a chore and I lacked any patience. My heart rate had normalised thankfully but my body temperature was still very low. I used a thermometer and my temperature was often lower than 97.0 degrees Fahrenheit (36.1 degrees Centigrade) and sometimes closer to 96.0 degrees Fahrenheit (35.5 degrees Centigrade).

More than any of these specific symptoms, I had this strange feeling of being less than my old self. This is quite difficult to describe but I felt like a shadow of the person I had been prior to developing thyroid disease. The T4 replacement therapy did not appear to have worked, even though my thyroid blood tests were normal.

THE ENDLESS BACK AND FORTH TO DOCTORS

After being on synthetic T4 for well over a year and still feeling very ill, I began to pay more frequent visits to my doctor's office. Due to the fact that my TSH, FT4 and FT3 levels all fell within the laboratory reference ranges, I was simply informed that my thyroid levels were fine. This was the point that I began to be referred to endocrinology specialists. I saw two different endocrinologists within the first eighteen months of being diagnosed. One of these I saw through the NHS and another I saw privately. The endocrinologists confirmed that my thyroid hormone levels were ideal and I was told that there was nothing further that could be done for me in terms of thyroid treatment.

My family doctor was very sympathetic but was clueless regarding a solution. This was very distressing because I continued to have most of the debilitating symptoms associated with hypothyroidism.

I began to understand more about T4 and T3. Through my own research, I became aware that T4 itself has little or no biological action but that some of it is eventually converted into the biologically active hormone T3. I asked my doctor and one of the endocrinologists, whether it was possible that my T4 might not be converting to a sufficient amount of T3. My family doctor did not know the answer to this question but the endocrinologist dismissed this idea. He said that it was not possible and that my thyroid blood test results were perfectly normal.

'Thyrotoxicosis'

Approximately eighteen months after my original diagnosis and after my synthetic T4 dosage had been slightly increased; I developed what appeared to be thyrotoxicosis.

Hyperthyroidism occurs when there are symptoms that appear which indicate the presence of too high a level of thyroid hormones. Thyrotoxicosis is a description of the toxic tissue levels of thyroid hormone that can occur in hyperthyroidism. A step beyond this is referred to as thyroid storm, which can develop if hyperthyroidism or thyrotoxicosis is left untreated. In thyroid storm the symptoms can be extremely distressing and life threatening.

My symptoms of thyrotoxicosis included very bad headaches, sweating, intense agitation, a very rapid heart rate over 130 beats per minute, severe physical tremors in my hands and, most disturbingly, bulging eyeballs. I was immediately given beta-blockers to control my heart rate and my T4 replacement was stopped temporarily. However, the thyroid blood tests that were done on same day that I rushed to see my doctor did not reveal a suppressed TSH or the elevated T4/T3 levels that would have been expected with thyrotoxicosis.

My family doctor could not explain why this problem had occurred and neither could the endocrinologist that I saw soon after this.

I was unable to work for nearly two months and eventually my synthetic T4 medication was started once more at a slightly lower level. I now suspect that this episode was not conventional thyrotoxicosis but in fact some form of severe reaction to the synthetic T4 that I was taking that my body could not effectively utilise. I have subsequently found information that suggests that these symptoms may have been triggered by a nutritional deficiency of some kind. For example, thyrotoxic-like symptoms can be caused by a thiamine deficiency (vitamin B1).[1]

I had been hypothyroid for a significant period of time before being diagnosed and given T4 replacement. It was therefore possible that my adrenal glands were not as healthy as I thought they were at that point in time. Low levels of adrenal hormones can result in low blood sugar and low cellular levels of glucose. Consequently, a further possibility is that my cellular glucose levels had become depleted due to adrenal insufficiency as a result of the wrong form of thyroid treatment being provided. This can sometimes give rise to symptoms that are similar to those of hyperthyroidism when thyroid medication is increased.

It did appear clear from my thyroid blood test results that this episode was unlikely to have been caused because my synthetic T4 medication was too high.

I mentioned that during the thyrotoxic episode described above that I had extremely bad headaches. It is also interesting that during the entire time that I was on T4 treatment, I had a low level headache in the centre of my forehead. I later began to refer to this as my 'thyroxine headache' as it only ever occurred when I was taking some form of T4 replacement.

T4 REPLACEMENT THERAPY CLEARLY FAILING

Over the next five years no dosage I was ever prescribed made me feel normal. My body temperature remained consistently low at 96.0 - 97.5 degrees Fahrenheit (35.5 - 36.38 degrees Centigrade) and I felt ill with many of the previously mentioned symptoms. My digestive problems worsened and I was permanently uncomfortable.

During this period of time I saw at least one additional NHS and another private endocrinologist and I also changed my family doctor. My T4 dosages were varied from 125 micrograms per day to 300 micrograms but I had no further episodes with symptoms similar to thyrotoxicosis.

Starting to feel awkward about visits to doctors

When you continue to return to your doctor's office and you complain about various symptoms and how you don't feel well, there comes a point in time when you start to feel as though you are not being believed. This may not be the doctor's actual view but it is a natural human reaction when you go back time and time again. It is natural to begin to wonder what the doctor, or indeed a friend or work colleague, is actually thinking about you. Over time I became conscious that I might be perceived as being a 'moaner' or a 'malingerer'.

After several years of living with thyroid disease and with an ineffective treatment, I began to feel that my doctor did not fully believe me any more. I liked my doctor and this view was probably not fair but it is hard for both patient and family doctor in these situations. I have read articles about doctors who have 'heart-sink patients', whose presence on the doctor's daily appointment list cause a moment or two of that sinking feeling. If I was a doctor who had struggled unsuccessfully over several years to treat a patient and they were due in my office that day, then I might feel exactly the same. I began to feel very nervous and stressed about the prospect of a doctor's appointment. I knew exactly what my symptoms were now and I also knew that I had been perfectly healthy prior to developing hypothyroidism but it didn't stop the anxiety that now accompanied medical appointments. It is bad enough to feel ill without also having to feel worried and apprehensive about how you are perceived. Yet so many thyroid patients feel exactly the same!

The impact of incorrectly treated thyroid disease

The consequences to my working life and career were profound. Anyone that has suffered from the symptoms of hypothyroidism will know how almost every system of the body may be affected. My job required clear thinking, decision-making and a lot of communication with many different people. Above all, it required tremendous energy and an ability to prioritise a large number of potential issues and activities. Coping with pressure was essential. All the natural skills that I possessed, that had made my career successful, were now severely damaged by the on-going symptoms of hypothyroidism. I had tried to keep on top of my work but to perform well in any full-time job is nearly impossible with this condition. I tried to do more work at home to compensate for everything I could not complete during the working day. This just made me more exhausted.

I began to have fainting episodes and the frequency of these increased. It was not unusual for me to pass out several times each week. I also began to lose weight. You may think that weight loss was a good thing but I lost so much weight and muscle that I became very weak indeed. My body weight dropped to just under 9 stones (126 pounds) compared with a normal weight for my height of around 12 stones (168 pounds). My suspicion now is that my adrenal glands were not being regulated correctly due to the ineffectiveness of T4 replacement therapy but I cannot prove that, because my adrenals were not fully evaluated at that time.

My work suffered because I could no longer perform my job as I had once done. I began to have more extended periods of time off work because I felt so ill. All of the above created a situation where my wife and I were uncertain as to how the steady deterioration in my health was going to end. My employers were unlikely to continue to employ me in my management role and my wife and I were very concerned about the future.

One of the consequences of the entire situation was that I was extremely difficult to live with.

My family life suffered. I had two small children who required a lot of time and attention and I had neither the energy nor the patience for them. I look back at this period of time and it makes me desperately upset to think about it. I was a poor father to my sons at that time. This was in large part due to the hypothyroidism that was still in full flower within me. My eldest son in particular suffered, as he was a small boy and very challenging.

If I were granted one change I could make throughout this illness then it would be to repeat this stage of my life and attempt to do things differently. If I had quit my job at this stage to allow more time for my children then this may have helped. It was a truly disastrous time in my life. The relationship between my eldest son and myself deteriorated and it is only now, nearly fifteen years later, that we are finally starting to have a good relationship.

The damage that this disease can do is immeasurable. It ruins lives. Thyroid disease that is not treated correctly may wreak havoc on an individual's life but the effects on other family members can be equally significant. I am not trying to imply that many other patients with other diseases are not having their lives devastated also, because I am sure that this is the case. Thyroid disease does tend to have the unfortunate tendency to undermine all the various systems of the body. Its effects are mental and physical and some of the damage done can have long-term health consequences, e.g. cardiovascular damage.

Like most people I did not discuss how my illness was having an impact at work and home with my family doctor or with the endocrinologists I visited. Maybe I should have done, as it might have made it more difficult for the various endocrinologists who saw me at that stage to have told me that there was nothing wrong with my thyroid hormones.

Starting to realise T4 was not working

I spent my working life involved in research and development projects. I have always been fond of using a technique known as Occam's razor. This is a method attributed to a fourteenth century logician and theologian called Father William of Ockham. He proposed that when faced with multiple, competing hypotheses to explain something in the natural world, you should generally select the hypothesis that fits the data and that makes the fewest new assumptions. In general, this means that you should pick the most obvious explanation that explains the data.

To put it another way, if it looks like a pig, sounds like a pig and smells like a pig then it probably is a pig! Don't go looking for a more complicated explanation. If you're dumb enough to look for an alternative explanation, then you'd better have a lot of data to support it.

So, applying Occam's razor to my thyroid problem was easy. I was healthy before my thyroid disease. When I was diagnosed with autoimmune hypothyroidism my symptoms were completely characteristic of hypothyroidism and I had the required levels of autoantibodies and low thyroid hormones. I was now on synthetic T4 replacement therapy and I still had all the symptoms associated with hypothyroidism. The simplest hypothesis I could come up with, that fitted all the available data, was that my T4 replacement treatment was not working.

Much to my disappointment, no doctor I saw concurred with this view! They were more preoccupied with talking about the nice levels of TSH, FT4 and FT3 in my bloodstream.

THE UNHELPFUL 'DIAGNOSES'

I was offered two alternative explanations of what was happening to me on several occasions by two different endocrinologists and my family doctor. These alternatives did not conform to Occam's razor, as they required additional new assumptions. The endocrinologists proposing these alternatives also had no data to back up these new assumptions. I knew immediately that these alternatives were based on bad science and flawed logic.

The first alternative I was offered was that I had developed a psychological problem that made me imagine that my symptoms were as bad as they were. This psychological problem was not given a name but depression was mentioned. I was unaware that depression could make you delusional and even more surprised that it was considered because I did not feel depressed and had no history of mental illness.

The 'you have a psychological problem' diagnosis is always a very handy one to pull out of the endocrinology cupboard, because it can be used to explain almost all problems that the endocrinologist has not managed to resolve. It does appear to be a very popular stock-in-trade favourite of many endocrinologists and doctors who find that their standard treatment for hypothyroidism is not working. Thyroid patients are often diagnosed with depression and given anti-depressant medication.

Depression may be one of the symptoms of hypothyroidism and unfortunately, it is often this depression symptom that doctors latch onto and prefer to believe is the underlying issue, rather than the far more complex problem of incorrectly treated hypothyroidism.

In my own case I had no history of mental illness. I was very concerned about my health and all the ramifications that my illness was having but I was not depressed. I was luckily able to avoid the depression diagnosis, which would have provided a very deep rabbit-hole to disappear down for a considerable time.

The 'some other disease is causing your symptoms' diagnosis was the second alternative I was offered. This diagnosis states there was that some other disease that was causing the symptoms and that this disease had no relationship whatsoever with thyroid hormones, because my doctors assured me that my thyroid blood tests were normal. This 'some other disease' diagnosis was indeed suggested to me by several doctors. The interesting thing about this 'diagnosis' is that it is rarely accompanied by any mention of what the other disease might be and what the investigation of this other disease is going to consist of. I find it interesting that no endocrinologist or doctor who suggested this alternative hypothesis to me felt any responsibility to investigate this as-yet unknown disease further and give it a name. The manner in which this alternative was offered was more of a 'washing of the hands'.

The second alternative diagnosis deserves even more attention. Because my blood levels of thyroid hormones appeared to be within a laboratory range, therefore it was assumed that it was more likely that some other condition was causing exactly the same set of symptoms that occur in hypothyroidism. This latter hypothesis is far from simple and assumes that one or more other diseases can masquerade perfectly as hypothyroidism!

I felt like I had just dropped into a universe where logic was faulty! I was well and truly down the rabbit-hole along with Alice and I knew it, which made it even worse. It was immensely frustrating to know that I was not being listened to or believed.

I have just written the above paragraphs. I know they are true. I know that this is what I was told. Some deranged medic did not tell me this. Several highly trained, supposedly intelligent endocrinologists gave me these explanations on several occasions. This still astonishes me. Yet it should not surprise me at all. I spend a lot of my time these days communicating with other thyroid patients in the UK and in other countries. This story is common. The simplest and most logical explanation that T4 replacement therapy does not always work is frequently rejected in favour of one or both of these far less likely explanations. For some reason my doctors appeared to be locked into a certain view of thyroid treatment that made them incapable of recognising the crystal clear fact that T4 replacement therapy was not working. It fitted every symptom that I was experiencing. It was also destroying my career and affecting my family.

I HAD TO TAKE RESPONSIBILITY FOR MY OWN HEALTH

I had been collecting daily information on my symptoms, my T4 dosages and any blood test results for several years at this point. I can say quite confidently that my symptoms did not appear to change with any changes of T4 dosage and the so-called improvements in my blood test results. T4 replacement therapy just didn't work.

Unfortunately, things got progressively worse and I began experiencing more weight loss as well as losing my leg hair. My energy level began decreasing and my overall health was declining so rapidly that I found I could no longer function at work. I was therefore forced to take long periods off work. I had to sleep for several hours during the day and, even after resting, my lack of energy and physical weakness were so severe, that I struggled to climb the staircase at home. Worryingly, I also began passing out more frequently. I am convinced now that my adrenal glands were not performing well due to the ineffectiveness of T4 replacement therapy. I believe my adrenal glands were working as poorly as the rest of my body.

During this period on synthetic T4 medication my TSH, FT4 and FT3 were monitored and they were always found to fall within the laboratory ranges. My life continued to fall apart. After each visit to a doctor and a blood test I was told to keep taking the synthetic T4. The process was uncannily identical each time.

I was offered counselling by one endocrinologist. He said that he thought I had myalgic encephalomyelitis (ME). This endocrinologist suggested that I joined a growing group of his thyroid patients that also had ME. The idea here was that I might get some solace and advice from others in a similar situation. I thought about this and my conclusion was that here was an endocrinologist who had patients for whom he had no effective treatment. He had labelled them with a diagnosis of ME, even though they were thyroid patients who had not managed to get well through T4 replacement therapy. I declined the offer from the doctor with the growing group of patients that remained unwell on T4 treatment.

We had moved house and because of this I had changed my family doctor. To add insult to injury my new doctor was so convinced that I had depression that he insisted that I went on a course of anti-depressants before he would consider referring me to anyone else! Eventually, I would end up having a full-blown row with this doctor and changing family doctors once again.

I was slow and stupid to realise the obvious. It should have been clear to me that my doctors and endocrinologists attributed greater value to my thyroid blood test results than to my presenting symptoms, clinical history and every other piece of information I was giving them. I collected data on my body temperature, which was consistently low. I assumed that this was important but not one doctor I saw at that time was even slightly interested in knowing that my body temperature was very low.

The doctors that I had seen up until then believed a successful treatment was one that resulted in the right thyroid blood test result numbers. One of the biggest issues that I encountered was that none of the endocrinologists I had seen were using improvements in my symptoms as the main measure of success of their treatment

It had taken me around six years to back my own judgement and believe that it was the T4 replacement therapy that was the failure. It was now obvious to me that I needed to get in the driving seat and work out not only what sort of treatment approach was needed but also how I was going to gain access to this treatment.

IS THAT AN ELEPHANT IN THE ROOM?

I now describe the rigid adherence to the belief that synthetic T4 is always an effective treatment for hypothyroidism as the 'elephant in the room'. Thyroid patients who feel desperately ill on T4 replacement therapy often appear to be the only group of people who know that synthetic T4 is not working for them. These patients can see the elephant.

Many thyroid patients go along to visit their family doctor or endocrinologist and they sit down in the doctor's waiting room and quietly rehearse what they are going to say, in order to try to get a more effective treatment than the T4 replacement therapy that isn't working. They know that their thyroid blood tests results aren't showing the whole story. For many of these patients the elephant in the room is clearly visible. The large grey beast may be sitting in one of the waiting room chairs, in heavy disguise. It may be wearing an extra large pair of shoes, a nice suit and a large hat and be reading a newspaper. The elephant's trunk may be tucked behind the newspaper.

However, some thyroid patients are able to see the elephant very clearly, even though every attempt has been made to not draw attention to it. Very few other patients appear to realise that the elephant is there. The doctor's office staff and nurses don't appear to have a clue that there is an elephant in the room.

If the patient were to ask the doctor or one of his staff about the elephant directly, then a range of reactions might be elicited, from total denial through to anger for describing one of the doctor's most valuable assistants as some sort of beast. The patient may even be 'diagnosed' as having a psychological problem and be offered anti-depressants!

However, make no mistake, the elephant is there. Once a patient has recognised the elephant in the room then it is very easy to spot from that point onwards. At some point a patient really has to have a very open and honest conversation with their doctor about the presence of the elephant (the failure of T4 replacement therapy). If the response is one of anger or denial, then it is probably time to find a more open-minded doctor. If a patient is lucky enough to have a doctor who simply winks back at them and says quietly "I know - let's see what else we can do", then maybe this is just the doctor that they need.

I NOW KNEW THAT I WAS RIGHT AND THE DOCTORS WERE WRONG

Why have I written about my story at all? What happened to me is not uncommon. My story is the story of so many other patients all around the world. A few of these patients eventually begin to join Internet forums dedicated to thyroid disease and share their own stories and look for help and advice from other patients.

Every week on Internet forums in various countries, I read the stories of other people who are struggling with severe symptoms of hypothyroidism, even though they have been told they are on appropriate treatment. Some men and women have already lost their jobs because of inadequate treatment. Others are not coping with their small children. Some have lost their partners because of the damage done to their relationships. Many are still searching for some solution and some appear close to giving up hope of ever feeling well again. The people that actually make it to the Internet forums are probably a small percentage of the total number of patients whose lives have been damaged by hypothyroidism. I find these stories and the knowledge that I am only aware of a tiny fraction of the real suffering to be deeply distressing.

By this stage in my own journey I now knew beyond any doubt that I still had hypothyroidism and the treatment that I had been given had failed. More importantly, I knew that T4 replacement therapy was never going to be the treatment that would help me become well again. I could see the elephant in the room very clearly now.

At this stage I began avidly reading books on endocrinology, as I realised that my existing knowledge was hopelessly inadequate. I needed to gain an in-depth understanding of how thyroid hormones worked and what could go wrong, if I was to have any chance of getting better. Before I could take the next step I needed to work out what this step should be.

NEED FOR A PARADIGM SHIFT TO FOCUS MORE ON PATIENTS' SYMPTOMS

Shortly I will begin to focus less on T4 replacement therapy and more on the use of T3. Before I do I must register a request to the medical profession to re-establish patients' symptoms as the paramount focus during all forms of thyroid hormone replacement therapy.

In the case of synthetic T4 and T4/T3 based treatments, thyroid blood test results clearly need to be an important focus during treatment. When a patient is diagnosed with hypothyroidism and undergoes a typical treatment with thyroid hormone, the patient's doctor reviews thyroid blood test results and the patient's symptoms. Over a period of time, the results of the patient's blood tests will change, usually in a direction of improvement according to some criteria. Over the same period of time, the patient's symptoms will also alter and in the majority of cases, hopefully, these will also improve.

However, for some patients, apparent improvements in thyroid blood test results are not matched by equivalent improvements in symptoms. My own experience and the experience of many other patients that I speak to, is that the paramount focus of family doctors and endocrinologists is on achieving improvements in thyroid blood test results.

The biggest issue occurs when the symptoms do not resolve, yet the thyroid blood test results have improved to the point that they are considered normal. In this situation many doctors are often satisfied that treatment has been a success. This is a fundamental problem in the way the measurement of successful thyroid hormone treatment is taught during medical training.

People, in any profession or line of work, orient themselves to the measures that are used to determine how well they are doing their job. Quality improvements in all types of services and industry are often achieved through placing appropriate measures on the goods and services that are being produced. The most effective measures are usually those that are most closely coupled to the desired result that the customer wants for the goods or service. I will use two totally different examples of this:

- Much of the improvement in production processes used in the automotive and electronics industries have resulted from the use of critical measures, or metrics, that are applied at each stage of the production process in order to measure the quality of the output of that process stage, prior to the component or sub-assembly moving on to the next stage in the process. By doing this it is possible to focus on improvement. By picking the right measures, substantial quality and efficiency improvements may be made.

- In the legal profession the number of cases that are won versus those that are lost may factor heavily in the assessment of the ability of the lawyer or barrister. In this example, the number of references to other similar cases, or points of law, that the lawyer makes during a given court case are insignificant compared to whether the case is won or lost, regardless of how clever the arguments that have been made are.

People and organizations have a natural tendency to change the way they operate in an attempt to be successful according to the measures that they are being judged by. Most people want to do good work. The measures used by a person's employer, or in the person's profession, to determine what is 'good work', often influences how that person performs their work.

Doctors tend to focus on blood test results not patients' symptoms

The strong impression that I and many other thyroid patients have, is that the symptoms of patients are not as important to how a doctor feels about the quality of their work compared with thyroid blood test results.

There is no formal assessment of patients' symptoms over time as thyroid hormone replacement dosage is adjusted. There is formal assessment of thyroid blood test results.

This point may seem trivial but it is fundamental. A simple change to formally track the status of patients' symptoms as part of every thyroid hormone treatment has the potential to make a profound change in emphasis during the treatment. One of the arguments against this is that any assessment of a patient's symptoms is likely to be subjective, whereas thyroid blood test results are not. My response to this is that **I don't care.** Even some subjective measures, done formally, will allow any progress or otherwise to be reviewed when plotted out over time.

A focus on patients' symptoms will yield many benefits

I also believe that even simple subjective measures of how thyroid patients are actually feeling will, over time, increase the focus of doctors on how patients are really responding to treatment. I believe that this would result in several real benefits:

- Improved patient doctor relationships.
- A shared view between the doctor and the patient on the progress regarding the patient's symptoms.
- Better outcomes during thyroid hormone replacement.

For example, six to ten basic symptoms associated with hypothyroidism could be selected and they could either be measured or given a patient rated score on a range of 1-10 (1 being very bad and 10 being perfect).

Examples of possible symptoms that could be tracked might include:

- Digestive performance.
- Body temperature (can be measured).

- Energy level.
- Normalising weight level (can be measured).
- Hair, skin and nails condition.
- Stamina.
- Mood.
- Muscle, joint aches and pains.
- Overall level of health.

These actual measures can be debated and modified but the important thing would be to routinely assess some simple, relevant measures and plot them to see if real progress is being made. They could even be captured and plotted with a computer program and incorporated into the patient's notes. This would allow both doctor and patient to have a common view on how the patient is actually feeling and what progress had actually been made. Patient and doctor would be 'on the same page'. If a computer program was used, then it might even be possible for the doctor and patient to select the top six to ten symptoms that the patient is most concerned about at the start of the thyroid hormone treatment and then monitor these particular ones over time.

Patients' blood test results are obviously still very important and will ideally be monitored and used along with patients' symptoms in determining appropriate treatment. This method, of course, would potentially make the elephant that I have already referred to quite visible in those cases when improvements in thyroid blood test results are not matched by similar improvements in symptoms. At the very least in these cases, the doctor and the patient will both have the same view of progress and be far more likely to continue to cooperate and work together to understand the problem and hopefully resolve it, even if it requires some other treatment than T4 replacement therapy.

I believe that it is essential that improvements in a patient's symptoms be placed centre-stage throughout their treatment for hypothyroidism. This needs to be done in such a way that both doctor and patient have a shared understanding of actual progress. It is the progress in how a patient actually feels that doctors should be primarily using to assess the quality of their own treatment. This request may seem somewhat backwards to some doctors who have come to trust the new thyroid blood tests. However, it would actually be a massive step forward for thyroid patients.

Chapter 8

Finding the Next Step

I decided that I was right. T4 replacement therapy was never going to work for me. So, I read as many books and articles on endocrinology and thyroid disease as I could. I used the library, borrowed and bought endocrinology books and, of course, used the Internet, as more information became available on it.

As time progressed, I began to formulate a clearer idea of what might be occurring in my body.

People require adequate amounts of the biologically active T3 hormone in their cells in order to feel healthy.

I still had a small amount of thyroid function left. This meant that my own failing thyroid gland was producing a very small proportion of both the T4 and the T3 in my bloodstream. The majority of the T4 in my bloodstream came directly from the synthetic T4 that I was taking. The remainder of the T3 in my bloodstream was being produced as a result of my body's conversion of some of the circulating T4.

A small fraction of the circulating T4 and T3 is not bound to proteins and is known as unbound or free thyroid hormone. A little of this free T4 and free T3 would be expected to enter my cells. Any remaining T3 that I required would need to be converted from the T4 that had already entered my cells. The T3 within my cells would then need to reach its intra-cellular targets - the thyroid receptors in the mitochondria and in the genes within the cell nuclei.

I SUSPECTED I DIDN'T HAVE ENOUGH T3

It is possible that my FT3 level may have been higher before I developed thyroid disease, despite the fact that my FT3 level now was still within the laboratory reference range. Even if my current circulating levels of FT4 and FT3 were the same as when I was healthy, if any problem stopped sufficient T3 from reaching its intra-cellular targets then this might account for my lingering symptoms.

I now know that many things can prevent adequate amounts of T3 from correctly reaching its targets within the cells. The more I looked at what had to work correctly, the more I realised that there are numerous potential points of failure. I began to find research studies that supported this concern. I also started wondering how the onset of an autoimmune thyroid problem could affect the way in which T4 was being utilised and how this could result in less than adequate T3 in the tissues.

DOUBTS ABOUT THYROID BLOOD TEST LABORATORY REFERENCE RANGES

Laboratories assess a wide population when calculating the reference ranges for TSH, FT4 and FT3. Several hundred-blood samples are typically collected in the process of calculating the ranges for a given laboratory. They try to avoid including people with known thyroid disease. What experts are coming to understand is that some people included in the laboratory reference range assessments may have undiagnosed health issues, including mild thyroid abnormalities.

The laboratory ranges for various thyroid hormones are therefore somewhat arbitrary, defined using statistical methods, which use 95% confidence limits. This means that 2.5% of the population are likely to have entirely healthy levels of thyroid hormones that would be higher than the reference range and 2.5% are likely to have lower levels of thyroid hormones that fall below the reference range.

In the process of calculating these laboratory reference ranges outliers are usually discarded first. Outliers are results that are on the extremes of a population and may be caused by measurement errors or by highly unusual individuals whose results are quite different to the rest of the population. Inclusion of outliers might skew the entire distribution and alter the reference ranges drastically.

Once the data samples are collected, analysed and outliers are removed then statistical methods are applied to derive a laboratory reference range that supposedly represents 95 percent of the population, i.e. if one hundred healthy patients were tested then hopefully 95 of these would have results that fall somewhere within this range.

The laboratory reference ranges for TSH, FT4 and FT3 therefore **cannot** represent all possible normal human thyroid hormone levels. A small number of completely healthy people may have thyroid hormone levels that fall outside one or more of the laboratory reference ranges. People do not go to their doctor and ask for thyroid blood tests if they are healthy. Consequently, if someone becomes ill with a thyroid condition then a blood test at this time will be incapable of revealing that this person ever had atypical thyroid hormone levels. They will be treated according to the laboratory reference ranges and their previously healthy but unusual thyroid hormone levels are unlikely to be replicated.

If an unlucky patient happens to be one of those people who requires a level of one of the thyroid hormones, at, or beyond, the laboratory reference range in order to feel healthy, then during thyroid hormone treatment this patient might reasonably expect to continue to feel unwell until this healthy level was duplicated once more. Simply telling the patient that their hormones fall somewhere within the laboratory reference range is no guarantee that they are being adequately treated.

In addition to all the above it is important to recognise that TSH exponentially increases as FT4 and FT3 levels decrease. There is an inverse logarithmic linear relationship between TSH and FT4. This has a bearing when a doctor says "your TSH of 2.0 is normal, you don't need a thyroid medication increase". In fact, it will take the same amount of T4 to reduce the TSH from 2.0 to 1.0, as it will from 10.0 to 5.0. So, a modest increase in thyroid medication at this stage will not suddenly result in a totally suppressed TSH. Some doctors may forget this log-linear relationship and be highly concerned about making further increases in thyroid hormone once the TSH begins to approach the lower end of the reference range.

Also the TSH distribution is skewed to the left with the median TSH being about 1.0. Similarly the FT4 and FT3 distributions are also skewed with most people being above the halfway point. Awareness of the shapes and relationships of these distributions is something that is critical to be aware of if commonsense is to prevail in the treatment of thyroid problems.

The application of an individual's thyroid blood test results, which concludes that the person's thyroid hormones are normal because they fall somewhere within the laboratory reference ranges is unlikely to be applicable to 100% of patients, because of the statistical methods used to create the ranges in the first place. Using laboratory reference ranges in this way may be a good practical approach because it treats many patients correctly but it is easily conceivable that some people will not be treated correctly with this approach.

The laboratory reference ranges for thyroid hormones are simply statistically derived reference intervals. They should never be confused with meaningful diagnostic ranges or therapeutic treatment ranges.

Technically we ought to be using the term 'laboratory reference interval' because it is an unambiguous statistical term, which reflects the methods used to create it. I am going to continue to use reference range in this book because it is in wider use than reference interval. I will **not** be using 'normal range' anywhere because this is very misleading, as it has nothing to do with an individual being 'normal' if their blood test results happen to fall within the range.

DOUBTS ABOUT FACTORS THAT AFFECT THYROID BLOOD TEST RESULTS

Thyroid function blood test results can be influenced by many factors, any of which should be taken into consideration, e.g.

- Labelling errors.
- Bacterial contamination.
- Yeast/Fungal contamination.
- Clotting.
- Sampling errors.
- Sample preparation errors.

- Sample storage errors.
- Thermal cycling.
- Anti-thyroid antibodies (any).
- Antibodies from any other cause.
- Presence of specific 'toxins' in the blood.
- Presence of pharmaceutical drugs (interferences) within the blood.
- 'Systematic' errors in analytical equipment or methodology.
- Composite errors.
- Carcinoma can also cause T4 and TSH values to be misleading.
- Low iron can also lower TSH values.[1]

The above are examples of some of the potential sources of errors, but they all add to the unquantifiable 'unreliability' of the final number that appears on a laboratory report; stated to be within/outside a reference range.

DOUBTS ABOUT THE USEFULNESS OF THYROID BLOOD TEST RESULTS

In a typical thyroid hormone blood test, the levels of TSH, FT4 and FT3 in the bloodstream are estimated from the blood sample. It is impossible for a thyroid blood test to reveal:

- The actual levels of T4 and T3 within the tissues.

- The efficiency of the conversion of T4 to T3 within the tissues.

- How successful the T3 has been in reaching its intra-cellular targets and whether cell function is actually being regulated correctly.

A blood sample cannot reveal any of these things, no matter how much we may want it to. In other words, thyroid blood tests can only, at best, provide a rough guide as to what *might* be happening with thyroid hormones within the tissues.

I now had serious concerns about how TSH was being used. Some may argue that because my TSH was in the laboratory reference range, my tissues were therefore getting an adequate supply of thyroid hormones. However, this would be making several, very large assumptions.

Firstly, my pituitary gland would have to be functioning correctly and accurately assessing the thyroid hormone levels that were present in my bloodstream and then reflecting this assessment with an appropriate level of TSH.

Secondly, the cells of my pituitary gland would have to be accepting T4 and T3 hormone at exactly the same rate as the cells in the rest of my body, in order for any resultant TSH to be representative of how much thyroid hormone the rest of the cells of my body were receiving.

Thirdly, the cells in the rest of my body would have to be able to use the T4 and T3 without any problems and as effectively as the cells of my pituitary gland.

These three assumptions have to be true in order to have any reliance on the results of a TSH laboratory test. They represent the never mentioned, but incredibly critical assumptions that underpin the TSH test.

In the extreme case, central hypothyroidism due to a pituitary or hypothalamus malfunction can cause TSH to be lower than it ought to be. There is no reason to suppose that various degrees of pituitary or hypothalamic malfunction cannot be present. So, it is possible for the first assumption to be invalid.

In terms of the second and third assumptions, there are published research studies that illustrate that these assumptions can also be flawed, including the biological fact that the pituitary gland converts T4 to T3 locally within its own cells. It is easy to see that TSH can be misrepresentative of adequate tissue levels of thyroid hormone.

I began to apply my concerns to my own blood test results. I knew that I was not responding correctly to T4 replacement therapy, even though my TSH, FT4 and FT3 were within the laboratory reference ranges. I therefore questioned whether these assumptions were accurate for me. Unfortunately, there was no practical method of testing the validity of any of these assumptions for a patient and, at the present time, there still isn't.

Although thyroid blood tests were providing my doctors with some estimate of my thyroid hormone status, they were incapable of determining whether I was adequately replaced with thyroid hormone at the tissue level. I reasoned that thyroid blood tests, no matter how 'normal' they may appear, cannot reveal the actual levels of thyroid hormones within the cells. **Blood tests are unable to indicate how well thyroid hormones are entering the cells and how much of the biologically active T3 hormone eventually reaches those critical parts of the cells where it is needed.**

MORE DOUBTS ABOUT SYNTHETIC T4

From the information I had managed to gather, I also had doubts about the efficacy of synthetic T4.

From the late 1890s until the 1960s and 1970s, physicians worldwide have treated hypothyroid patients with tablets containing desiccated (dried and powdered) animal thyroid glands. These tablets contain both natural T4 and natural T3.

In 1958, the first synthetic T4 tablets were marketed in the United States. There is evidence that suggests that many of the doctors who were successfully using natural thyroid at the time when synthetic T4 was introduced, found that the synthetic medication was not as effective at treating patients' actual symptoms.

It is also important to remember that money is involved - a lot of money. The pharmaceutical industry is one of the biggest and most profitable worldwide businesses. Synthetic T4 is a major drug for many of the world's biggest pharmaceutical companies. In the Guardian newspaper of 15/March/2011, it was stated that synthetic T4 is now third on the list of the most prescribed drugs in the UK. Synthetic T4 is financially very important to these companies. It is no surprise that pharmaceutical companies pay lobbyists to work on their behalf with governments, make targeted donations to political groups and to hospitals and medical schools. Pharmaceutical companies do not employ smart-suited drug company representatives to work with doctors and endocrinologists out of the goodness of their heart. Big business operates in exactly the way that you would expect it to.

There are already a number of excellent books available that extensively discuss comparisons between synthetic T4 and the arguably superior natural thyroid preparations.

NEXT STEP DECISION - A TRIAL OF T3

No matter how hard I tried, I failed to get any doctor that I consulted to consider any of my deep-seated concerns, or my ideas on why T4 replacement was failing. In any of these discussions, my own ideas and concerns were immediately discounted and I was offered no opportunity to have any serious discussion about them.

The results of my TSH, FT4 and FT3 blood tests were being used almost exclusively to determine whether I was hypothyroid or not and I had little hope that any of the doctors that I had seen so far would change their blinkered approach.

It was clear to me that something had changed in the way that my body was utilising thyroid hormones and it was highly unlikely that any blood test could identify the problem.

After extensive research and a great deal of thinking I reached a conclusion. It would be a very useful experiment to try taking T3 on its own. My idea was to eliminate the T4 from my system entirely and see if I would respond better to T3 alone. I believed that this would eliminate several potential issues at once. By using only T3 medication I would be providing my body with the biologically active thyroid hormone, in sufficient quantities, to prove beyond doubt whether my symptoms were due to thyroid hormones or not.

If taking T3 alone did not resolve my symptoms, then the doctors were probably right and something else might be responsible for my ill health. If the use of T3 succeeded, then it would provide the proof that I needed to confirm that the advent of Hashimoto's thyroiditis had altered the way my body was utilising T4, or, that at the very least, synthetic T4 was a poor replacement for naturally produced thyroid hormones.

Taking T3 would be a valuable diagnostic exercise and if T3 actually resolved my problems, then it might be the solution I had been looking for. A short trial of T3 was a very sensible approach and was the only viable way of collecting more data. My life was already in chaos and I was close to losing my job, so I needed to try something different in order to learn more about my health problem.

MY ENDOCRINOLOGIST REFUSED T3 TRIAL

I had hoped that my doctor and endocrinologist would share the same viewpoint but I was naïve again of course. Why would I expect a perfectly rational approach to be thought of as a good idea? How stupid of me!

My family doctor was unsure of what to do and wanted my endocrinologist to make the decision but my endocrinologist informed me that he would not prescribe T3 and that the T4 treatment was doing an adequate job already. However, they did not know what was causing my symptoms and I was told that they had no further ideas on any alternative treatments. Amazingly, neither of my doctors knew what was causing my symptoms but they still refused a short trial to learn more about the problem!

My health had deteriorated so much that I was off work for extensive periods of time. My career was irreparably damaged, so I decided to resign my position and take a less senior management role. I couldn't do the job, as I knew it needed to be done, which wasn't fair on my colleagues or the people who worked for me. So, I stepped down and hoped I could hang on to a job until I found some solution to my health problem. Unfortunately, shortly after doing this, I became so ill that I began to spend more time out of work than in work.

I couldn't persuade my doctors to allow a trial of the T3 thyroid hormone, even though I was quite happy to take the risk that it would not work and I had fully explained the reasons for wanting to try it. It defies understanding that this can be allowed to happen. I was asking for a short trial of T3 to determine if it was my thyroid hormone metabolism that was in some way flawed. My job was at risk. My family was being affected by my ill health and yet this trial was still being refused.

Most of my naivety had gone at this point. I knew time was my most precious resource. I knew I was right and that the doctors that I had seen were wrong, or had no ideas about what to do.

I HAD TO FIND ANOTHER DOCTOR - T3 TRIAL WAS A GOOD PLAN

I began looking for a doctor who might prescribe the T3 thyroid hormone and even considered going to the USA and would have gone, had I not managed to locate a doctor in the UK who was prescribing T3 occasionally for some thyroid patients.

During my first appointment with this doctor I spent half an hour going through my medical history with him. He made careful notes and was very interested in my symptoms. Surprisingly, he was actually interested in the fact that my body temperature was still consistently low. This was the first physician of any kind that had actually paid attention to my low body temperature. My new doctor waited until he had my laboratory tests back and then he told me that he felt that my symptoms were due to a lack of response to T4 replacement therapy.

Consequently, approximately seven years after my initial diagnosis of hypothyroidism, I eventually succeeded in finding a medical professional who was prepared to let me try alternatives to synthetic T4 thyroid hormone replacement. This doctor threw me a lifeline for which I will always be grateful.

Chapter 9

The T3 Trial

Having now found a doctor, who appeared to share some of my views and seemed interested in exploring solutions that might actually help me, I was determined to try T3 replacement therapy. My new doctor pointed out that there were several more practical alternatives to be explored first.

Prior to any new thyroid hormone treatment I needed to be assessed for adrenal insufficiency and for some basic nutritional problems that can undermine thyroid metabolism or even masquerade as hypothyroidism.

ADRENAL ASSESSMENT

It was advisable to find out if I had low cortisol or not prior to commencing T3 treatment. If thyroid hormone treatment is started in the presence of low cortisol it can sometimes fail to resolve symptoms and it may even cause new unpleasant symptoms. Consequently, being aware of the status of the adrenal glands at the outset is very important, although there are different ways of handling any adrenal insufficiency if it exists. If any nutrient deficiencies have been ruled out or dealt with, then one of the biggest diagnostic clues to low cortisol is when the patient's body temperature remains low, even when the patient is receiving an adequate level of T3. Even in the absence of any other symptoms, if the patient's body temperature does not consistently stay above 98.0 degrees Fahrenheit (36.6 degrees Centigrade) then there is the possibility of an underlying adrenal insufficiency issue (or a previously undiagnosed nutrient deficiency or blood sugar metabolism issue).

An ACTH stimulation test was organised to measure the stress response of my adrenal glands and the results confirmed that my adrenals appeared to be working well and no fundamental damage was present.

However, in truth, I did have some evidence of low cortisol. My belief now is that I may have had some adrenal insufficiency but this was only due to inadequate thyroid hormones that were not allowing my adrenals to work correctly, rather than any fundamental issue with the adrenal glands themselves.

The decision was taken to move forward with no adrenal support to begin with and see how things went.

VITAMIN AND MINERAL TESTS AND SUPPLEMENTS

At this stage I had some basic tests done, which included a serum iron and serum ferritin test to assess my iron storage level and a B12 test. Both of these were completely normal. If I had been aware of the importance of having tests for transferrin saturation % (iron), folate and vitamin D at this time, then I would also have had all of these tested.

I visited a nutritionist and was put on a range of vitamin and mineral supplements designed to support both the thyroid and adrenal metabolic pathways. These supplements were the start of the supplementation regime that I have already described.

This discussion about nutrients is brief but it is extremely important. If there are nutritional deficiencies then these may undermine any treatment that is given and may make the thyroid hormone replacement appear to fail even though it is a vitamin or mineral deficiency that is responsible. Having a few basic tests, beginning a sound supplementation regime, as well as maintaining a healthy diet, are all important, if a patient wants to improve the chances of a swift recovery.

T4/T3 REPLACEMENT THERAPIES

Trial of natural thyroid

My new doctor was keen to see how I responded to natural thyroid prior to any trial of T3 on its own.

Natural thyroid, also known as desiccated thyroid, generally consists of a powdered form of porcine (or a combination of porcine and bovine) thyroid gland. Natural thyroid preparations were developed in the late 1800s and are still used today to treat hypothyroidism.

Natural thyroid preparations predominantly contain the hormone T4 but they also contain a small amount of naturally produced T3. In addition to T4 and T3, natural thyroid contains all the other hormones that you would expect to find in a thyroid gland. These include the T1 and T2 thyronines and calcitonin. Due to the fact that natural thyroid contains T3, it is common to divide the daily dosage into separate doses spread evenly throughout the day. This divided dose approach enables smaller amounts of T3 to be delivered during the day. Depending on the amount of natural thyroid being used, this might mean dividing a daily dosage of natural thyroid into two, three or even four divided doses per day.

The importance of calcitonin found in natural thyroid preparations is often discounted, as it is destroyed by stomach acid. As a result it may prove to be an irrelevant ingredient in natural thyroid preparations, unless you attempt to take it sublingually (which some people do). The effects of T1 and T2 are yet to be ascertained; however there is some evidence to suggest that they may be biologically active and that T2 may have some, as yet unknown, effects on gene transcription. This makes the argument for using natural thyroid preparations, instead of synthetic combinations, more compelling.

It became apparent that the natural thyroid preparation was not going to be able to resolve my symptoms. In fact I felt increasingly worse when my natural thyroid dosage was raised, which was a similar result to my experience with synthetic T4.

Short trial of adrenal support

One concern that my new doctor had, was whether I might have low cortisol that may be interfering with treatment. For some people, long-standing health issues might give rise to adrenal insufficiency. If my cortisol levels were too low during parts of the day, then this might be hampering the production of cellular energy and limiting the ability of thyroid hormone to correct my symptoms.

Consequently, for a short period of time, I was prescribed a low physiological dose of adrenal hormone, to see if this made my natural thyroid replacement work more efficiently. I was prescribed several very small doses of hydrocortisone, spaced by three to four hours during the day, alongside my natural thyroid medication. This made absolutely no difference to my symptoms and so the hydrocortisone was stopped and replaced by two low doses of prednisolone. I couldn't detect any beneficial effects from this form of adrenal support either and so this was also discontinued.

It was evident, from the ACTH stimulation test and from my response to actual adrenal hormones, that adrenal insufficiency was not the significant issue - it was the natural thyroid hormone replacement, itself, that was not working.

Trial of Synthetic T4/T3

The next step was to try a combination of synthetic T4 with the addition of a small amount of synthetic T3. This was the synthetic equivalent of the natural thyroid I had already tried but with the flexibility of varying the ratio of T3 to T4. I spent a few months trying combinations of synthetic T4 and T3. The results were very similar to natural thyroid. My symptoms remained, although as the ratio of T3 to T4 was increased, there seemed to be some slight evidence that the T3 may actually be helping.

Decision to prescribe T3

Eventually, after these treatments were tried and found to offer no significant improvement in my symptoms, my new doctor decided to prescribe T3 on its own, in an attempt to improve my health. Even if the T3 failed it would provide the vital diagnostic information that I desperately required.

INCORRECTLY TREATED HYPOTHYROIDISM SCREWS YOUR LIFE UP

When I use the term 'incorrectly treated', I mean the prescribed treatment did not resolve the symptoms that it was intended to correct. I don't give one fig if a thyroid hormone medication I was taking resulted in levels of TSH, FT4 and FT3 in my bloodstream that fell beautifully within the laboratory ranges. I was still incorrectly treated because I still had the majority of the symptoms that were present when first diagnosed with hypothyroidism, nearly seven years earlier.

At least I was now working with a doctor who was prepared to try alternative treatment options. I did not blame him for my lack of response to natural thyroid or T4/T3 treatment. It was simply that the treatments we had tried so far were not correct.

At this point my career ended. My employers were decent to me but there was no avoiding the inevitable conclusion. My life was utterly changed by having hypothyroidism left incorrectly treated for so long. All I could do was accept the situation and concentrate on trying to get well. Only after recovery would I be able to re-evaluate my life.

THE START OF THE T3 TRIAL

When I began using T3 I found very little useful information regarding the use of this medication as a full thyroid hormone replacement therapy. There were small pieces of information, scattered in various places on the Internet but these were not comprehensive enough, even when gathered together, to guarantee using T3 successfully.

My new doctor realised that it was important to divide the T3 taken each day into divided doses, rather than taking it all at once. However, he thought splitting the T3 into two separate divided doses would be sufficient. It is still common for doctors and endocrinologists to recommend splitting T3 into two divided doses each day.

With very little initial information it took me two to three years to fully understand the complexities of using the T3 thyroid hormone. I will describe what happened when I began using T3 hormone replacement therapy and I will spend more time later discussing all the lessons I have learned over the years and the process that I eventually developed to determine my T3 replacement dosage.

When I began this trial I could not find sufficient practical information about the use of T3. All I had was the symptoms of hypothyroidism, a supply of T3 tablets, an organised mind, a sympathetic doctor and a certain amount of bravery.

No information on T3 dosages used by patients like me

In particular, I had no information on the range of T3 dosages used by patients who had not responded to T4 treatment. Neither did I have information on how many divided doses per day might be needed or any guidelines on individual dose sizes or timings. I will share some of this information later but, when I first started to use T3, I had to guess and use trial and error.

The one piece of information I was given by my new doctor and I also found referred to on the Internet, was that a typical person's full replacement dosage of T3 was usually in the range of 40-60 micrograms per day. These days I have a lot more information and some personal views on this range, all of which I will discuss later. When I began using T3 though, this was the only information on the range of T3 replacement dosages that I was aware of.

Guided by caution, I decided to take a very conservative approach and I began using only a very small amount of T3 to ensure that I had no adverse reactions. My rule regarding the use of T3 is that safety always has to come first. Finding the correct dosage can therefore require a great deal of time and patience. Even if I had been aware of the wide ranges of T3 dosages actually being used by patients around the world today, I would still have exercised extreme caution when beginning to use T3 replacement, starting with a very low daily dosage, e.g. 10-20 micrograms of T3 per day.

From the beginning, my goal with regards to my T3 replacement therapy was always to find the lowest possible dosage that fully addressed my symptoms and made me feel well, without triggering any adverse symptoms.

In achieving my goal, I was prepared for the fact that I might end up with a fully suppressed TSH (< 0.1 mU/L). I knew that some doctors might interpret this to mean that I was thyrotoxic and experiencing tissue over-stimulation as a result of excess thyroid hormone. I was not concerned about this because I had already concluded that thyroid blood test results do not reflect what is actually happening inside the tissues, where thyroid hormone function actually counts.

Stopping all T4 and starting to use T3

My doctor advised me to stop taking any medication that contained T4 and wait as long as I could tolerate before taking any T3 on its own. I managed to last for about one week before commencing to take some T3.

I began by taking only 20 micrograms of T3 divided into two doses, i.e. 10 micrograms of T3 in the morning and 10 micrograms in the afternoon.

Due to the 7-day half-life of T4, it may take around eight weeks before most of the remaining T4 medication clears from a patient's body. After around eight weeks, any circulating T4 that a patient still has, will be coming from the residual function of the patient's own thyroid gland.

Because of the problem of waiting for any T4 medication to clear over an eight-week period, it is difficult at the start of T3 replacement therapy to ascertain if the remaining T4 is affecting the T3 treatment and compromising its effectiveness. I felt that it was necessary to try to limit any T3 dosage increases until the T4 had been given an opportunity to clear, believing that this would give the T3 the best opportunity to work effectively and reach its intra-cellular targets.

I was unable to wait for eight, or even six weeks before I had to increase my T3 a little. However, keeping any T3 dosage increases to the bare minimum during this period is important. The approach worked well and within a few weeks I was able to increase my T3 dosage with ease and without major issues.

I needed to use at least three divided doses of T3

At this stage I was still taking 2 divided doses of T3 every day, which was how I had been advised to use the T3. As each divided dose of T3 rose above 15 micrograms I began to get some side effects, such as a rapid heart rate and a feeling of anxiety. Worryingly, in between the two T3 divided doses, I felt that my symptoms of hypothyroidism returned, as though the T3 had been used up. Two divided doses did not seem to sustain me throughout the day but when I increased one of the divided doses it became too potent and caused side effects.

I also tried to use a single dose of T3, large enough to get me through the day, but this also increased my heart rate far too much. T3 acts much more quickly on the cells of the heart and the liver. Consequently, I found that it was quite easy to spot if I had taken a little too much T3 and then it was simple to correct.

Through trial and error I discovered that I needed to take my daily dosage of T3 in at least three and possibly four or five divided doses. Two divided doses per day were not going to work for me.

Initially I took my first T3 dose at 8:00 am and my last T3 dose at 5:00 pm, with any other T3 divided doses spaced out evenly in between. I started with much lower individual divided doses than I could reasonably expect to provide me with enough thyroid hormone each day. However, this meant that I could carefully increase the divided doses over a period of several weeks, which gave me a good level of control over my treatment and also provided a high degree of safety.

Due to the shorter half-life of T3, I found it was far easier to make more frequent adjustments to T3 doses, than it was with T4. With T4 replacement therapy patients need to allow at six weeks to determine what the full effect of a T4 dosage change may have been. With T3 however, some of the results can be apparent within a day or two.

T3 BEGAN TO WORK

Once my T3 daily dosage reached 35 - 40 micrograms per day, a lot of my symptoms began vanishing. My body temperature returned to normal within forty-eight hours and I no longer felt cold. My memory reverted to normal. My digestive symptoms were totally eliminated during the first few weeks. My hair and skin condition improved and my ability to think clearly returned. This transformation occurred so quickly it was as though a switch had been pressed. The correlation in the improvement of symptoms to the T3 dosage increases convinced me that T3 was going to be the solution that I had hoped it would be.

During the years on T4 replacement therapy my doctors had continued to tell me that my thyroid levels were normal and that my symptoms were nothing to do with the thyroid hormones at all. However, I never believed this and now, for the first time, I had real data that illustrated that T4 replacement therapy had indeed failed.

How could T3 replacement therapy resolve most of my symptoms, if these symptoms weren't being caused by a lack of the right thyroid hormone in the first place?

I went back to see my family doctor, feeling healthier than I had done for many years. I explained the trial with natural thyroid and synthetic T4/T3 and what had now happened on T3 replacement therapy. My family doctor was pleased for me but wanted confirmation that this treatment was appropriate.

FURTHER ENDOCRINOLOGIST AND FAMILY DOCTOR PROBLEMS

So, I was referred back to the endocrinologist I was seeing at that time. I was severely disappointed with the response I received from this specialist. I was told that I should not be taking T3 and that the standard treatment of T4 replacement therapy was suitable in my case, despite a detailed explanation of my clinical history. I was then told that because my thyroid blood test results were in the laboratory reference range when I was taking synthetic T4, this meant that I had been responding well to the T4 treatment and that I should revert back to it. The fact that I was actually responding to T3 treatment, feeling healthier with many of my symptoms resolved, did not appear to make any difference.

I had landed in the universe of broken logic once more. The endocrinologist refused to acknowledge that I was recovering because of the T3 replacement therapy. I was astounded by the endocrinologist's view that my T3 treatment was not a viable option, despite the fact that I was actually recovering at a remarkable rate! Once again I was not being listened to, when I actually had something useful to say.

My family doctor decided to prescribe the T3, based on what I had to say about the T3 trial results and a letter from the doctor who had given it to me. I continued to take the T3 and have never had any cause to regret this decision.

At this point I wish to make it very clear to any reader that it was never my intention to self-medicate, i.e. to determine my own T3 dosage. I wanted to find both a family doctor and an endocrinologist who I could work with effectively to manage my T3 replacement therapy. Ideally, I would have liked my treatment managed by a doctor who knew all that there is to know about using T3 and about my own problems with T4 replacement therapy. This was not possible at the time - because of the limited information available on the practical use of T3. I was forced into having far more involvement in the management of my treatment than I would have liked but I also still wanted an empathetic doctor who would work with me, listen to me and support me.

Shortly after discovering a T3 dosage that appeared to eliminate the majority of my symptoms, I was referred to yet another endocrinologist. This began a short but extremely difficult period, during which I received a number of very unhelpful diagnoses and suggestions.

I was given a variety of feedback, including that my problems were psychological in nature, that I had been suffering depression and that I had ME. The fact that my health had improved on T3 appeared to be irrelevant. I was told that I should be taking T4 replacement therapy.

SWITCHING DOCTORS AND FEELING HEALTHIER

This forced me to switch to a different family doctor and fortunately she was extremely easy to work with and supportive (and at a later date she suggested I write about my experiences). My new doctor referred me to a more sympathetic, more open-minded and more capable endocrinologist. Having supportive doctors that I could easily work with made a really big difference to the level of support that I felt I had. Both the new family doctor and the new endocrinologist had no issues with the use of T3 replacement therapy, as I appeared to be doing so much better on it. I continued to have the T3 prescribed by my family doctor from that point onwards.

Around this time, my employer and I finally parted company officially. There was nothing that could have been done to avoid this. I harbour no bitterness towards the company that I worked for.

I had a lot of work ahead of me yet to fully resolve my T3 dosage and to completely regain my health, due to the long number of years of hypothyroidism and loss of fitness and general health. It did take nearly three years to completely fine-tune my T3 dosage, in terms of the number of divided doses, their sizes and when to take them. However, throughout this adjustment phase, I still felt significantly better than when I was on T4 replacement therapy.

Once the T3 began to work properly, the difference this treatment made to my life was indescribable. It was the discovery of the **Circadian T3 Method**, which I will discuss in Chapter 16 and then 25, which finally enabled me to completely recover.

For the first time in many years I enjoyed the feeling of being healthy. I was able to go up and down my own staircase with ease and begin exercising properly. I started to build some muscle and lose fat. I felt a lot more like my old self. It is difficult to convey what a difference T3 replacement therapy made to me. You would have to experience it yourself, to fully appreciate it.

Chapter 10

Living Well on T3

So, am I still well? How effective has T3 replacement therapy been over the years? These are questions that I get asked, from time to time, by other thyroid patients.

The answer is that it did take a few years to fully understand how to use T3 correctly and I intend to describe everything I have learned in the coming pages. Fortunately, I had a really supportive family doctor, who helped me to get the right laboratory tests done, when I needed them. She also encouraged me and helped me to remain positive when I occasionally felt low. I also had a new endocrinologist, who has proven over the years to be highly capable and easy to work with. I didn't visit him very often but he was terrific when I did.

How am I now, after nearly thirteen years of using only T3 replacement therapy? I am healthy. I play tennis regularly and I use the gym. I have no issues with my weight and I have a reasonably consistent and normal body temperature. My energy level is good for my age and my mind is still very active. I have no obvious symptoms of either hypothyroidism or hyperthyroidism. I also have no requirement to take any form of adrenal support. I do take a good range of nutritional supplements that I have already described.

As a result of taking only T3, I now have very low levels of T4 and this has not caused any problems. There has been no need to combine any synthetic T4 medication with the T3 so far, although I have never ruled out this possibility as my thyroid ceases to produce any T4.

T3 MAY BE USED SAFELY AND EFFECTIVELY

I regularly communicate with other thyroid patients. Some live locally and others are scattered across the globe. Some people remain doubtful as to whether T3 replacement therapy is a viable long-term solution for treating hypothyroidism. This scepticism may arise from the fact that very few people use only pure T3 and so the evidence to support its safe and effective use is somewhat scarce. All forms of thyroid hormone, used incorrectly, can negatively affect the body, not just T3. If the correct dosage of any thyroid hormone is being taken, then the body should not be under any stress and there should be no symptoms of thyrotoxicity. If a patient responds well to T3, after T4 treatment has failed, it is likely to help to reduce the risk of heart and cardiovascular disease and other long-term health issues.

I certainly am not a T3 only zealot. Quite the opposite, because T3 dosage management is quite complex, I actually believe T3 should be the thyroid hormone of last resort. However, when other thyroid hormone replacement therapies have failed to resolve a patient's symptoms, then, with appropriate knowledge, T3 may be used safely and very effectively.

The best quotation that I have found, that both accurately and elegantly describes why this should be, is from Dr. John C. Lowe in his Question and Answer section on his website. [1] This was his reply to a patient who was asking whether it is mandatory to take T4 as a thyroid patient:

> "Studies indicate that T4 is of no use to anyone except, figuratively, as a storage unit for the metabolically-active thyroid hormones T3, T2 and possibly T1.
>
> When T4 ends its long ride through the circulating blood, it enters cells. There, enzymes convert it to T3 and, after a while, other enzymes convert T3 to T2. The T2 becomes T1 and eventually T1 becomes T0 (T-zero). T0 is just the amino acid backbone (called "tyrosine") with no iodine atoms attached. Because it has no attached iodine atoms, T0 is no more a hormone than is T4.
>
> Rather than being a hormone, T4 is a pro-hormone. That means that enzymes have to convert T4 to T3 before T4 benefits us.
>
> T4 is no more a hormone than beans in an unopened can are a food. For all practical purposes, canned beans become food only when a can opener frees them so you can eat them.
>
> Hence, T4, like canned beans, only potentially benefits us, but actually does so only after being freed from its metabolically unusable form.
>
> Your endocrinologist may say that T4 is a gentler way to get T3 into your body.
>
> This to me, however, is a specious argument. When taken properly, T3 can affect one as gently as T3 derived from T4."

T3 is the main biologically active thyroid hormone and does not require any biochemical conversion, unlike T4. If the right dosage of T3 is provided then an adequate amount is able to reach the tissues, allowing the body to function normally and the individual to feel healthy.

In my opinion, the main disadvantage of using T3 has nothing to do with its effectiveness or its safety as a thyroid replacement therapy. It is the complexity of dosage management, especially in the early weeks and months, that is the main disadvantage of T3. The initial dosage management for T3 replacement therapy does require more support by the patient's doctor than that required for T4 replacement therapy. However, when all T4 replacement therapies have failed, T3 may be the only thyroid hormone that is able to help a patient recover from hypothyroidism.

MY CURRENT T3 DAILY DOSAGE

For completeness and clearly **not** as a recommendation to anyone, the following table shows my current dosage of T3, with details about the divided doses of T3 that I take and the times that I take them. The rationale for some aspects of this dosage, which has been tailored for my personal requirements, will become obvious in the following chapters.

Time	T3 Dose	Comment
4:30 am	25 micrograms	One 20-microgram liothyronine sodium tablet and a further 1/4.
11:30 am	20 micrograms	One 20-microgram liothyronine sodium tablet.
5:30 pm	10 micrograms	One half of a 20-microgram liothyronine sodium tablet.

Please note that my regime does **not** constitute a recommendation for anyone else because, as discussed, patients' T3 replacement dosages vary considerably.

The above regime provides me with a total daily dosage of 55 micrograms of T3. For the past ten years I have been on a very similar total dosage of T3. Over the past two years I have reduced my T3 dosage a fraction and increased the interval of time between each divided dose. These necessary changes have occurred at the same time as my thyroid autoantibodies have reduced, my thyroid gland has atrophied and my FT4 level has fallen. I cannot be certain what change has necessitated the alteration of my T3 dosage but it may be associated with my immune system, my thyroid gland, improving adrenal glands or my vitamin and mineral supplements.

For the rest of this book, when I refer to *T3 dosage*, I mean the size of each divided dose of T3, the number of divided doses being used and the time that each one is to be taken per day, i.e. all the information required, to fully describe the T3 dosage. In any reference to *T4 dosage*, I simply mean the size of the dose of T4 that is taken each day.

ATTEMPTING TO USE T4 REPLACEMENT AGAIN

There have been occasions when I wanted to discover whether anything had changed in the way T4 worked in my body. However, whenever I have attempted to use T4 replacement therapy again, it still failed and I quickly became very ill.

However, after many years as I complete this book, I now appear to be able to tolerate 12.5 micrograms of T4. I have chosen for the moment to not use the 12.5 micrograms of T4 in practice but I do appear to be able to tolerate this amount of T4 now. This new tolerance may or may not be related to my thyroid autoantibodies falling to zero or the lack of any T4 production by my own thyroid gland.

THE END OF MY STORY

I have now completed my personal story. It should now be clear why I was compelled to use T3 replacement therapy and that it worked.

The focus in the coming chapters will now move on to the practical use of T3 replacement therapy, based on my own experience with T3, information from other patients who also use only T3 and various other sources.

SECTION 3

LESSONS LEARNED ON T3 USE

Chapter 11

Information About T3

LESSON #1: INFORMATION ABOUT T3

The thyroid hormone triiodothyronine contains three iodine atoms in its molecular structure, hence it is referred to as T3 for short. T3 is the biologically active thyroid hormone that controls almost every physiological process in the body, including growth and development, metabolism, body temperature, and heart rate.

T3 comes in tablet form as the compound liothyronine sodium. Common brand names are Liothyronine or Tertroxin in the UK (available as 20-microgram tablets) and Cytomel in the USA (available as 50, 25 and 5 microgram-tablets). Liothyronine sodium is a synthetic isomer of natural triiodothyronine.

I use the term T3 to refer to both T3 produced naturally and synthetic T3 but it should be clear to which I am referring from the context. In tablet form, T3 is sometimes referred to as 'standard T3', 'pure T3' or liothyronine.

T3 dosage ranges for patients that have not responded well to T4

Before I began to use T3 replacement therapy, I was hoping to gather as much information as possible regarding the range of daily T3 replacement dosages, used by thyroid patients with a similar clinical history to mine. Unfortunately, at that point in time, I failed to find any relevant information.

Endocrinologists have told me that the typical daily T3 replacement dosage for adults is between 40 and 60 micrograms per day. I have also seen these figures written in some endocrinology texts.

Two very well known endocrinology texts suggest that 75 micrograms of T3 may be the upper end of the replacement dosage range and that more than this may be required.[1, 2]

However, I can find no scientific research evidence to support the recommended 40 to 60 micrograms per day range. I speculate that these figures may have been calculated from the T3 needs of people who may have had their thyroids removed, despite being healthy in all other respects. It seems likely to me that this 40 - 60 micrograms per day range has been generated using a sample population of adults that are not representative of patients that have failed to recover their health through T4 replacement therapy. Therefore, this data may not be based on patients with bio-chemical problems that have forced them to use T3 to resolve their symptoms.

I needed to know the range of T3 replacement dosages used by other patients who had not responded adequately to T4 treatment. I did **not** want to know how much T3 a person with normal thyroid hormone metabolism would require. In fact, I would have preferred to exclude any sample data like this and just look at the sample data from patients who have had similar problems with T4 replacement therapy as myself.

My concern arises from my belief that some patients, who have a biochemical issue that prevents thyroid hormones from working normally, may require larger amounts of T3 in order to fully restore their health.

Over the years I have continued to search for any information regarding replacement T3 dosages and fortunately, I have managed to acquire some useful figures based on actual treatments of patients with T3. In one of my referenced texts, the author shares the results of a large number of case studies involving patients who were given T3 thyroid hormone replacement therapy.[3]

The patients in these case studies required daily dosages of T3 in the range 75 - 162.5 micrograms in order to correct their symptoms. However, the author has seen other patients requiring as much as 250 micrograms of T3. The T3 dosage range encountered by other physicians is also referred to, the lowest was 10 micrograms of T3 and the highest was 300 micrograms of T3.

This case study data suggests that the upper range of T3 required by representative patients, who have not had their symptoms resolved by T4 treatment, might be between closer to 175 or 200 micrograms of T3 rather than 60 or 75 micrograms. It also suggests that the lower range of 40 might be too high for some people.

I have also seen one report of an individual who required 500 micrograms of T3 per day in order to restore their health, with no evidence of tissue over-stimulation.[4]

What is clear to me from the above is that the potential range of full replacement dosages of T3, for patients who have failed to respond to T4 replacement therapy, may be wider than I was previously led to believe. On a more anecdotal basis I have spoken to many patients who also have eventually been given pure T3 and a few of these have indeed required dosages of over 100 micrograms of T3 and in a few cases over 175 micrograms of T3 before their symptoms finally vanished.

Most of the thyroid patients I have communicated with that are on T3 replacement therapy and use a T3 dosage management process similar to that described in this book use between 30 and 80 micrograms of T3 per day, with a few requiring much higher T3 dosages. The T3 dosage management process described in 'Recovering with T3' tends to discover the minimum T3 dosage required for good health and one that does not cause issues with tissue over-stimulation. It is important to recognise that these are patients for whom T4 replacement therapy simply did not work. I believe that it is the nature of the bio-chemical problems that drove these people to use T3 in the first place that may account for the wide range of T3 replacement dosages.

The process that I used to determine my T3 dosage has its entire emphasis on safety and caution. A T3 dosage far lower than 30 micrograms has always been my starting point and any increases beyond that may be done very slowly and carefully, with the ideal T3 dosage being 'crept up on', thus avoiding any risks. Any small T3 dosage increase may be completely assessed before any further increase is contemplated. Even had I required a much larger amount of T3 to achieve good health, there would have been no need for any risks to be taken, because I have adopted a sound approach to T3 dosage management.

T3 absorption rate and half-life

In the human body, the biological half-life of T4 is approximately seven days, which means a patient could take their entire daily dosage of synthetic T4 in one go, without any issues, because it is used up relatively slowly.[5, 6]

In contrast, the biological half-life of T3 is believed to be twenty-four hours.[5, 6] Therefore, a dose of T3 remains in the body for a far shorter period of time than T4. If the twenty-four hour half-life of T3 were accurate, then half of the existing T3 would still be in the body twenty-four hours later.

T3 is absorbed, like synthetic T4, within the gastrointestinal tract. However, T3 is almost totally absorbed within the gastrointestinal tract (approximately 95%), within a few hours. This compares with significantly less absorption of T4 medication (approximately 75%), if taken on an empty stomach. In addition, T3 binds poorly with the thyroxine-binding globulin (TBG), which partially explains why T3 remains in the bloodstream for a far shorter time than T4.[1]

A single dose of T3 is rapidly absorbed and reaches peak circulating concentration in just two to three hours after ingestion.[1, 5] Blood serum concentrations of T3 are elevated for six to eight hours.[5] After this, blood serum concentrations then decline again, unless another dose of T3 is ingested.

T3 and blood test results

Therefore, patients who are receiving T3 replacement therapy should expect unusual laboratory tests of thyroid hormone levels. Low FT4 levels should be expected. FT3 results could be low, normal or elevated, depending on how much T3 is being prescribed and the exact time of the thyroid blood test, in relation to the time that the last divided dose of T3 was taken.[7] TSH may also be rapidly suppressed when using T3.[8]

The above information, on the rapidity with which T3 achieves peak serum concentrations and then declines again and the potential variation of TSH and FT3 results, is very important. This means that laboratory tests that attempt to assess the adequacy of replacement with T3 are extremely difficult to make sense of, because of the wide and rapid fluctuations of T3 in the bloodstream.[1]

It is the concentration of T3 in the tissues that really counts. This is far more significant than how much T3 can be measured in the bloodstream. Currently the only way to judge what is occurring at the tissue level is to consult our symptoms and signs and assess how we actually feel.

How fast T3 appears to work and how long its effect lasts

In terms of the effect of T3, I have found that I can begin to feel some minor improvements within one hour of taking a single dose. Within two to three hours I feel my body is able to perform at its absolute best. However, I physically feel that I need to take more T3 after about five to ten hours following my previous dose, depending on the size of that previous dose. If I did not take more T3 at this stage, then my body temperature would drop, my energy level would deteriorate and several other symptoms and signs would indicate the need for me to take more T3. Some may argue that I simply do not take enough T3 at any one time but that is not the case. My doses of T3 are ideally tailored for my needs and any more would give rise to indications of tissue over-stimulation. I have tried larger doses of T3 and I know this for certain.

During the day when I am active, I require more T3 after a maximum of ten hours has passed since the previous T3 dose. This is a significantly shorter period of time than the twenty-four hour T3 half-life and the blood serum elevation period of six to eight hours would tend to imply. I am actually able to detect subtle changes that suggest that some of my tissues no longer have an adequate supply of T3 after just five or six hours.

Therefore, I have found the documented data regarding the twenty-four hour half-life of T3 and the six to eight hour period of T3 serum elevation to be of little help when trying to manage my T3 replacement therapy. This may be due to the fact that I cannot tolerate individual doses of T3 much higher than 25 micrograms. In fact, if I had been told that the half-life of T3 was only eight hours, I would have found this more credible. People who can successfully use much higher doses of T3 may find the physiological information on half-life and blood serum levels to be more useful than I have done. It is also possible that what I experience is more driven by the effect of T3 on the mitochondria, the energy producing elements within the cells, rather than the effects on the cell nuclei but this is just a possibility.

How T3 is usually taken each day - divided doses

Someone new to T3 replacement therapy may believe that the medication can be taken in a single daily dose, just like synthetic T4. This may work for a few people but for others, the daily dosage of T3 will need to be split up and taken in smaller doses, known as divided doses. This divided dose approach enables T3 to be taken at various intervals throughout the day, in order to provide a steady supply of T3 to the body. The use of divided doses also ensures that no single dose of T3 creates an exceptionally high peak level of T3 in the tissues of the body. Through the careful use of divided doses, it is possible to avoid the risk of tissue over-stimulation by T3 (T3 thyrotoxicosis). Some people refer to the taking of divided doses as multi-dosing.

In the UK, T3 is only available in 20-microgram tablets. Unfortunately, this makes matters rather difficult for the patient.

In order to achieve a divided dose strategy, the UK-based patient may have to carefully break the tablet in half (to create two 10-microgram doses), or into quarters (for a 5-microgram dose). If a 2.5 microgram T3 dose is required, as is often the case, then the tablet has to be broken up even further, which can be difficult. The USA patient has a range of T3 tablets available, which includes a 5-microgram tablet.

In the USA, some doctors use specialist companies, known as compounding pharmacies, to tailor a specific dosage of sustained release T3 for given patients, in order to avoid potential issues caused by large peaks and troughs in the circulating level of T3 throughout the day. Sustained release T3 is sometimes referred to as 'slow release T3'. I have asked several endocrinologists whether it would be possible for me to have a trial of sustained release T3. I have always been told that it is not available in the UK. There are mixed reports from the USA concerning sustained release T3. I have heard that the variability in the various compounding processes may lead to a lack of consistency in the way that the T3 is released. If this were true, then it would make dosage management very difficult. I have also heard that, for those patients who require a full replacement of dosage of T3, sustained release T3 does not appear to work as well as pure T3, as patients appear to need the rapid rise of T3 in their bodies that a pure T3 dose provides. These reasons could explain why many of the patients who have tried to use sustained release T3 have chosen to go back to using pure T3.

When he initially prescribed T3, my doctor recommended that I split the daily dosage into two divided doses. I quickly discovered that two divided doses were not going to provide a steady enough level of T3 for me during the day. This is just one example of how limited the existing information on T3 was, as there were no recommendations to try smaller, more frequent doses, if the larger, less frequent doses caused side effects.

I have now communicated with many patients who use T3 replacement therapy. There are a small number of patients who do manage on **two** divided doses of T3 per day and a very small number, for whom **one** large dose of T3 appears to work perfectly well. **However, the vast majority of patients using T3 replacement therapy appear to be using between three and five divided doses of T3 per day.** I have also heard of some patients who use even higher numbers of divided doses but I would consider higher numbers of divided doses to be bordering on impractical.

I cannot emphasise how important it is for many people to employ T3 in divided doses. For a small proportion of people one or two divided doses of T3 apparently works very well.

3-5 doses a day is best for most people

However, the careful use of three to five divided doses of T3 appears to suit many people extremely well. This is presumably because these people cannot tolerate high levels of individual T3 divided doses and therefore, they need multiple smaller divided doses of T3 in order to feel healthy.

T3 may be used safely

I will be discussing some of the misconceptions about the risks of using T3 in a later chapter. I will say that many of the rumours and misconceptions surrounding the use of T3 are unsubstantiated by scientific studies. The majority of the genuine concerns over T3 do not take account of the experience that has been gathered by patients and doctors, all over the world, from long-term T3 usage. If the T3 dosage is carefully managed, there should be no risk at all in its use. An effective dose should allow the cells of the body to function as they did before thyroid hormone problems developed.

It is important to recall that T3 does most of its work once it has entered the cell nuclei. There it binds to the thyroid hormone receptors on the genes within the nuclei, in order to activate certain genes and inhibit others, which in turn controls the number and types of proteins synthesised by cells. In this way T3 regulates cell function. This genomic action can take days or weeks to be fully realised. In this way some of the effects of T3 are actually 'softened' or 'buffered' and therefore some of the effects of T3 will not be felt immediately.

Taking T3 on an empty stomach and interaction of T3 with iron, calcium

On far more practical terms, T3 should ideally be taken on an empty stomach, at least one hour before any food is consumed and ideally several hours since the last meal. This will maximise the absorption of T3, which may be very important for someone who has impaired digestion due to prolonged hypothyroidism.

T3 should be taken at least one hour before any iron or calcium supplements, as both iron and calcium may interfere with the absorption of the T3 and the effect will be as though slightly less T3 has been taken. If iron or calcium supplements are taken then ideally no more T3 should be taken for a further four hours, to allow the iron and calcium to digest. It may make sense to take any iron and calcium supplements with an evening meal, after most, or all, of the T3 divided doses have been taken for the day.

I tend to ignore this advice. I simply chew up my T3 into powder in my mouth and swallow, to enable the fastest possible absorption. I haven't noticed any effect from any supplement taken in proximity to my T3 but the above advice is probably sound and will enable maximum possible absorption of the T3 thyroid hormone.

However, I have no digestive system issues. If I had suffered with any gastrointestinal issues or I had found that the T3 did not appear to be very effective then I would have taken my T3 on an empty stomach. To be absolutely confident of maximum absorption I would have ensured that two to three hours had passed since my last meal prior to taking the T3 and I would have allowed two to three hours after the T3 dose before eating my next meal. I would also have applied the guidelines above with regard to iron and calcium supplements. There is some evidence that some people find that these measures make a difference to absorption and effectiveness of their T3 medication.

T3 Replacement Therapy is Not Physiological Thyroid Hormone Replacement

There are a lot of doctors who use what they call 'physiological hormone replacement', which means replacing hormones to match 'normal' levels. The idea being that if a hormone is low as measured by a laboratory test then by replacing it until the laboratory test indicates it is at a 'normal' level then the person will get well. This is an admirable concept, especially when the entire range of hormones and nutrients are considered. There is a flaw though. This approach assumes that all thyroid patients have the same type of problem and will respond to correcting one or more hormones or other chemicals. However, for those people who have been forced to use only T3 in order to get well this approach may not work well at all. In some cases when T4 thyroid hormone replacement is used then thyroid and other hormone levels may appear perfectly normal but the patient may still be very ill with many of the symptoms associated with hypothyroidism.

I need to use T3 replacement. If I take even a small amount of T4 then my symptoms return very quickly. There is little point in any doctor attempting to replace my hormones using a physiological replacement methodology because I have something 'broken' at a cellular level. The only way that I have been able to maintain excellent health is to use only T3 with no T4 at all. This creates an unusual balance of my thyroid hormones within my bloodstream in order to ensure that normal levels of T3 become active at the appropriate receptors in my cells. I required a replacement that is far from physiological in the bloodstream to ensure that it is physiological at the cell nuclei and mitochondria.

I am not arguing that patients who can benefit from the physiological replacement of T4 and T3 should not do so. In fact, I am a strong believer that thyroid patients should indeed be offered T4 and T3 where possible (either synthetic or in the form of natural desiccated thyroid). This is obviously how the body was originally intended to work and all efforts should be made to resolve a thyroid patient's issues using this method. I always say that T3 replacement therapy is the thyroid treatment of last resort.

Once it is clear that physiological replacement of thyroid hormones is of no use to a thyroid patient then some enlightened doctors may offer a trial of T3. If the patient begins to respond well to T3 then why would anyone expect the same laboratory reference ranges of thyroid hormones to be of any use during T3 treatment? These laboratory ranges were based on the thyroid blood tests of people with no known thyroid issues, for the use of the majority of patients who do respond to T4 and have nothing broken at a cellular level. It is nonsense to manage thyroid patients to the standard laboratory reference ranges for TSH, FT4 or FT3 once they are using only T3 or predominantly T3 (in a T4/T3 based replacement).

I know many patients who have been frustrated and annoyed because their health has been improving on subsequent T3 dosage increases, yet after reviewing TSH, FT4 and FT3 results their doctors have panicked and reduced their T3 dosage or even insisted on adding T4 to their treatment. In some cases, some patients have been told to switch back to T4 treatment even though it was obvious from how the patient was feeling that they were actually improving. I've heard many stories like this and they make no logical sense to me.

For those people who have been forced to use T3 only to get well 'physiological replacement' should mean replacing T3 until people feel normal and display healthy symptoms and signs. This isn't what is happening in some cases and some patients are being left with inadequate treatment due to the flawed belief that conventional approaches using thyroid laboratory tests may continue to be useful in an unconventional situation. I discuss thyroid blood tests when on T3 replacement therapy in far more detail in Chapter 15.

Long-Term Use of T3 Replacement Therapy (and is there a need for T4?)

I have seen some arguments that insist that T4 is essential to good health and that there are properties specific to T4 that cannot be obtained via T3 alone. I have also seen it argued that T3 on its own cannot provide good health in the long-term.

There is very early research that suggests that T4 may be active in its own right, potentially in unique ways, such as encouraging hair growth or regulating the heart rate. The research is in the early stages and as yet I am yet to see any information that worries me. Even the possible heart regulatory effects of T4 do not make a great deal of sense based on the information from the many people who use T3 who have no such issues. When T3 is titrated carefully people do not have raised heart rates. If it turns out that there are some slight benefits to hair growth of T4 then I have so far to meet anyone who has noticed any issues due to a lack of T4.

However, it is not beyond the bounds of possibility that future research may find some unique benefits of T4, as more research is required in many aspects of thyroid hormone metabolism.

The view that is sometimes expressed that T3 replacement cannot be used as a long-term treatment is nonsense. These views often incorporate the hidden assumption that too much T3 is being used. If too much T3 is provided to the tissues then clearly this will cause problems. This is true of T3 or T4. However, T3 may be titrated safely and very effectively without providing too much T3 to the cells. The later chapters on the T3 dosage management process will explain how this may be done. I know many people who have been on T3 only for many years and they are a good deal healthier than many of the so-called 'properly treated' thyroid patients that are trying to get through their lives, still suffering the symptoms of hypothyroidism.

I've seen arguments that T3 causes ECG issues, memory or cognitive issues, osteoporosis, heart problems, muscle weakness, insulin resistance, intolerance to exercise, shortness of breath, insomnia, brain fog, hair quality issues etc. Many of these assertions are not based on actual research but on reports of some people who have been on T3. T3 may be used incorrectly and I would fully expect some of these issues to occur if a T3 dosage was too high. However, properly titrated T3 can be used safely and effectively and there are ways of doing this systematically, as I will explain in later chapters.

For those who simply cannot use T4, T4/T3 or NDT, because T4 does not work well for them, then there is no alternative but to use T3. Life is too short to suffer with terrible symptoms of hypothyroidism. I have been well for over a decade on only T3. I have virtually no T4 in my body. My vital signs are normal. My body temperature is usually around 98.4-98.6 Fahrenheit, I have no ECG issues, I have no weight issues, my cognitive function is as good as it has ever been and I am reasonably active and fit for my age (playing tennis as often as I have time to). I am not unusual. I know many people who have arrived at a T3 dosage that is safe and effective and are completely well with none of the side effects that are sometimes used to scare people.

Finally, I see no reason why people who simply cannot get well with T4, T4/T3 or NDT cannot identify their ideal T3 dosage and then attempt to find the maximum amount of T4 that they can tolerate alongside it. However, I genuinely believe that from the research material available today and from speaking to many people who have used T3 for a long time that T3 is a perfectly legitimate thyroid hormone replacement for the long-term and does not need to be used with any T4, although there is no reason why T4 should not be added to tolerance.

Chapter 12

General Lessons Learned on T3 Use

LESSON #2: WE ARE RESPONSIBLE FOR OUR OWN HEALTH

I spent several years after the initial diagnosis, going back and forth to two different family doctors and about four different endocrinologists and other specialists. Like many people, I placed my trust in the medical professionals I consulted. After a short while I began to prepare written notes about my symptoms beforehand and I brought these with me when I saw a doctor. This helped me to cover all the points and ask all the questions that I needed to.

During these early years I carried with me a stereotypical view of the patient-doctor relationship. This view was that I, the patient, had to tell my doctor what was wrong with me and then the doctor would take complete responsibility for deciding how to investigate, diagnose and treat me. At this time I felt that all doctors I saw were more knowledgeable than me and I would never have insisted on debating any aspect of my treatment, let alone arguing with a doctor about the approach to diagnosis or treatment.

It is this implicit handing over of the responsibility for our own health, when we enter a doctor's office, that I have learned can be a mistake with a complex illness like hypothyroidism. I believe my own slowness to recognise this caused me to waste a significant amount of time and remain ill for far longer than I needed to. Once I had recognised this and could see how it was hampering my progress, I was able to move forward more rapidly.

I began to view myself as the person responsible for my health. I knew that I was in charge of trying to understand and diagnose the nature of my health problem. Yes, I would need to select and work with appropriate health professionals to do much of this work but the responsibility was fundamentally with me.

To do this properly I had to learn more about thyroid disease. This is the cost of being responsible for your own health - you must, on occasion, be prepared to do some work. I also knew that sometimes it would be necessary to present a sound argument and be prepared to defend this. There were also occasions when I had to back my own judgement on what was wrong with me and on what the next step in the investigation or treatment should be. However, I was always prepared to give my doctors a chance to make their own proposals, I just no longer felt that I had to agree with them.

If the differences of viewpoint between a doctor and myself were too great and there was no cooperation or compromise, then I was prepared to go and find a new doctor. I also began to realise that there might be times when I would have to do some research to locate a doctor that I could work with, rather than simply taking the easiest option available.

This lesson was probably the first and the hardest that I learned. It was also the most important and empowering. If I hadn't learned this lesson then I would never have recovered.

LESSON #3: TIME IS OUR MOST PRECIOUS RESOURCE

More time can be lost due to our slowness to recognise that we need to take responsibility for our own health, than for almost any other reason. During the diagnosis and treatment of hypothyroidism there are many opportunities for vast amounts of precious time to be wasted. In my own case and in the cases of many patients I have communicated with, many years can go by, whilst alternative dosages of synthetic T4 are tried. Often, far too long is allowed to go by on a dosage of synthetic T4 that is not effective before, yet again, it is modified in the hope that it may help. It is often very clear to the patient after a year or so has passed by, that the synthetic T4 being given is not making any difference at all. Before long, six, eight or ten years may have gone by. A large percentage of a person's life may be spent living with unnecessary ill health.

Time spent feeling dreadfully ill, is time that is being cut out of our lives. It is also time that in some ways, lessens the lives of our children, partners and other family members or close friends. It is the 'death by a thousand cuts' because the time just disappears in small pieces, until eventually, a significant part of a lifetime has slipped by.

It is important for a patient to recognise whether their doctor is able to help them get well or not. If a doctor refuses to adjust medication by any method other than thyroid blood test results, or will not consider using thyroid replacement hormones other than synthetic T4 then it may well be time to begin looking for a more knowledgeable and supportive doctor.

If a different family doctor or endocrinologist does need to be found, then obtaining a personal recommendation that provides confidence in the potential new physician is the preferred option. If this were not possible then it may be worth trying to communicate with the doctor prior to making the decision. I would want to find out some relevant information about any potential new doctor:

- How does the doctor track the progress of thyroid hormone treatment? If blood test results were the primary method, then what is the doctor's attitude to tracking symptoms?

- Does the potential new doctor believe that synthetic T4 treatment always resolves hypothyroidism or not? If the doctor believes that T4 always works, then this doctor would be unlikely to prescribe any other treatment.

- Knowing explicitly if the doctor would consider prescribing a combination of T4/T3, natural thyroid or pure T3 is very important.

- In the case of using T4/T3, or just T3, it is important to gain some insight into how the doctor would manage the dosage of medication and how a patient's symptoms might be taken into account in managing dosage.

- I personally prefer to be an active partner and discuss how my symptoms are progressing and what the best treatment options are. It may be important to know if the potential new doctor is comfortable in working in a manner that suits the patient.

It may be difficult to find out all the answers to the above. Ideally, this information will come from another thyroid patient who has had a good experience with the doctor that is being considered. However, if this information is not easily available then at the very least knowing that the doctor is empathetic and supportive is essential.

This lesson may seem trivial but once you begin to see time itself as a critical resource, then it will change your actions and your attitude to ineffective or slow treatment practices.

LESSON #4: T3 IS THE THYROID REPLACEMENT OF LAST RESORT

I believe that T3 replacement should only be considered when all the other treatments have failed and when all other causes of remaining symptoms have been eliminated.

Many thyroid patients are able to recover using T4 and T4/T3 replacement therapies. Each of these therapies, possibly including synthetic combinations of T4/T3 or natural thyroid preparations, should be given some time to see if they may have a benefit for a patient.

The single biggest difficulty with using T3 is the complexity of dosage management. For some people it can take a considerable amount of time and effort to tailor a final T3 dosage that meets their needs.

Managing a predominantly T4 dominated therapy may require some use of divided doses if there is any T3 also being used. However, aside from continuing to monitor the patient's symptoms, the doctor may also use FT4 and FT3 as a guide during a T4 based treatment. There is little requirement with a T4/T3 therapy to split the daily dosage of T3 into more than two or three divided doses and each of these T3 doses can usually be of the same size.

If the T4 based replacement therapies have failed to resolve a patient's symptoms, then in this case and, if no other medical condition is responsible, the extra effort in using T3 is well worth it. Used correctly, T3 is highly effective. There may only be a small percentage of patients that a doctor ever has to consider placing on a trial of T3. However, not having T3 treatment available as an option is to fail to make available one of the most effective treatments for hypothyroidism.

I have seen statements by endocrinologists that T3 should never be used for long term thyroid treatment, because of issues with patient compliance, i.e. the patient may not take their tablets exactly at the right times or may miss some or take too many. For those patients who are sick and tired of being sick and tired, compliance is a non-issue. I have also seen comments that suggest that some doctors are concerned that T3 will be used with patients for whom it is not appropriate. Clearly, T3 replacement therapy should only be used in the right circumstances.

Therefore, my firm opinion is that T3 should be the treatment of last resort but T3 replacement therapy absolutely has to be available as an option.

LESSON #5: RISKS OF USING T3 - THE REAL STORY

Any patient reading the following views on the risks of T3 use should clearly discuss any perceived risks with their own personal physician, as individuals may have particular health issues that their doctor needs to take into account.

My personal opinion is that the majority of the issues that people claim are present with the use of T3 are either false or highly misleading. Almost all of the comments, or articles, that I have read concerning the risks of using T3, have at their heart the implicit assumption that a patient will be using T3 incorrectly.

A careful process of dosage management to tailor a T3 dosage to the specific needs of a patient will result in no single divided dose of T3 ever causing tissue over-stimulation. I mean that no collection of tissues in the body will become over-stimulated due to T3 thyrotoxicity. This is not the same as having a high FT3 level in the bloodstream or having a suppressed TSH, because both of these may exist at the same time as ideal levels of T3 within the cells.

Any patient that wants to undergo a trial of T3 replacement therapy has probably tried and failed to get well on all the other available treatments. It is completely unreasonable to bar a patient's access to a potentially viable treatment and, possibly, the only hope of recovery, because of the silly assumption that T3 will be used improperly.

There may be one exception to the above. People who have a pre-existing serious heart condition are generally not advised to use T3. However, it is also important to remember that if a patient is not receiving an adequate level of thyroid hormone, or if their T4 therapy is failing, then heart and cardiovascular problems can arise due to the lack of appropriate levels of thyroid hormone. So, it is important for the patient's doctor to assess whether any heart issues could be adversely affected by too little circulating thyroid hormone and whether T3 could be helpful or unhelpful in this situation.

I have seen no scientific studies that indicate that, when used correctly, T3 is harmful in the long-term. No extended studies have been done on patients that only use T3. So, there is no evidence of thyrotoxicosis, tissue level over-stimulation, heart problems, bone loss issues or any other issue for that matter, based on the study of patients on T3 replacement therapy.

There are reports of patients being rushed to hospital with thyrotoxicosis due to excess thyroid hormone but these are based on patients who have either been taking too much synthetic T4, or have developed hyperthyroidism due to over production of hormones by their own thyroid gland. Certainly, too much thyroid hormone in the tissues, such that there is tissue over-stimulation, is a bad thing. No one would argue with this point. But to assume that simply having the ability to take too much T3 from a bottle of tablets, is an extremely poor argument for not allowing the correct, effective and safe use of the T3 thyroid hormone.

Some specific areas of concern are sometimes raised with respect to the use of T3. It has been suggested that excess thyroid hormone is potentially a risk for the development of osteoporosis and fractures and that the use of T3 might induce heart abnormalities, including cardiac arrest. Let me deal with these issues one by one, dealing firstly with one of the main measures that some doctors use to conclude that there is risk of tissue over-stimulation - a suppressed TSH.

Risks - TSH Suppression

Some doctors might argue that if a thyroid blood test result revealed that my TSH was suppressed below 0.1 mU/L, then this would mean that I was hyperthyroid and at risk of having adverse effects due to thyroid hormone. I would argue differently. If my body temperature is normal, I have no adverse symptoms, my heart rate, blood pressure and ECG are normal, my digestive system is working well, my skin, hair and nails are normal, my energy level is ideal, I have no excessive weight gain or loss, my mind is active and at ease, my mood is good and I feel well, then, regardless of my TSH, or any other thyroid hormone blood test result, I am not taking too much thyroid hormone.

If I had adjusted my T3 dosage, so that it was too high, then I would expect to have several of the following symptoms and signs: nervousness; anxiety; heart palpitations; weight loss; loose bowels; hyperactivity; raised body temperature; sweating; higher than normal systolic blood pressure; fatigue; feeling weak; irritability; nausea; shortness of breath; staring eyes and shaking hands or tremors. One or more of these may indicate the presence of over-stimulation in some tissues.

If T3 dosage management is performed correctly then any unusual or adverse effects will be quickly noticed. It is actually quite easy to recognise symptoms associated with tissue over-stimulation and quickly correct the T3 dosage.

In later chapters I will review medical research that illustrates how misleading TSH may be regarding tissue levels of T4 and T3 and the highly suppressive effect that T3 replacement has on TSH. Because of this last point, it will become obvious that for any patient on T3 replacement therapy, the TSH blood test result only becomes of use for occasionally checking that the pituitary gland is functioning correctly. On T3 replacement therapy the TSH is unreliable and potentially highly misleading if it is being used in the assessment of the patient's T3 dosage.

Typically, on T3 replacement therapy, a patient's TSH will be low or suppressed, but this may depend on how long prior to the blood test the patient took any T3. It will also depend on how much of the patient's own thyroid function is left. TSH blood test results for a patient on T3 treatment are a bit of a lottery. I have had TSH results that are suppressed and other TSH results that are high. In each of these cases, my T3 dosage has been the same.

One of my well-used texts is littered with information and powerful arguments for ignoring a suppressed TSH if the patient feels well and has no adverse symptoms.[1] The text also illustrates how misleading a TSH result may be in the initial diagnosis of hypothyroidism.

Two recent scientific papers have been published that provide logical, coherent and scientific analyses based on many years of clinical practice that also help us to further understand how TSH may be grossly misinterpreted.[2, 3] The papers clearly and logically illuminate the flaws in the thinking that a suppressed TSH means that a patient is suffering from excess thyroid hormone and that thyroid medication dosage should be reduced. The authors present compelling arguments that for some thyroid patients, particularly but not exclusively those patients that have been on calorie restrictive diets, the thyroid system has maladapted such that a lower TSH 'set point' now correlates with healthy thyroid hormone levels. The authors argue that FT4, FT3, rT3 results and the symptomatic response of patients should be of primary focus during thyroid hormone treatment rather than the TSH, even if the TSH is totally suppressed.

A suppressed TSH is not something that concerns me at all. In fact, I would rather have laboratory test results with a fully suppressed TSH and FT3 above the top of the laboratory reference range, because results like this have corresponded to the times when I have felt really well. In general, since being on T3 replacement therapy I no longer pay any interest to TSH results.

TSH is not an indicator of tissue levels of thyroid hormone, especially in T3 replacement therapy, so something else will need to be used, such as clinical presentation and some actual physiological measures of effective tissue levels of T3.

Risks - Bone Loss

Let me discuss the concerns that some doctors may have about the use of T3 and bone loss. The process of bone-loss, if it continues, can ultimately lead to osteoporosis.

I know of no research studies performed on patients who use only T3 replacement therapy, which suggests that there are any more risks associated with using T3 than for any other form of thyroid hormone replacement. No thyroid hormone replacement therapy should present a problem with bone-loss if there is no evidence of tissue over-stimulation.

However, there is evidence that untreated or under-treated hypothyroidism is linked to bone-loss.[4] Therefore, there must be a risk of bone-loss from synthetic T4 thyroid hormone treatment that has left a patient with the symptoms associated with hypothyroidism. To put it another way, both hypothyroidism and hyperthyroidism, or too little or too much thyroid hormone, of any kind, can cause bone-loss.[5]

I refer you to a well-organised analysis on this whole topic, which gathers together most of the recent research about the effect of TSH-suppressive and non-suppressive dosages of thyroid hormone.[4] The author concludes that the views of some doctors, that TSH-suppressive dosages of thyroid hormone results in osteoporosis, is based on early flawed studies and is simply false.

A lot of evidence now indicates that the risks of bone-loss in thyroid hormone replacement have been extremely exaggerated. This is supported by the fact that fractures are not a normal feature of correctly treated hypothyroid patients.

In my own case, I adopt a sensible approach to bone health. I have used serum calcium blood tests from time to time, if I had any concerns that my T3 dosage may be too high, to see if any calcium leaching is occurring. I take magnesium, calcium, vitamin D3 and a broad range of other mineral supplements every day. I do regular, weight bearing exercise. I have a Dexa bone density scan every few years, in order to see if any change has occurred. More importantly, I use a good T3 dosage management process that is designed to provide only the level of T3 needed to be healthy and not a microgram more. If someone had any particular risk of bone-loss, then a more frequent bone density scan could be performed and interventional medication could be used, if required.

Risks - Heart Problems

I wish I had a pound for every time I have heard someone say that T3 might be linked to heart problems.

There is no published research that links the correct use of T3 containing medications, or of T3 on its own, to heart attacks or other heart related issues. In fact, in 2003 a group of respected endocrinologists published a paper, which included the comment '... the possible long-term risks of elevated or fluctuating T3 levels have not been evaluated.'[7]

As already stated, if someone has a pre-existing heart condition, then they may be advised not to use T3, because of the increased risk of any adverse effects due to a dosage change that is incorrect. Although, it may be possible to locate a doctor with the practical experience and track record of good results in prescribing T3 to people with this type of condition.

There is research that clearly shows that untreated hypothyroidism causes elevated cholesterol, homocysteine levels and heart attacks.[8, 9] Untreated, or incorrectly treated hypothyroidism, is also associated with strokes and peripheral vascular disease. Any thyroid hormone medication, if taken in too high a dosage, will lead to tissue level over-stimulation and may result in a variety of heart related symptoms or events. A proper dosage management process that leads to an ideal T3 dosage for a patient, will not create tissue level over-stimulation and, by definition, cannot give rise to heart related issues.

One recent research study has concluded that T3 may in fact help the heart to repair after a heart attack and that low levels of T3 are actually associated with increased morbidity and mortality in patients with heart conditions.[10] Rather than being a risk, T3 may turn out to be very important to the health of the heart. This research may be the first of many that help us to understand why untreated hypothyroidism has been found to be associated with heart attacks.

During the process of adjusting a T3 dosage it is possible, very occasionally, to take a little too much T3. These occasions are few and a sound dosage management process will ensure that only a little extra T3 will be involved, because only small increases will be made at any given time and therefore, any symptoms will be mild and very short-lived.

I have always asked my doctor to provide me with a small supply of propranolol (beta-blockers), which may be used, if necessary, for the few hours that any effect lasts. Asthma sufferers should not use propranolol. If T3 is handled correctly, then these occasions are incredibly rare and only involve a very mild elevation in heart rate for a few hours. I have only used propranolol on a few of occasions due to this situation and that was many years ago. In fact, I had far more issues with heart rate elevation during my time on T4 replacement therapy.

In the case of a patient who may have a heart condition, cardiovascular problems or is elderly, then the doctor should be wary of prescribing T3. At the very least, in this circumstance, the patient should be thoroughly investigated by a cardiologist, prior to commencing treatment with T3.

From a practical point of view, I have a blood pressure monitor at home that I use. I regularly monitor my heart rate and check that it is normal. When I see my family doctor my heart is listened to and my blood pressure is checked. I have had the occasional routine ECG, and at my age I would do this whether I was on T3 or not. I also take Vitamin C, Vitamin E, Coenzyme Q10 and L-Taurine, which are thought to have beneficial effects on the heart. Most importantly, I do regular exercise and I do not smoke. I have no concerns that T3 will have anything but positive effects on my cardiovascular system.

There is a situation during the early stages of dosage management of T3 where it is possible that some people may experience an elevated raised heart rate and not be sure if this is being caused by too much or too little T3, or deficiency of some nutrient or other hormone. I have dealt with this specific case when I talk about the process I use for T3 dosage management. My experience has been that these situations are often caused by problems with low nutrients like iron, by low levels of cortisol (sometimes correctable by careful use of T3), or by other factors like blood sugar imbalances rather than the T3 itself.

Risks - Conclusions

I hope I have gone some way to alleviating some of the fears surrounding the most misunderstood thyroid hormone, T3.

What would I do if I did develop heart problems or osteoporosis? What do you think? Is it likely that I would put myself back in the condition that I was in when I was using T4 replacement? No, I would not wish that for myself or anyone else. With a family history of heart disease, if I did develop a heart condition, I would continue taking my T3 and have any heart problem managed in the normal way. I do not consider T3 replacement therapy to be providing me with anything other than benefits and, hopefully, it will lessen my risk of developing any form of cardiovascular disease.

T3 was the only solution that corrected my original symptoms, so it must be exactly what my body requires. My overall goal has always been to find the lowest T3 dosage that addresses my symptoms and makes me feel well, without inducing any new adverse symptoms. Therefore, since my dosage of T3 is performing extremely well, at the lowest dose I can determine and since it is producing no adverse symptoms, then it must be safe.

There is no reason why anyone who decides to use T3 thyroid hormone replacement, cannot work with their own physician to ensure they are also on a safe and effective dose.

I do not support self-medication. I believe it is important for a patient to find a doctor that they are comfortable working with, so that proper medical advice may be provided and the appropriate tests can be performed when required. We just need more doctors who provide a wider range of thyroid hormone treatments and are fully aware of how to use them effectively and safely. Once a sufficient number of endocrinologists and doctors are providing T3 replacement therapy and can do this effectively and safely, then this should reduce the number of patients that feel the need to self-medicate. This will further reduce the perception of risk associated with the use of T3 replacement therapy.

Chapter 13

Lesson Learned on Clearing T4 Prior to T3 Use

LESSON #6: CLEAR THE T4

The T4 needed to be allowed to clear, before I could evaluate the effectiveness of T3 or invest effort in fine-tuning my T3 dosage.

T4 has a half-life of 7 days. I calculated various timescales for the T4 medication that was in my body to be used up, based on different daily dosages of T4 medication. For a patient who had been taking 100 micrograms of T4 for many months, it would take around sixty days for the T4 medication be used up by the body, leaving only the residual level of T4 produced by the patient's own thyroid, i.e. about eight weeks. For a patient on 150 micrograms of T4, the clearance time would be about sixty-five days (nine weeks). For someone on 200 micrograms of T4, this increases slightly to about sixty-eight days (ten weeks) and on 300 micrograms of T4, the clearance time might be around seventy-five days (nearly eleven weeks). The effect of T4 half-life causes the clearance time to be slightly longer if the T4 dosage is higher but the difference is not great.

In most cases, it is safe to assume that once all T4 medication is stopped then the majority of any T4 medication that has been taken will clear in around eight weeks, regardless of the T4 dosage that the patient was taking. If someone wanted to be absolutely confident that all the T4 medication had cleared, then twelve weeks would be a very safe estimate. Many hypothyroid patients still have a little T4 production from their thyroid gland. The level of T4 may be quite high if the patient does not have Hashimoto's thyroiditis, or their autoantibodies have fallen to low levels before their thyroid gland was destroyed. Consequently, it is often impossible to clear all the T4; hence I have assumed that eight weeks is a reasonable amount of time to wait for the T4 to clear.

The advice I was given was to wait as long as possible after stopping the use of T4, before starting to use T3 replacement therapy. One of the potential issues is that the addition of T3 to an already high level of T4 replacement might possibly result in a bad episode of hyperthyroidism as the body begins to function better and this must be avoided at all costs.

Managing only to wait around one week before starting to take any T3, I then used only the minimum amount of T3 that I could survive on, until the eight weeks for T4 clearance had passed. I did need to increase my T3 dosage during this time but didn't reach a fully satisfactory dosage of T3 until much later. This required quite a lot of patience and acceptance that some symptoms would remain during this period.

During the years that I was taking T4 replacement therapy, I often had a slight headache in the centre of my forehead, which I referred as my 'thyroxine headache'. When I first began using T3 and before the T4 had cleared, my thyroxine headaches actually grew worse. As I tried to raise my T3 dosage during the first few days, my heart rate increased and I felt quite anxious and tense. These initial adverse side effects were bad enough to prevent me from increasing my T3 dosage further.

Over the past ten years, I have experimented several times with combinations of T4 and T3. Whenever I try to take a dose of synthetic T4, higher than 25 micrograms, the unpleasant symptoms and the thyroxine headaches soon return.

During the first few weeks of T3 use, I also noticed that the beneficial effects of the T3 did not appear to last for very long. I guessed that the limited effects of T3 were probably being caused by the remaining T4 in my body. Thankfully, I was proven correct. Over a period of just a few weeks the beneficial effects of each T3 dose increased and lasted longer.

When the remaining T4 reduces to a low level, it is possible to experience even worse symptoms of hypothyroidism, even if a low level of T3 replacement has already started. This began to happen to me several weeks after having stopped taking T4. I was then able to increase my T3 dosage, with no further issues from T4. Further T3 increases began working effectively without any side effects.

Therefore, during the initial eight-week phase of allowing the T4 medication to clear, T3 should not be used at all until the symptoms of hypothyroidism are too difficult to cope with. Even when T3 replacement therapy has started the T3 dosage should be kept to the lowest level required to provide some relief. This may be a little uncomfortable but it is the safest way to proceed and it also reduces the number of potential problems and confusion that might occur when T3 replacement therapy is started in earnest.

T4 May be Optionally Added Back to Tolerance After Determining T3 Dosage

I was not able to get well using T4 replacement and needed to begin using only T3. I knew that it was essential to clear all the T4 to ensure the T3 had the best possible chance of working effectively. I have never excluded the possibility of adding some T4 medication once my T3 dosage was determined. The T3 dosage management process is capable of adding T4 back in to tolerance once a safe and effective T3 dosage has been determined. In my own case I can still only tolerate about 12.5 micrograms of T4. Some people who have been driven to use T3 replacement therapy may not be able to tolerate any T4 and other may be able to tolerate more than I can. Every person is unique and for those that have a concern that they need some T4, the option exists to add T4 back in to tolerance once the T3 dosage is stable.

Chapter 14

Lessons Learned on Divided Doses of T3

LESSON #7: WAVES OF T3

For each divided dose of T3, I discovered that there was definitely a 'threshold level' that had to be exceeded before any real benefit was experienced from the hormone. As I increased the dose beyond this threshold level then the effects were greater. If I exceeded the threshold too much then I experienced symptoms of tissue over-stimulation. My threshold level tended to be lower as the day progressed. So, later in the day I required lower doses of T3 to achieve the same effect. This perception may be due in part to some cumulative effect of the previous doses of T3 but the interaction with other hormones, which reduce in level during the day, may also be relevant.

I often use a specific analogy to describe to other people how T3 appears to behave:

Imagine a sandy beach, which is sheltered from the sea by large rocks. Only a wave that is large and powerful enough is capable of striking the rocks and sending a spray of seawater over them to drench the sand beyond.

Each T3 divided dose is like a wave, the intra-cellular targets of T3 are akin to the beach and the rocks represent all the possible bio-chemical barriers that the T3 has to overcome. I do not believe that this is just some idle analogy. This is definitely how T3 replacement appears to feel and work within my own body.

T3 BEHAVES VERY DIFFERENTLY TO T4

T3 operates completely differently to T4. T3 has a much shorter half-life. T4 medication can be taken in a single daily dose, which the patient won't feel the effects of immediately. T4 achieves its effect by building up slowly in the body over time.

Once T3 reaches my cells, I begin to feel the positive effects almost immediately. These last for a few hours and then I distinctly feel the effects wearing off, which makes me aware that I require my next dose.

I have found that other hormones and chemicals, including some medications, can interfere with the intensity and the duration of the effects of each divided dose of T3.

When a T3 dose is large enough to become noticeably beneficial, then further increases may produce far greater effects than might be expected. Even small increases at this stage may produce a significant improvement in symptoms. Therefore, great care must be taken when making increases to a T3 divided dose, once the T3 begins to correct symptoms. At this point, much smaller T3 divided dose changes should be used.

The above illustrates how divided doses of T3 feel and appear to work for me. I have done no studies to attempt to establish whether this is the way that many patients experience T3. However, I do know that some other patients I have communicated with experience T3 in a similar way.

I do not know whether the wave-like feeling that I experience, with each divided dose of T3, is linked to the mitochondrial action of T3, or the genomic action of T3, or both.

Those patients who do better with one or two doses of T3 per day may not experience T3 in the same way as I have described. These patients often need to be able to take much larger divided doses of T3 before any symptomatic improvement occurs and the effects of these may extend for a longer period. This would suggest that they don't experience the same wave effect of T3 that I do or that it is less pronounced. This may be closely linked to the differences in metabolic issues between patients.

LESSON #8: USE DIVIDED DOSES OF T3 TO MANAGE THE WAVES

In a healthy person, some T4 is being constantly converted to T3 and, through this process, relatively stable levels of T3 in the bloodstream and the tissues are maintained.

The use of divided doses, or multi-doses, of T3 has two distinct purposes:

1. Avoiding tissue over-stimulation. T3 medication is absorbed rapidly into the bloodstream and then into the tissues. Too large a divided dose of T3 will cause symptoms of tissue over-stimulation. To avoid this, most patients using T3 replacement therapy use several divided doses of T3. Whilst this method of using T3 cannot replicate the steady levels of serum and tissue T3 that comes as a result of correctly processed T4, it can feel nearly the same, if the divided doses of T3 are chosen carefully.

2. Overcoming the bio-chemical problems that caused T4 to fail. Most people who eventually resort to using T3 to recover from hypothyroidism do this because something, somewhere within their body has misbehaved or broken, such that normal thyroid hormone metabolism no longer works. I will discuss this in far greater detail later. The use of pure T3 allows each divided dose to be carefully adjusted in size, or titrated, so that it is just high enough to be perfectly effective but without producing symptoms or signs of tissue over-stimulation. This titration of each individual divided dose of T3 was critical for me, as it enabled me to overcome the problem that was causing T4 replacement therapy to fail. I

have spoken with many patients who have also been successful in making T3 replacement therapy work and they too have found that it is important to get exactly the right level of T3 in order for their symptoms to go.

I have also discovered that the contents of an individual T3 dose needs to be delivered at once. If I attempt to take 4 quarters of a single T3 divided dose spread over two hours then it is not effective at all. I need to swallow the entire divided dose all at once. I have drawn one other very important conclusion from all of this experience. I believe that it is only via the use of pure T3 that a sufficiently high level of the hormone may be delivered to the thyroid hormone receptors within the cells. I believe that it is these individual waves of T3 that saturate the cells with enough T3 that enable some of it to be effective. For me and for many T3 users this latter point is crucial. I do not believe, for instance, that the use of timed release T3 could easily duplicate the excellent results that carefully titrated divided doses of pure T3 can achieve. This may well be the reason why some T3 users who have tried timed release T3 have returned once more to the use of pure T3. These views are my own and are only relevant to those people with biochemical problems that prevent the successful use or processing of T4.

T3 DIVIDED DOSES - HOW MANY PER DAY?

The majority of patients, experienced in using T3, use between three and five divided doses of T3 per day. However, some patients use only one or two doses of T3 per day and some use more than five divided doses per day. Any patient, who is contemplating the use of T3 replacement, may want to begin with using between three and five divided doses of T3 and explore the other options, if required, as the treatment progresses.

I have talked to many thyroid patients who have been placed on trials of T3 thyroid hormone by their endocrinologists. The recommendation of two divided doses of T3 per day still appears to being taught in medical schools, as this is frequently what patients are being told to use. This needs to be updated, as it is not the best way to start to use T3.

A T3 dosage should have carefully selected divided doses that ensure that:

• The number of T3 divided doses per day and their sizes make the individual feel healthy throughout the entire day.

• Each T3 divided dose is only just large enough to make the individual feel well.

• No divided dose should create any evidence of tissue over-stimulation.

By using divided doses it should easily be possible to avoid providing too much thyroid hormone to the cells, i.e. any risks of using T3 should be easily avoided.

T3 DOSAGE - VARIATION IN SIZE FOR DIFFERENT PATIENTS

It is also worth mentioning that when I speak to other patients, who use T3 replacement therapy, it is evident that there is a large variation in T3 dosage. The wide range of T3 dosages being used is probably due to the varying degrees of biochemical problems that patients have. These biochemical problems caused T4 replacement therapy to fail for these patients and drove them to using T3 replacement therapy.

I know of people who have completely recovered by taking 30 micrograms of T3 per day in divided doses. I have communicated with thyroid patients on total daily dosages of 40 micrograms of T3, whereas others take 60 or 75 micrograms per day. A smaller number of patients appear to require between 120 and 150 micrograms of T3 per day and I have spoken to a few on 200 micrograms of T3 per day. I take significantly less than this, as my total daily requirement for T3 has varied only between 45 and 60 micrograms of T3 during the past ten years. Some people do well on several very small divided doses of T3 per day and so require a rather modest daily T3 dosage.

I believe that the underlying cellular problem that an individual has dictates the number of divided doses that appear to be ideally suited to that person. It is clear to me that some people do appear to be healthier on one or two divided doses and others need three to five divided doses. There is need for far more research into this.

Regardless of the amount of T3 taken by different patients, the objective is always the same - to take just enough T3 in each divided dose in order to feel well with zero adverse effects and not a microgram more. I have learned to be extremely wary of anyone who believes that a certain total dosage or individual divided dose size of T3 is required for good health. T3 dosage must be fine-tuned to the needs of the individual with each person obtaining just enough T3 from their gastrointestinal tract to make them healthy and no more. I do not trust any individual or physician who says otherwise. The type and severity of metabolic issues that people can experience are too varied for any fixed ideas to be held about T3 dosages.

T3 DIVIDED DOSES - SAME SIZES OR DIFFERENT?

The simplest assumption would be that each of the divided doses of T3 would be of the same size - this would be a 'level-dose strategy'. For example, in a level-dose strategy with four divided doses, if a patient were taking 60 micrograms of T3 per day, then each T3 dose would be 15 micrograms.

The slightly more complex scenario is a 'tailored-dose strategy', which would allow each of the T3 doses to be different. In a tailored-dose strategy, it may be more common for the earlier doses to be slightly larger than the later doses. An example, for a patient who uses 60 micrograms of T3 per day, then the four divided doses might be: 20 micrograms, 15 micrograms, 15 micrograms and 10 micrograms. Clearly, it is more complex to adjust each divided dose of T3 to a unique and optimal size. However, for some people this amount of tailoring of divided doses may be required for an ideal, effective and safe T3 dosage to be established. Incidentally, some patients appear to do better with a smaller first T3 divided dose first thing in the morning. People have their own individual requirements.

Some individuals may find that a level-dose strategy works perfectly well and others may find that they require a tailored-dose strategy. Trial and error will be the only way to determine this. I will discuss this further in section 5.

Some factors that tend to support a tailored-dose strategy are:

- The first T3 divided dose may need to be a little larger than the ones that follow. This is because the interval preceding the first T3 dose is generally the largest interval. Patients usually haven't taken any T3 since the previous day, so the first T3 divided dose may need to act as a 'kick-start'. Sometimes this first T3 divided dose may need to be smaller than the others, perhaps because of the interaction with the adrenal glands or other hormones early in the morning. However, the need for a larger or smaller first T3 divided dose does require a tailored-dose strategy for some people.

- T3 has a short half-life but there may be a cumulative effect of doses during the day. Therefore, this may require lower doses of T3 as the day progresses.

- Various hormones have high levels in the morning and tend to reduce during the day. I believe that these can also influence the effectiveness of T3, perhaps contributing to the need for slightly higher divided doses of T3 in the morning and lower doses later in the day.

In the world of T3 replacement therapy, everyone has his or her own unique needs that must be met. The most important thing is to have the right sized T3 divided dose at the right time for the individual.

T3 DIVIDED DOSE TIMINGS

These will be discussed in detail during the chapters on T3 dosage management but to satisfy the curiosity of some people, typical dose timings for four divided doses might be:

8:00 am, 11:00 am, 2:00 pm and 5:00 pm.

While, typical timings for three divided doses might be:

8:00 am, 11:00 am/12:00 noon and 5:00 pm.

The above are just sample timings and, in practice, people work with their own doctors to identify timings that suit their own needs.

I FOUND I COULD NOT 'TOP UP' DIVIDED DOSES OF T3

During the initial work of determining my T3 dosage, I often found that I had taken a divided dose of T3 that was too small. If I tried to correct this by taking a small 'top up' T3 dose, half an hour or an hour later, it appeared to do nothing at all. I found a similar result when trying to take a greater number of smaller divided doses of T3 - they just didn't work. My experience has been that each divided dose of T3 needs to be big enough to deliver the correct amount of T3 at any given time.

This may only apply to those people with some form of bio-chemical issue that impairs the cellular response to thyroid hormone. It was impossible for me to just 'top up' a divided dose of T3. I had to take a large enough divided dose of T3 in the first place.

This experience with small 'top up' doses of T3 also fits with the idea that a wave of T3 needs to be large enough to reach its intra-cellular targets.

MORNING AND EVENING DOSES OF T3

Most people will take their first T3 dose between 7:00 am and 9:00 am. I will discuss the idea of taking the first T3 dose earlier than this and how this might sometimes assist the adrenal glands in a later chapter.

Taking T3 in the evening after 6:00 pm used to prevent me from sleeping at night, although I am more tolerant of evening T3 now. Other patients also appear to have problems if they take T3 late in the evening. However, everyone is different. I know of some people who take a small dose of T3 late at night or before they go to bed, because they feel that this helps them to sleep.

COMPLIANCE

This is a term used by doctors to describe whether a patient will remember to take their medication on time each day. I have had reports of doctors who do not wish their patients to take more than two divided doses of T3 per day because they are concerned that the patients will not remain compliant.

For those patients that have eventually got to the stage of using T3 replacement therapy, then I believe that whether two, three, four or more divided doses of T3 per day are required, the patients are likely to remain compliant if they feel healthy once more.

No patient who uses T3 replacement therapy that I have spoken with has considered this to be an issue. Moreover, if three, four or more T3 divided doses are required to be effective then it is likely that on two divided doses that either the T3 dosage will be too low or there will be some evidence of tissue over-stimulation.

Therefore, compliance will be a non-issue for most patients and the management of the T3 dosage is simply something that has to be addressed head-on. In fact, it is quite easy to do.

LESSON #9: SMALL DOSE CHANGES, SENSIBLE FREQUENCY

I never make more than one change to my T3 dosage at any time. Only one divided dose will be changed and this will be a size or timing change but not both at the same time.

When I started to use T3 replacement therapy and still had the symptoms associated with hypothyroidism, any increases or decreases to the size of a divided dose tended to be only 2.5 or 5 micrograms. Unless I had made an obvious blunder, then I only changed my T3 dosage every three to fourteen days. Even allowing only three days, to observe the effect, can often be enough to confirm whether the dosage change is positive or not. If I remained comfortable, then I would wait longer, before making another change.

The small changes may have continued to leave me feeling hypothyroid but my emphasis was always on caution and, in order to be cautious when you still have symptoms, you also have to be patient. Patience and caution go hand in hand, when determining the correct T3 dosage.

If I made a dosage change that caused any adverse symptoms, I immediately reversed it.

Once closer to a working T3 replacement dosage, I grew even more cautious, only increasing or decreasing the size of a divided dose by 2.5 micrograms. I also increased the time between changes to allow more time for observations. Allowing two to four weeks between dosage changes was quite common when getting close to a final T3 dosage.

Chapter 15

Lessons Learned on Thyroid Blood Tests

LESSON #10: DON'T USE TSH, FT4 AND FT3 FOR T3 DOSAGE MANAGEMENT

Doctors are used to using blood test results to determine how T4 replacement therapy is progressing. Different doctors have different approaches. During T4 replacement therapy some doctors place more emphasis on FT4 and FT3 and less emphasis on the TSH. The majority of doctors still place a great deal of emphasis on ensuring that the pituitary hormone, TSH, is maintained in the low part of the laboratory reference range but is not completely suppressed.

In T3 replacement therapy however, none of these thyroid blood test results are of any use in determining if the treatment is progressing well, or whether the current T3 dosage is adequate. In fact, attempting to use TSH, FT4 or FT3 to determine whether to increase or decrease the T3 dosage may result in extremely bad decisions being taken and the patient being harmed as a result.

This is radically different to T4 and T4/T3 replacement. Why should this be the case? Let me consider FT4 and FT3 thyroid blood test results during T3 replacement therapy before reviewing TSH blood test results.

FT4 AND FT3 THYROID BLOOD TEST RESULTS IN T3 REPLACEMENT THERAPY

I have already discussed the rapid absorption of T3, how quickly it raises the serum concentration of T3 and its subsequent decline. The conclusions that follow this knowledge, that are well documented in endocrinology texts, are simple and clear:

- Patients who are receiving T3 replacement therapy should expect unusual laboratory test results of thyroid hormone levels.[1]

- Low FT4 levels should be expected.[2]

- FT3 results could be low, normal or elevated depending on how much T3 is being prescribed and the time of the blood test, relative to the time that the patient most recently took any T3.[2]

• Laboratory tests that attempt to assess the adequacy of replacement with T3 are extremely difficult to make sense of, because of the wide and rapid fluctuations of T3 in the bloodstream.[1]

Low levels of FT4 are possible and should be anticipated

Patients taking pure T3 often question the low level of FT4 in their blood test results. In my own case, due to my highly atrophied thyroid and a full replacement dosage of T3, I naturally have a very low level of FT4 appearing in my blood test results.

The popular belief is that T4 is an inactive hormone, which is then converted into the active hormone T3 as and when it is needed. However, some doctors have suggested that T4 itself may have some, as yet unknown, mild biologically active role. These doctors still acknowledge that T3 is at least ten times more potent than T4. Medical research will hopefully one day reveal the truth about the biological activity of T4. At the moment, the most widely held view is that T4 is a biologically inactive hormone, or pro-hormone, that only exists in order to provide a reservoir ready to be converted into T3.

I know that it is possible for me to feel completely healthy with very low levels of T4 in my system. If T4 proves to have some biologically active role, then I seem to be managing exceedingly well without it and so do countless other patients using only T3.

Expect very high levels of FT3

I can also confirm the view that any FT3 blood test is dramatically affected by its proximity to the most recent T3 divided dose that was taken before the test and by the size of that dose. The timing of my blood test has more impact on the value of FT3 than the size or effectiveness of my overall T3 dosage. If my last T3 dose is taken within two to four hours of my blood test, my FT3 level may be elevated well above the top of the laboratory reference range. However, if my last T3 dose is taken eight hours prior to my blood test, then my FT3 level will be significantly lower and may be within the reference range. There is absolutely no useful information in this FT3 blood test that gives any clue as to how appropriate my T3 dosage actually is.

Some patients may also find that they require a very high level of T3 before their symptoms abate. Some patients who take T3 dosages of 60 micrograms or more may have extremely high FT3 results, even though they feel perfectly well.

Therefore, the FT3 test result during T3 replacement therapy should not be used to draw any conclusions about the effectiveness or safety of the T3 replacement dosage. In fact, should any doctor attempt to draw some conclusions from the FT3 result and make changes to the patient's medication based on it, this is very likely to result in the wrong T3 dosage being prescribed.

Here are three of my FT3 test results:

- In May 2004 my FT3 was 6.9 nmol/ L (3.5-7.8 nmol/L).

- In August 2009 my FT3 was 9.3 nmol/l (3.5-7.8 nmol/L).

- In March 2011, my FT3 was 8.9 nmol/L (3.5–7.8 nmol/L).

In all the above blood tests I was taking very similar levels of T3 (give or take 2.5 micrograms). My FT3 results tend to be at the top end of the laboratory reference range or above the top of the range. These results are quite unhelpful in managing my T3 dosage. The timing of the blood test in relation to when I last took T3 is the major factor in the result. My doctors and I have never been able to use the FT3 blood test result to usefully guide any change in my T3 dosage.

TSH THYROID BLOOD TEST RESULTS IN T3 REPLACEMENT THERAPY

Has the TSH blood test provided me with any valuable information during T3 replacement therapy?

It should be obvious from the previous section that there may be a high degree of variability of FT3 levels within the bloodstream and low FT4 levels should be expected. This means that FT3 may be the predominant input to the pituitary gland. Since FT3 could be low, normal or highly elevated, this will necessarily mean that TSH will may have a much higher degree of variability than for a patient on T4 replacement therapy.

For a very short period of time, at the start of using T3 replacement, my family doctor and I did attempt to use my TSH test results as an indicator of how to adjust my T3 dosage. It quickly became obvious that this was futile and dangerous.

TSH is produced by the anterior part of the pituitary gland. Thyrotroph cells in the anterior pituitary are able to detect a decrease, below a certain level, of the combined level of FT3 and FT4 in the bloodstream. The thyrotroph cells then secrete TSH in response to thyroid hormone levels being too low. The secretion of TSH is known to be pulsatile, which means that TSH is released in short bursts rather than in a steady stream. TSH secretion also exhibits a circadian rhythm, i.e. a twenty-four hour cycle. The TSH level is characteristically lower during the day and higher at night, peaking around midnight. This increase in serum TSH at night can be as much as 100-200% of the level during the day. Once in the circulation, TSH attaches to receptors in the thyroid, which responds by producing more T4 and T3. When the circulating level of thyroid hormone rises, the pituitary then produces less TSH as the demand diminishes.

Expect a totally suppressed TSH or for some people a fluctuating TSH

For a patient feeling well on T4 replacement therapy, their circulating FT4 level is fairly stable and, as a result, their circulating FT3 tends to be relatively stable too, as it is produced by ongoing and regular conversion of the FT4. Due to this stability, the TSH should remain relatively steady as well, with the exception of the natural circadian rhythm.

However, a patient taking T3-only replacement therapy is likely to have a highly fluctuating level of FT3 throughout the day. This is most likely to result in a completely suppressed TSH for most thyroid patients on T3 treatment. However, occasionally some people find that their TSH actually fluctuates during a 24-hour period. I have observed significant fluctuations in TSH in my own case and I believe this is due to the fact that I only require a very modest amount of T3 and my thyroid gland has been virtually destroyed by Hashimoto's thyroiditis so I have almost zero FT4. As mentioned previously, a single dose of T3 is expected to achieve peak circulating concentration within a couple of hours after it has been taken. Blood levels of T3 are expected to remain high for around six to eight hours and then decline again, unless another dose of T3 is taken.

In my case, I feel the effects of T3 within a couple of hours after each divided dose and can even detect changes in heart rate, body temperature, mental sharpness, muscle strength and energy level. These changes indicate that the T3 has not only been absorbed into my bloodstream but more importantly, my cells have also taken up the hormone. Within six to eight hours, depending on the size of the last T3 dose, I can feel some of the more obvious effects of T3 start to reduce.

The use of T3 can rapidly suppress TSH.[3] For this reason, as well as the widely fluctuating level of FT3, those patients on a full replacement dosage of T3 may find their TSH is either totally suppressed of they may have more variation in their TSH level than someone using T4 replacement therapy. In particular, there may be considerable impact on TSH as a result of the divided dose of T3 taken immediately prior to the blood test. This property of T3 may be one of the reasons that it is sometimes used with patients who have conditions that require pituitary TSH suppression. Consequently, patients who need to use high T3 dosages to resolve their symptoms may find that they have a permanently suppressed TSH.

Pituitary response to T3 medication is different to T4 - so don't expect the same TSH result when taking T3 compared to taking T4

There have been a number of very interesting experiments with animals, that provide more insight into the pituitary suppression of TSH in response to T4 and T3. [4, 5, 6] In these studies with thyroidectomized rats, that were given a small amount of T3, the TSH significantly and rapidly reduces.[4] After two hours, the TSH level of the T3 infused rats, dropped to its lowest value and then returned to its previous value within seven hours.[5] Interestingly, the same study showed that when the experiment was repeated with T4 infusions, the TSH remains suppressed for nearly a whole day. There was not the same level of TSH fluctuation as was seen with the T3 infusion.

What is interesting about the studies is that the researchers found that at the seven-hour point, after infusion with T4, the rats had too low a level of T3 in their bloodstream to account for the TSH suppression.[5] An additional experiment was performed and the thyroidectomized rats were treated with a drug that prevents the conversion of T4 to T3 in the liver and kidneys and then the T4 infusion was repeated. The T4 infusion still completely suppressed the TSH for a long period.[6]

The pituitary is known to be able to convert T4 to T3 within its own tissues and the drug used to suppress the conversion of T4 to T3 does not have the same effect within the pituitary gland. These studies suggest that the TSH suppression by T4 was not due to conversion of T4 to T3 in the liver and kidneys, i.e. the T4 does not have to be converted to circulating levels of T3, in order for the suppression of TSH to occur. The T4 can act locally, within the pituitary, converting to sufficient T3 to cause the pituitary to suppress TSH.

What should be clear from the above studies is that the effect of T3 on the pituitary suppression of TSH is quite different to that of T4, although the scale of the fluctuation of TSH due to T3, might possibly be modulated over time, as the pituitary is thought to be able to make some adjustment to produce a less violent fluctuation of TSH.

The studies begin to highlight the uniqueness of the pituitary response to T4 and T3, compared to other tissues in the body. In particular, because the pituitary can respond independently to changes in bloodstream levels of T4 and T3, compared to other tissues, it also begs the question: **is TSH representative of tissue levels of thyroid hormone?**

The timing of the blood test relative to the most recently taken T3 divided dose can be more important than how much total T3 is taken in a day

I discovered from blood test results that my TSH was significantly affected by the size and time of my last T3 dose prior to the test. I take my first dose of T3 at the same time each day but it was the varying blood test appointment times that were responsible for the variation in my TSH results. Sometimes the TSH results came back fully suppressed and at other times it was above the top of the laboratory reference range. As already mentioned though, I have almost zero FT4.

Some examples are appropriate:

- In April 2002 my TSH was 0.25 mU/L (0.1 - 5.0 mU/L). TSH was 'normal'.

- In May 2004 my TSH was 0.17 mU/L (0.4 - 4.5 mU/L). TSH was suppressed.

- In September 2006 my TSH was 7.5 mU/L (0.4 - 4.5 mU/L). TSH elevated. Clearly not suppressed.

- In September 2007 my TSH was 0.1 mU/L (0.4 - 4.5 mU/L). TSH was suppressed.

- In March 2011 my TSH was 9.1 mU/L (0.4 - 4.5 mU/L). TSH was elevated even though my FT3 was also elevated, which I described earlier. This result is likely to be related to further atrophy of my thyroid gland, rather than just a blood test timing issue.

In 2002 I was taking around 5 micrograms less T3 than from 2004 onwards. Since 2004 I have been taking a very similar T3 dosage. The variation that may be seen in TSH is not due to changes in my T3 dosage. It is likely to be linked to how many hours before each blood test that I had taken any T3, combined with some degree of thyroid gland atrophy. What I can say with confidence is that the variations of TSH are not due to lack of compliance, because I am rigorous in taking each of my divided doses on time.

My most recent thyroid blood test results, in March 2011, that I had done partly to illustrate the points in this chapter were:

- TSH was 9.1 mU/L (reference range 0.4–4.5 mU/L).

- FT4 was 0.3 pmol/L (reference range 9.0–25 pmol/L).

- FT3 was 8.9 nmol/L (reference range 3.5–7.8 nmol/L).

These results show an elevated FT3 and largely non-existent FT4. TSH this time is high because of the timing of the blood test and possibly the effect of thyroid atrophy, i.e. I now have almost no T4 being made by my thyroid gland.

Any doctor who attempts to manage my T3 dosage based on these thyroid blood test results is going to struggle. In order to make my results look like those of a patient on T4 replacement therapy, my T3 dosage would need to be reduced significantly and I would need to take a substantial amount of synthetic T4. If either of these changes were made then they would make me extremely ill.

My doctor and I gave up trying to use TSH at all for dosage management

It became obvious to my family doctor and me that TSH was highly variable and of no value in deciding if the treatment was effective or not. It wasn't possible to draw any useful conclusions at all from the TSH test results. My doctor and I quickly realised that relying on the TSH blood test as a guide to help me adjust my T3 dosage would be pointless and could be potentially dangerous.

To illustrate this, the only time, in twelve or thirteen years of T3 replacement, that my family doctor suggested that I might want to increase my T3, was based on the 2006 TSH result above. I did increase my T3 slightly and I had some immediate symptoms of tissue over-stimulation, which meant I had to quickly reduce my T3 dosage to the same level it had been for a long time.

A low TSH is desirable for people with Hashimoto's thyroiditis. This is because a low TSH level tends to reduce the activity of the thyroid gland and as a result the autoimmune response tends to become less severe over time, resulting in declining levels of autoantibodies. The reduction of autoantibody levels will reduce the rate of thyroid damage.

My doctor and I decided that achieving a low TSH level should be a side effect of T3 replacement therapy and not a goal in itself, because we could not rely on the TSH result.

In T3 replacement therapy the TSH result is not a reliable indicator of the adequacy of the T3 dosage and it should not be used to determine changes to the T3 dosage.

CONCLUSIONS ON TSH, FT4 and FT3 FOR T3 DOSAGE MANAGEMENT

In addition to all the above information, as far as I can tell, there are no published scientific studies that have looked at a population of patients on T3 replacement therapy and determined:

- The variation in TSH level throughout twenty-four hours.

- The variation in FT3 level throughout twenty-four hours.

- How TSH and FT3 fluctuations relate to the number, sizes or timings of the T3 divided doses being used.

It is likely that some patients on T3 replacement therapy, like me, have highly atrophied thyroid glands. This has the potential, depending on the T3 dosage that these patients require, to result in either a suppressed or fluctuating TSH, the FT4 level extremely low and FT3 levels extremely high. So, within a population of patients on T3 replacement therapy there may be many different patterns of thyroid blood test result, depending on the T3 dosage they require and how much their thyroid gland has been destroyed.

I doubt very much that any population of patients who are taking a safe and effective T3 dosage have been studied. The devil is in the detail, or in this case, the scientific evidence.

Impaired cellular response to thyroid hormone makes a nonsense of blood test results

The arguments I have used do not take into account that some patients on T3 replacement therapy may have problems at a cellular level, which prevent the normal utilisation of T4 medications. I will discuss this far more in section 6 but I believe that after the onset of Hashimoto's thyroiditis, I began to have some problems at a cellular level, which impaired the utilisation of T4.

If there is impaired cellular response to thyroid hormone that has necessitated the use of T3 replacement therapy then the standard thyroid hormone measures of TSH, FT4 and FT3 are even less likely to be of value. Thyroid blood test results will not be representative of what is occurring within the cells of the body. The pituitary gland, with its ability to convert T4 locally, is a rather special case and it may continue to function perfectly well, even though other tissues may be suffering with low thyroid hormone levels and poor regulation of cell function.

This is the final and, perhaps most telling reason, why TSH, FT4 and FT3 test results are of little use to me. Many patients, who find that they require T3 replacement therapy, may also have this type of issue and find that thyroid blood test results do not have any bearing on how they actually feel.

Some doctors are still trying to manage T3 dosage through blood test results

However, I have talked to some patients on T3 replacement therapy, whose doctors appear to be committed to the use of TSH, FT3 and even FT4 to determine if the patient's T3 dosage is adequate or not. As I complete writing this, two more patients have just told me that their T3 medication has been reduced, based on low TSH, high FT3 and low FT4 blood test results. Both people were improving in terms of symptoms and signs and beginning to feel well. These inappropriate medication changes will cause these patients to feel ill again but the T3 dosage changes may induce thyroid blood test results that conform more closely to the laboratory reference ranges. This highlights a large problem with the approach of some doctors and perhaps with medical training. Fortunately, my family doctor and endocrinologist did not fall into this trap.

For any patient on T3 replacement therapy, it should now be clear that TSH, FT4 and FT3 are unreliable and inappropriate in determining if the T3 dosage is adequate and in making dosage change decisions.

WHERE TSH, FT4 AND FT3 DO HAVE VALUE

Undoubtedly, the TSH, FT4, FT3 and thyroid autoantibody blood tests were critical during the diagnosis phase of my thyroid condition. Diagnosis is not what I am discussing here though.

I have TSH, FT4 and FT3 blood tests performed only once per year. My family doctor is keen to occasionally check these in order to ensure that the results are somewhat as we might expect them to be. I fully support this use of the thyroid blood tests. In particular, it is useful to ensure that no highly unexpected value of TSH is present because this might suggest the development of a pituitary problem.

Thyroid blood tests are also very useful as an assessment of how my thyroid gland is deteriorating - the level of FT4 provides some indication of this. In my most recent blood test results, in March 2011, there is more evidence that my thyroid has almost been completely destroyed, because my FT4 was only 0.3 pmol/L.

Occasionally, I have a blood test for the two main thyroid autoantibodies (TPO and Tg). Several years ago, my autoantibodies fell to a virtually negligible level. Every few years, my family doctor runs these routine blood tests again, to ensure that the autoimmune response remains quiescent.

THYROID URINE TESTS

Before I complete this chapter I need to briefly discuss the use of urine testing to assay thyroid hormones.

I have already mentioned that thyroid hormones may be measured through the collection of urine and that some doctors believe that this is a more sensitive test that may be more effective in the detection of previously undiagnosed hypothyroidism.

However, it should be clear by now that, like thyroid blood tests, thyroid urine tests do not establish how much T3 has successfully reached its intra-cellular targets. Therefore, thyroid urine tests, like thyroid blood tests, are unable to reveal how thyroid hormone is actually regulating cell function. For those patients like me with a problem that affects the cellular action of thyroid hormone then thyroid urine tests provide no better identification of this problem and therefore, offer little benefit.

This does not take away the potential benefit in increased sensitivity that this type of testing may offer to many thyroid patients who have a more typical form of hypothyroidism.

HOW IS THE EFFECTIVENESS OF T3 REPLACEMENT THERAPY MONITORED?

FT3 can fluctuate widely in the bloodstream and is unrepresentative of cellular activity of thyroid hormone during T3 replacement therapy. TSH may be suppressed or might even fluctuate and FT4 has little relevance to a patient on T3 replacement. So, what can be used to determine if a patient's current T3 dosage is adequate and what changes, if any, are required?

Basal Metabolic Rate (BMR) is defined as the daily rate of energy metabolism an individual needs to sustain, in order to preserve the integrity of vital functions in the body. The BMR test is rarely used these days. Any patient undergoing a BMR test needs to be completely at rest for some time before the test and may have needed to fast for some time also. The measurement of BMR requires specialised equipment to assess oxygen consumption over a sufficiently long period of time during which the patient is resting. A few decades ago measuring BMR was one of the main means of determining if a patient had a thyroid problem.

Referring to Werner and Ingbar's *The Thyroid*, David V. Becker discusses the decline in use of the BMR measure.[7] He writes, 'The BMR remains unique and irreplaceable as the only quantitative measure of total body energy production readily available to the clinician.' He goes on to state, '... the BMR remains the most satisfactory index of the overall metabolic effect of thyroid hormone on the organism.'

The use of BMR is exceptionally rare today but this last point begins to hint at what might be helpful in establishing a safe and adequate T3 replacement dosage.

To a certain extent, we must turn back the clock and use some measures of peripheral thyroid hormone activity that are actually representative of how any prescribed T3 is affecting the body.

I am not suggesting the use of the BMR but **far simpler, cruder and easily available measures,** whilst we wait for medical research to provide more appropriate laboratory tests. I will discuss this specific topic of monitoring T3 replacement therapy in section 5 on T3 dosage management.

Chapter 16

Lesson Learned on T3 Effect on Adrenal Glands

LESSON #11: T3 EFFECT ON ADRENAL GLANDS

Various hormones in the body have a circadian rhythm. This means that they are not secreted in a steady way throughout the day. Their secretion follows a set pattern that is repeated every twenty-four hours and is typically linked to our patterns of sleeping and waking, or daylight and night. One example is testosterone secretion in males, which is linked to the cycle of night and day and rises during the early hours of the morning, typically from around 4:00 am, peaking at around 8:00 am.[1]

My main interest is in the secretion of the adrenal glands and cortisol in particular. Cortisol is secreted by the adrenal glands, with a steady rise in production during the last four hours of sleep, usually between the hours of 4:00 am and 8:00 am. It is the rising level of cortisol that helps us wake up in the morning, with the highest level of cortisol in the bloodstream at around 8:00 am.[2] Cortisol levels then fall gradually during the day and are at their lowest between midnight and 4:00 am in the morning.

The level of cortisol in the bloodstream does not fall smoothly during the day. There are mini-spikes of cortisol associated with food and exercise, which is why people with low cortisol are advised to use appropriate supplements, eat regularly, have small healthy snacks and do some exercise to help raise it.

TIME WHEN MAJORITY OF CORTISOL IS PRODUCED

Cortisol production is linked to our sleeping and waking cycle. This means that cortisol production increases during the last four hours of sleep, which for most people is between 4:00 am and 8:00 am, hence the timings discussed above. For other people, perhaps shift workers, or people with a different pattern of sleeping and waking, this rise in cortisol will occur during their last four hours of sleep, whatever that time period happens to be.

In order to make this discussion a little simpler, I will assume that I am talking about people who have a typical sleeping and waking cycle. Therefore, I will assume that the highest level of cortisol production will be between the hours of 4:00 am and 8:00 am. I will refer to this period of time, during which the adrenals produce the highest volume of cortisol, as the ***main cortisol production window.***

During the first year or two of using T3, my health improved but was not ideal. I did not know exactly why this was. I tried various options with my T3 medication but could not discover quite why I did not feel completely healthy. Eventually, it dawned on me that some of my hormones had a circadian nature and I found out about the cycle of cortisol and testosterone secretion. I also discovered from endocrinology books that TSH typically reaches its highest level around midnight or 1:00 am in the morning and subsequently T4 reaches its highest level in the early hours of the morning as a result of the peak level of TSH. Consequently, I became highly suspicious that the T3 thyroid hormone may normally reach quite high levels in the body during the night and given what I had learned about the circadian rhythm of cortisol I wondered whether I needed to make a radical change in my T3 dosage.

Based on this knowledge and these ideas, I began to experiment with using doses of T3 early in the morning before I got up. When I found that I felt better with a T3 dose at 5:30 am, what was happening started to become clear to me.

I believed that because my adrenal glands were trying to do most of their work during the main cortisol production window, they would be trying to work at their maximum rate during the time when my body was at its lowest ebb, in terms of T3. My last dose of T3 on the previous day was around 5:00 pm, so by 4:00 am nearly eleven hours had passed with no further T3 medication.

TIME OF FIRST T3 DIVIDED DOSE AFFECTED MY CORTISOL PRODUCTION

I decided to ask my family doctor to support me with an experiment involving a series of twenty-four hour urinary cortisol tests, taking the first T3 dose of the day at different times throughout the main cortisol production window and also after it. My family doctor was incredibly helpful and agreed to support me. Through this experiment, it soon became apparent that the size and timing of the first T3 dose had a very significant effect on cortisol production. Here are a couple of actual test results that illustrate this effect.

In March 2008, with my first T3 dose of 20 micrograms taken at 3:30 am, the results showed that my total cortisol output was 349 nmol/sample (reference range 50-319 nmol/sample) and my free cortisol index was 74.0 nmol/l (reference range 20-100 nmol/l).

In July 2008, when I had moved my first dose of T3 to 8.45 am, the results were startlingly different. Total cortisol output had dropped to 81.0 nmol/sample and free cortisol index had dropped to 27.0 nmol/l.

The only difference between the first and second test was the time that the first dose of T3 was taken, in relation to the main cortisol production window. The size of the dose remained exactly the same. Adjusting the timing of my first T3 dose, in relation to when the adrenal glands were trying to do their hardest work, caused my total cortisol output to rise just above the laboratory reference range in the first test and fall close to the bottom of the reference range in the second test.

These two tests show just how much the timing of the first T3 dose may affect cortisol levels and how by adjusting the size and the timing of the first dose of T3 in the morning I was able to make a very significant change to my body's production of cortisol. The timing of this first dose of T3 affected my testosterone level in a similar way. **Even a timing change to the first T3 divided dose of half an hour was capable of changing cortisol levels.** The twenty-four hour urinary cortisol test is not sensitive enough to be able to determine a target cortisol level and a suitable first T3 dose change. However, as a rough guide to how much cortisol is being produced, the twenty-four hour urinary cortisol test worked well.

I realised that I had a choice, either changing the timing of my first T3 dose, to attempt to increase my cortisol output until I felt better, or consider some form of adrenal support. However, I did not know if I could adjust my first T3 dose sufficiently to feel completely well.

TAKING MY FIRST T3 DIVIDED DOSE EARLIER RAISED MY CORTISOL

My approach was simple, using how I felt, in conjunction with the changes in the twenty-four hour urinary cortisol results, I attempted to see whether I could alter the timing of my first divided dose of T3, in order to feel completely well and establish reasonable cortisol levels. It was a judgement call but one based on some data.

In terms of my health this was a turning point, because I found that the size and timing of the first dose of T3 provided an excellent and unexpected degree of control over both cortisol and testosterone. By taking my first T3 divided dose between 4:00 am and 5:15 am I began to feel really healthy for the first time since my thyroid problems started. I managed to do this without any requirement for additional adrenal support. Note - I did try to take this T3 dose at bedtime but this not only affected my sleep but it also did not provide my adrenal glands with enough T3 when they actually needed it.

Part of the reason that I felt healthier was probably because, by establishing a normal level of cortisol, my blood sugar metabolism may have been working more normally and thus the chemical energy, in the form of ATP, which is produced by the mitochondria, may have been at a healthier level. Unfortunately, this process had taken nearly three years from the start of using T3, because I was unaware of this technique of adjusting my cortisol level.

Even at the time of writing, I can still find no reference to this method being used elsewhere. However, a relatively new research study has found that in healthy people T3 levels have a circadian rhythm, related to the cycles of TSH and T4.[3] This results in T3 typically reaching a peak in the body around 4:00 am. **Perhaps it is not so surprising that this novel method was as successful as it was because it was actually emulating nature.**

It is also worth noting that only by ensuring that the adrenal glands work as closely to how they did in good health can the numerous adrenal hormones be produced at the appropriate levels. This can never be achieved by using hydrocortisone or other methods, although of course sometimes this is the only approach that is possible, e.g. in Addison's disease, hypopituitarism or when the low cortisol is very severe and will not adequately respond to this approach.

I was not taking any form of adrenal hormone or adrenal glandular when I did these experiments and it would have made clear analysis impossible. The purpose of taking an early divided dose of T3 within the main cortisol production window is to feel healthier and remove the need to take any adrenal support or at least to minimise it. So, if I had been taking any adrenal support before I did any of these experiments then I would have to have done one of two things:

- Ideally, I would have slowly weaned myself off the adrenal support over a period of time and under the guidance of my doctor.
- The alternative would have been to slowly reduce the adrenal support as I was beginning to use T3 within the main cortisol production window. If I had been on a lot of adrenal support and my doctor was concerned about reducing this, then slowly weaning the adrenal hormones as this method was applied may have been the only viable method.

The entire purpose of my investigation was to determine how capable my own adrenals were and for my purposes I needed to have no adrenal support. Fortunately, I was able to get a rapid response from using an early morning T3 dose. If I had needed some adrenal support at the end of this investigation then it would have been likely to be at the lowest dosage required as I had already enabled my own adrenal glands to work as well as they were capable.

Reducing adrenal support should only be done slowly and in consultation with a qualified medical practitioner. It should certainly not be considered if someone has diagnosed Addison's disease or hypopituitarism or any other condition that may cause a dangerously low cortisol level as a result of removing adrenal support.

IT MAY TAKE SEVERAL WEEKS FOR ADRENALS TO ADJUST

During all this testing, I found that it could take several weeks for the adrenals to completely re-adjust after a T3 dosage change and for the final cortisol output level to become apparent. My cortisol levels took around six weeks to fully adjust to a new first T3 dose timing.

People who have success with T4 replacement therapy do not tend to have the above dosage timing issues. Their bodies are able to convert enough T3 from a relatively stable level of T4 and so they usually have enough T3 available for their adrenal glands to function well.

I also found that as my own adrenal glands worked more effectively I had to fine-tune my other T3 divided doses. I often found that the subsequent T3 divided doses were more effective and needed to be reduced a little and spaced out further.

I also had to adjust the timing of the first T3 divided dose and its size to ensure that my adrenal glands did not produce too high a level of cortisol. It takes months for under-stimulated adrenal glands to become highly effective again. Consequently, I needed to fine-tune my first T3 dose for some time after I realised my adrenal glands were functioning well once again.

I ONLY USED T3 TO RAISE CORTISOL LEVELS WHEN I KNEW IT WAS NEEDED

Had I felt completely well without taking the first T3 dose within the main cortisol production window of 4:00 am - 8:00 am, then it would have been prudent to take no divided dose of T3 any earlier than 8:00 am (when I woke up), in order to avoid causing an elevated cortisol level. If I already had a normal cortisol level then taking the first T3 divided dose earlier than 8:00 am may have actually created an unhealthy level of cortisol. Consequently, great care and attention needs to be taken to gather sufficient information on cortisol levels prior to using this approach.

THIS MAY NOT WORK IN ALL CASES OF LOW CORTISOL

I am not suggesting that taking the first dose of T3 just before or during the main cortisol production window will correct adrenal insufficiency in all patients who have a low cortisol or low aldosterone problem (some patients still refer to adrenal insufficiency as 'adrenal fatigue'). In the case of someone with permanently damaged adrenal glands, e.g. because of autoimmune destruction, hypopituitarism, or other disease then even providing adequate T3 in the main cortisol production window will not help and the use of adrenal hormone medication may be essential. This approach may also fail in the case of someone who has other serious blood sugar metabolism issues and in this case, after everything else has been tried, some adrenal support may still be required as determined by the patient's own doctor.

However, the above approach worked exceptionally well for me and it has become increasingly apparent that this approach does actually work extraordinarily well for many people. I now believe that some people with low cortisol levels may actually have a form of adrenal insufficiency brought about by hypothyroidism. In these cases it may simply be that this is due to the need for more T3 in the tissues of the adrenal glands when they are trying to work at their maximum rate.

I have incorporated all of these findings within my T3 dosage management process, which I will discuss later.

I have become aware that many thyroid patients have now tried this approach and found that it frequently works extremely well and may remove the need for many forms of adrenal support or reduce the level of adrenal medication required. I have also been told of many thyroid patients who have applied this approach when they are on natural desiccated thyroid or on T4/T3 combination therapy and that they have removed or reduced the need for adrenal medication. **Typical early doses of T3 containing medication need to have at least 10 micrograms of T3 and often 15 micrograms of T3 before this begins to help promote better adrenal function**. It is also advisable that no adrenal medication is taken at the same time as this early dose of T3 because doing this would tend to suppress the adrenal glands.

This is quite exciting as it is now obvious that this is a more widely applicable technique than I originally suspected it would be.

LAST FOUR HOURS OF SLEEP

It is important to remember that the majority of cortisol is produced during the last four hours of sleep. Consequently, the references to the main cortisol production window of 4:00 am to 8:00 am throughout this chapter assume that someone wakes up around 8:00 am in the morning. For someone who wakes up later or earlier then these times would need to be adjusted and the appropriate four-hour period identified.

It should also be realised that when trying to provide the adrenal glands with enough T3 to function normally it is important to start carefully by placing the first T3 divided dose only about one and a half hours inside the main cortisol production window, e.g. 6:30 am for an 8:00 am riser. Over time this first T3 divided dose may be moved earlier in steps of half an hour. This careful process will avoid too much cortisol or other adrenal hormones being produced.

In order to encourage a healthy adrenal output, the first T3 divided dose appears to need to be eventually placed somewhere in the first three hours of the main cortisol production window time period. So, for a 4:00 am to 8:00 am time period this would be somewhere in the 4:00 am to 6:30 am timeframe. Finding the correct time is a process of trial and error.

FIRST T3 DIVIDED DOSE ADJUSTMENT OPTIONS

There are two options that may be used to attempt to adjust the amount of cortisol being produced by the adrenal glands:

1. The first T3 divided dose may be moved either half an hour later to reduce adrenal output or half an hour earlier to increase adrenal output. Further changes should continue to have an effect as long as the first T3 divided dose remains within the main cortisol production window. This adjustment in the time of the first T3 divided dose appears to be the most predictable and simplest option to use to influence cortisol levels.

2. The first T3 dose may be increased if it does not appear to be sufficient for the adrenals or decreased if it appears to be too much. This adjustment in the size of the first T3 divided

dose should only be used to make changes when the T3 divided dose size is clearly wrong. The changes to cortisol or aldosterone output are very difficult to predict using this method. However, both increases and decreases in first T3 divided dose size may need to be tried. Symptoms of adrenal insufficiency may be present when the first T3 divided dose is too low or too high. **In the case of a first T3 divided dose that is too low** then clearly the adrenal glands may have insufficient T3 to perform their task correctly and low levels of cortisol may be a consequence. I have had feedback from people that have had success in increasing the size of their first T3 divided dose and eradicating their symptoms of low cortisol, e.g. by increasing their T3 divided dose from 15 or 20 micrograms of T3 to 20, 25 or 30 micrograms of T3 the adrenal insufficiency has been corrected. **In the case of a first T3 divided dose that is too high,** then the adrenal glands may be driven too hard and asked to do more than they are capable of and this can also result in **low levels of cortisol** and in this case the first T3 dose should be reduced. In other cases **far too much cortisol** may be produced after a first T3 dose increase that is too high and it should be reduced.

Often a timing change to the first T3 divided dose will be sufficient to correct any adrenal symptoms. As I have made clear, in some cases no amount of T3 dosage titration will compensate for adrenal issues and some form of adrenal support will be essential.

SUMMARY OF USING T3 IN THE MAIN CORTISOL PRODUCTION WINDOW

There is a lot to digest in this chapter. I've summarised the conditions that I believe are required before an early morning T3 dose may be considered to have some possible benefit and additional important information regarding this method:

1. Standard T3 should be used for the first T3 divided dose and not slow release T3. However, I know of many thyroid patients who have successfully applied this method using only natural desiccated thyroid (NDT).

2. There is adrenal insufficiency. This needs to be proven first, in order to be confident that cortisol won't be raised to too high a level. Chapter 3 outlines the available testing methods and symptoms and signs associated with adrenal insufficiency. Ideally an adrenal saliva test would have been done which clearly highlights cortisol insufficiency. Thyroid patients should consult their own doctor or a specialist before reaching firm conclusions that they have adrenal insufficiency.

3. There must be no fundamental adrenal damage. Adrenal damage may be due to Addison's

disease or other disease. Hypopituitarism will also invalidate this technique, as it won't be possible to stimulate the adrenal glands because they will not be receiving sufficient stimulus from the pituitary in the first place. This does not mean that the use of this method would be dangerous - it just would not work, and this would soon be apparent, as no significant benefit would be seen.

4. This technique may be used and then any existing adrenal hormones could be slowly weaned as the first T3 dose is carefully titrated. These adrenal hormones may include: hydrocortisone, prednisolone, adrenal glandular products or drugs like florinef designed to replace aldosterone. Clearly, any weaning of any of these prescription adrenal drugs should be done with the full support and involvement of a patient's doctor. Because of the critical importance of aldosterone in regulating blood pressure the patient's doctor is likely to advise that any medication designed to replace aldosterone is weaned slowly and carefully and perhaps last of all. In some cases this weaning may take many months and complete weaning may never be entirely possible for some patients. Patients should work closely with their own doctors on all of this. No adrenal medication should be taken at the same time as the early (circadian) dose of T3 because this would suppress the natural adrenal production of hormones.

5. There should be no issues with blood sugar balance. Pre-diabetes or undiagnosed diabetes may result in low insulin, high blood sugar and low cellular glucose levels. This will undermine the T3 replacement or any thyroid hormone replacement, as it is likely to result in insufficient cellular energy (ATP) being produced by the mitochondria, due to the low cellular glucose levels. Any other issues with blood sugar may also have this effect and can disrupt thyroid hormone treatment, e.g. insulin resistance. Consequently, blood sugar levels may need to be investigated by a medical professional if there is any concern about them.

6. It must is done slowly and carefully in order to avoid excess cortisol or aldosterone being produced, which can raise blood pressure. I found that a good starting time was one and a half hours before the end of the main cortisol production window, which was 6:30 am, in my case. I could then move it back by half an hour every few weeks in order to find the optimal time. If I had found an optimal time but the method was still not working well enough then I increased (or possibly decreased) my first T3 dose by 2.5 or 5 micrograms. If I was unsure that I had found the optimal time to take this first t3 dose then I started again at 6:30 am and slowly repeated the process of moving it earlier in time in half hour steps. Some form of cortisol testing is required at least when the T3 divided dose and timing has been finalised in order to verify that the adrenals are not producing too much cortisol.

7. Fine-tuning of the times and sizes of the T3 divided doses that follow the first T3 divided dose may be required as a result of applying this technique and improving the performance of the adrenal glands. My experience has been that once the adrenal glands are regulated correctly and begin to work normally then everything changes. Much less T3 may be needed. Individual T3 divided doses may become ferociously potent and may need to be reduced in size. The changes required may be substantial. I was not prepared for this but hopefully any doctors who are open minded enough to consider this method might prepare their patients for this possibility.

I hope that over time this technique is investigated by the medical profession, as it appears to offer promise and makes sense in terms of the natural circadian rhythms of thyroid and adrenal hormones. All medication changes should of course only be done under the guidance of a qualified medical professional.

THE CIRCADIAN T3 METHOD

I have described my story to many thyroid patients over the past several years and now realise that my method of using the first T3 divided dose to provide enough T3 for the adrenal glands may be very important for thyroid patient. I have started to use the term the *Circadian T3 Method* (or CT3M or T3CM) to refer to this technique to make it easier to refer to.

It may only be done by using standard or pure T3 only (or natural desiccated thyroid) and it attempts to approximate to the natural T3 circadian rhythm. The intention of the Circadian T3 method is to provide a healthy amount of T3 in the main cortisol production window that healthy people with no thyroid problems would expect to have. If adrenal insufficiency is present due to a lack of T3 in the adrenal tissues then the CT3M can be of great help.

The typical range of the T3 required to successfully apply the CT3M is between 10 and 30 micrograms, with 15 to 25 micrograms often being more common. This T3 could be pure T3 or the T3 contained within natural desiccated thyroid.

Some people appear to be surprised at how well this method seems to work. It should not be surprising at all. The adrenal glands in many people are not damaged and are simply under supplied with T3. When T3 is provided at the right time and the right dosage then the adrenals may be able to produce the full range of hormones at healthy levels. It is simple but effective.

There is no magic in the Circadian T3 Method at all. It is simply the application of scientific understanding of the natural circadian rhythm of our hormones in order to mirror nature as much as possible. The only surprise is that it hasn't been used until now.

Chapter 17

Lessons Learned on Records/Detective Work

LESSON #12: KEEPING EXCELLENT RECORDS

I recorded the following information each day on A4 sheets of paper:

- The current day's date.

- The medication I was taking. For T3, I recorded the exact details of the sizes and times of each divided dose of T3 and the total daily dosage. As an example I may have written 20T3@5:00am, 17.5T3@11:00am, 10T3@5:00pm. Total 47.5 T3. *Example of timing*

- Any new supplement that was added or any that I stopped taking and the date this occurred.

- A list of the symptoms that I still had and how bad they were. I recorded the time of the day that I observed these, so that if any changes occurred during the day that were related to any T3 divided dose then it would be possible to correlate the symptoms to the T3 dose. This list of debilitating symptoms was probably the most important information that I recorded. When my thyroid problems were at their peak I would pick my most significant symptoms and score them on a scale of 1-10, with 10 being totally normal and 1 being dreadful. Scoring these symptoms and recording how they changed over time as my medication or supplementation was altered really helped to identify whether I was making improvements or not.

- Any body temperature measurements I made and the times that these readings were taken.

- Any blood pressure and heart rate readings (via a home blood pressure monitor or my family doctor). All these results were recorded with the time of the day that they were measured. It is important to note that when taking a home blood pressure reading the upper arm that the BP cuff is on should be aimed away from the body (approximately at right angles to the body) and the arm should be supported on a chair arm or pillow to get an accurate result.

- When I was trying to understand a very confusing problem I would record more information on symptoms and signs. In this case, I typically considered a day as if it was divided up into segments of time that followed each T3 divided dose. I tried to take measurements at the start of each segment of time, several in the middle of the segment ant least one towards the end. This enabled me to see how each T3 divided dose appeared to be performing. I could also use this data to compare the performance of the T3 within each segment of time and look for trends or revealing responses. This involves a lot of data collection. I only did this thorough data collection from time to time or if I did not know what was causing some change in symptoms or signs.

- Any thyroid blood test results with all the specific result numbers, the units these were measured in and the relevant laboratory ranges. Getting these details often required having to ask one of the doctor's staff to provide them, as usually they only said whether a result was normal or not. This information is critical and it is important to be **assertive** and keep asking for it until you have all the results. I recorded the date that the test was actually performed so that it was possible to see what T3 dosage I was on at the time.

- Any twenty-four hour urinary cortisol or twenty-four hour adrenal saliva test results and other test results, with the dates that the tests were done.

- Any reports from doctors were filed within this chronological record.

Recording this information during each day was very useful. It allowed me to present a credible history of how I was responding to treatment, to any doctors I saw. It also enabled me to look back over time and recognise relationships between the T3 dosages I had been taking and any improvement or deterioration in my symptoms. Time and time again, I have found these daily records to be extremely helpful. I have often looked back through my records, which date back many years, in order to find some critical piece of information.

As time went on and my treatment was successful, I began to have to record information less frequently. Sometimes I would go weeks or months with no further entries. When I began to make a new record I just wrote down that particular day's date and recorded what I needed to. Over time, my records began to have very large gaps in them and required almost no effort at all to maintain.

I recommend that any patient using T3 replacement therapy adopts this type of method - it works. **Trying to manage the T3 dosage management process without comprehensive records would be extremely difficult and swift progress to a healthy T3 dosage would be far less likely.** The other use of the records was to help me to perform some detective work when it was needed.

LESSON #13: DETECTIVE WORK

I have been using T3 for many years now. I have also communicated with hundreds of thyroid patients via Internet forums. It is immensely clear to me that during T3 replacement therapy symptoms and issues can arise that at times seem extraordinarily hard to understand. It should be clear by now that thyroid blood test results will be of no value in determining if the T3 dosage is responsible for these issues or not. Symptoms and signs may provide the necessary insight but sometimes some issues can be most puzzling.

My conclusion is that it is mandatory to do thorough preparatory work prior to commencing the use of T3. Only through this preparatory work can large numbers of potential pitfalls be avoided. This preparatory work includes a number of things but high on the list are a comprehensive range of nutrient tests and the commencement of a nutrient supplementation regime.

It is critical to ensure that all the essential vitamins and minerals that can hamper thyroid or adrenal hormone metabolism are fully supplemented. This is not optional in my opinion because during T3 replacement it can be extremely hard to ascertain whether any issues are related to T3, adrenal hormones or nutrients. If nutrient deficiencies can be completely side stepped by thorough laboratory testing and optimum levels of supplementation then this will remove an entire class of problem during T3 replacement.

In Chapter 19 these mandatory preparatory steps are explained and some of these steps will require referral back to Chapter 3 and Chapter 4.

During the early years of using T3 replacement therapy there were times when I had symptoms that were confusing. This confusion arose if a T3 dosage change that I thought was going to be beneficial, produced an unexpected result. Some detective work was occasionally required. Some of the common sense approaches that I used to resolve confusing situations were:

- It was far more valuable to get to the root cause of the problem, rather than just make a knee-jerk change to my T3 dosage.

- Use a systematic approach. This might involve testing several hypotheses, regarding the cause of symptoms, before finding a permanent solution. I feel that this approach saves time in the long run.

- Sometimes I needed to take extra measurements of body temperature, heart rate and blood pressure during the day - even as often as every half an hour. This enabled me to go through the results with a fine-tooth comb, in order to find any subtle patterns that might have been missed if fewer readings had been taken. This was especially useful if I wasn't sure if a specific divided dose of T3 was too high or too low. The studying of results immediately before the T3 dose was taken and then over the following hours, often helped to clarify the situation.

- Occasionally, the process of elimination is a valuable tool, i.e. by adjusting a T3 divided dose in order to eliminate a dosage that definitely doesn't work. Over time, answers regarding dosage can become more apparent as more potential solutions are ruled out.

- Sometimes a particularly difficult problem just has to be answered using the most powerful tool available to a patient - the human brain. I found that on one or two occasions, I had to spend a lot of time thinking about a particular problem I was experiencing. This was how I eventually realised that the timing of my first T3 dose was so critical to my cortisol production.

- If, after thorough investigation, a situation was still confusing, my dosage was altered to either a previous dosage that appeared to work better, or to a much lower dosage, which enabled the T3 to be raised again slowly, in order to find an optimum solution.

- Sometimes this process is just difficult and you have to let the information mull around for a while until some inspiration comes. Avoiding too many rigid assumptions about what might be causing problems is important as occasionally these may turn out to be entirely wrong. Being flexible, adaptable and looking for inspiration from other people or sources can also be helpful.

Problems can arise during T3 dosage management that appear to be confusing. Many of these may be eliminated with sound preparatory work. However, if a few problems still occurred then I found that the combination of patience, good records and detective work always succeeded in the end.

Chapter 18

Lesson Learned on Practical Aspects of T3 Use

LESSON #14: SOME PRACTICAL ASPECTS OF T3 USE

I want to share some of the practical tips that have enabled me to successfully organise and manage my T3 replacement therapy:

- I bought a small, multi-compartment pill container to store my medication for the day. This enables me to split my T3 tablets in the previous evening and carry them during the day.

- Remembering to take each divided dose of T3 can be a challenge, especially after the initial novelty of taking T3 and feeling healthier has worn off. I found it essential to purchase a watch that had multiple daily alarms, to avoid forgetting to take a divided dose on time. Some modern mobile phones may also provide a multiple alarm facility.

- It was important for me to take my first T3 divided dose on time, as I was using the Circadian T3 Method to ensure my adrenal glands performed well. To avoid missing this first T3 divided dose I invested in a very loud alarm clock, set about five minutes later than my watch alarm. If I ever missed taking my first dose on time then I took it as soon as I remembered. If I had family members in my house that I could not afford to wake up then I would have used a vibrating mobile phone or an alarm clock designed for deaf people.

- Splitting of T3 tablets can be a challenge at first, especially if there is a need to split beyond quarters, i.e. splitting to create one eighth of a 20-microgram T3 tablet (2.5 micrograms). I have found that it is easier to split the tablets using my thumbnails rather than a knife, which tends to make the tablets crumble. If there are slight imperfections then I accept this, assuming that over a typical week these will average out.

- T3 tablets are tasteless and can easily be crunched up in the mouth between the teeth. This makes them very easy to take, even if a drink is not available to wash them down. The other advantage is having broken them up so thoroughly, they tend to be absorbed into the system faster, which will reduce the chance of interactions with supplements like iron.

- I purchased a battery operated blood pressure monitor that I could use at home. These are reasonably inexpensive now and I found that it was definitely worth the money to have the reassurance that my blood pressure was normal. This does not constitute a replacement for consultations with my family doctor, who always checks my heart and blood pressure during any routine visit. I have concluded that this is an essential piece of equipment when T3 replacement therapy is being used.

- My doctor prescribed propranolol tablets (beta blockers), which I kept in my medicine cabinet just in case I ever took a little too much T3. In the rare case of experiencing any problems with a slightly elevated heart rate due to increasing a T3 dose incorrectly the propranolol would quickly resolve this. It is important to note that if I suffered from asthma, or any other contra-indicated conditions, I would not have been able to use propranolol.

- In the UK all of our clocks are adjusted twice per year. In the spring we move them forward by an hour to adopt British Summer Time (BST). In the autumn, at the end of BST we adjust them back by an hour to Greenwich Mean Time (GMT). After a clock adjustment, I discovered that my body clock wasn't able to change overnight with the clock change. Therefore, at the end of BST (in the autumn) I move the timing of my first dose of T3 by between half an hour and one hour earlier. At the start of BST (in the spring) I do the opposite and move the timing of my first dose of T3 later by half an hour to one hour. Anyone who is affected by seasonal clock changes might need to consider this. **This can be especially critical for someone using the Circadian T3 Method.**

- I never adjusted the time I tale my first T3 divided dose (circadian dose) if I got out of bed later at a weekend. It appears to take 4 - 6 weeks for the adrenals to fully adjust to a timing change, such as getting up later and consequently, the adrenals continue to produce most of the day's cortisol at approximately the same time even if I got up later for a couple of days.

- Some women have reported to me that during certain phases of their menstrual cycle they have found that they appear to require a little more T3 each day, e.g. 5 to 10 micrograms extra per day. The suspicion is that hormonal fluctuations may sometimes act to interfere with the action of T3 in some manner. These fluctuations and the way that it affects women may vary from person to person depending on their own hormonal balance and on how T3 performs for them. Consequently, I am not making any specific recommendations. Women need to be watchful for more than just temperature fluctuations during their monthly cycle. Some women may experience changes in the effectiveness of their T3 medication at certain times of the month. An allied point specifically relevant to women is that even those who do not take iron supplements during the entire month often take them during menstruation to avoid lowering their iron storage.

These tips are simple but do make life a little easier.

SECTION 4

PREPARATION & GOALS

Chapter 19

Preparation for T3 Replacement Therapy

There are a few steps that summarise the preparatory work that I believe is **essential** to perform prior to starting T3 replacement therapy:

- Ensure you have an excellent family doctor and/or endocrinologist to work with and ensure that the full range of thyroid hormone and thyroid autoantibody tests have been done.

- Assess the status of key nutrients that can undermine thyroid hormone metabolism and establish a good nutritional regime prior to starting T3 replacement therapy. This step may appear to be quite minor or even optional but because of the level of difficulty associated with solving issues when T3 replacement therapy is being used I believe that this step is mandatory.

- Assess adrenal status before taking any T3, so that any low cortisol problem is known about.

- Investigate any other suspected issues prior to using T3.

- Begin regular daily exercise, to improve cardiovascular fitness and increase muscle tone and muscle mass.

Let me now clarify these preparatory steps in a little more detail.

FIND A GOOD FAMILY DOCTOR AND/OR ENDOCRINOLOGIST TO WORK WITH AND HAVE THOROUGH THYROID EVALUATION

Having a good working relationship with a family doctor and/or endocrinologist makes progress significantly easier and far less stressful for all concerned. In many cases, there will be no T3 replacement therapy or any useful progress with it, until the right medical professionals are found. There were many occasions early in my treatment when I visited my family doctor with some request for her but with the real aim of just being able to express my frustration with how things had been going. I also found that my endocrinologist was tremendously supportive and helpful if I had a specific issue or question that I needed to have resolved. This wasn't always the case, as I have already explained.

This step is potentially a critical requirement for many patients. A few patients, who are strong-willed and well informed, may be able to cope with poor working relationships with their physicians. For the majority of patients who still feel dreadfully ill, finding supportive and knowledgeable doctors will be essential. It is difficult enough to deal with thyroid disease without having to do battle during each visit to a doctor. To achieve this, it may mean having to change doctors. This may cause some initial stress and turmoil but, if it needs to be done, it is better to do it as soon as possible.

Having good doctors helped me a great deal, even though I was well armed with information and quite determined. This may need to be the first step that a patient needs to focus on.

I have spoken to many people with thyroid problems over many years and I have heard many tales of people who have only had a partial evaluation of their thyroid and thyroid hormones. I believe that before any patient and their doctor considers the use of T3 replacement therapy the full range of thyroid tests should be performed: TSH, FT4, FT3 and the TPO and Tg autoantibodies.

It should be very clear from the information in this book that I am convinced, that during T3 treatment, thyroid laboratory tests are of little use to manage T3 dosage. However, there is substantial diagnostic value to be gained by having the full range of thyroid laboratory tests prior to the start of T3 treatment. This is a non-optional requirement in my view. Knowing whether autoantibodies are elevated will help enormously in setting expectations about the future development of the disease and the likely need for more thyroid hormone as time goes on. The presence of elevated autoantibodies may also suggest that a higher priority should be given to calming the immune system. The values of TSH, FT4 and FT3 may also provide useful insights into further diagnostic work or the treatment itself, especially if any unexpected results are present.

The full range of important laboratory tests are more likely to be performed when the patient is working with a capable family doctor and/or endocrinologist who they have a good working relationship with.

ASSESS KEY NUTRIENTS AND ESTABLISH A NUTRITIONAL REGIME

This is also a critical step in the preparation prior to commencing T3 treatment. If problems occur during T3 treatment then it may be extraordinarily difficult to determine if these are being caused by T3 or by something else. Consequently, doing thorough nutrient testing beforehand is essential. Many thyroid patients find it beneficial to ask their family doctors to run tests on at least the following nutrients:

- Iron. The comprehensive range of iron tests need to be performed, which would include complete blood count, serum iron, transferrin saturation % and serum ferritin. A patient's family doctor can gain an excellent insight into the patient's iron status from these tests. Unfortunately, transferrin saturation % often remains untested. See Chapter 4 for more information on these tests and the meaning of various test results.

- Vitamin B12.

- Folate (folic acid).

- Vitamin D (via 25-hydroxy vitamin D test).

It is essential to avoid taking supplements that contain any of the above nutrients prior to these tests in order to obtain an honest and accurate test result that reflects the actual levels of these key nutrients in the patient's body. I usually try to avoid taking the relevant nutrients for a **week** prior to a laboratory test just to be absolutely certain that a truly representative result is obtained but at least several days is advisable. It is sensible to discuss how long to stop taking supplements with a family doctor prior to any tests.

If there are problems with any of the test results then the patient's doctor can provide the correct supplementation and then monitor progress.

I would definitely advise patients to ask for the specific test results for each of the above, including the units used and the laboratory reference ranges. These should be recorded in the patient's own records. It is also common for a patient to be told that their results are normal simply because the results creep above the lower end of the laboratory reference range. Consequently, it is only sensible for the patient to also check their actual test results and ensure that each of the critical nutrients is at a healthy level. See Chapter 4 for more details on what to look for in the results of the above tests.

I have discussed some important vitamins and minerals in Chapter 4. Patients have multiple ways of handling this, including working with their doctor or a qualified nutritionist. It is very important to ensure that all the important vitamins and minerals that are critical to thyroid and adrenal hormone metabolism are in the diet at the levels required or being taken as supplements.

The supplements that I have personally found **absolutely essential** to establish prior to using T3 in order to reduce or eliminate problems that can occur are:

- Strong B complex. All the main B vitamins at high levels, e.g. 50 mg B1, B2, B3, B5, and B6. These B vitamins are **crucial** for the adrenal and thyroid pathways to function correctly.

- Vitamin B12. How much depends on the result of the B12 test. If B12 is deficient then the patient's doctor will establish a treatment. If the B12 test was normal then some low level of B12 supplementation may still make sense to ensure it cannot develop into a problem during thyroid treatment, e.g. 500 ug or 1000 ug.

- Vitamin C. Taken 4 to 6 times per day in divided doses of 500 mg each.

- Vitamin D3. How much depends on the result of the vitamin D test. If the vitamin D was low then the patient's doctor will advise treatment. I have successfully used vitamin D3 supplementation of 2500 IUs of vitamin D3 during the months when there is less natural sunlight (October to March in the UK) and I stop taking vitamin D3 in the months when there is more natural sunlight available.

- A good quality chelated multi-mineral with a wide range of macro and trace minerals.

- Magnesium. Supplementation of magnesium at 400-1000 mg per day. I have found that chelated magnesium is easier on the digestive system and I now use 200 mg of chelated magnesium twice a day (as well as the small amount in my multi-mineral). When I say 'easier' I mean that I can't take any other form without having major digestive issues!

- Any other specific nutrients that have been found to be deficient from the nutrient testing (iron, B12, folic acid, vitamin D3).

These are some of the nutrients that I have found to be essential for my own health. Please refer to Chapter 4 for more details on the above and other nutrients. Readers should also consult their own personal physician and ensure that any supplements they are considering taking are safe and are being taken in safe quantities and will have no adverse interactions with other medications or conditions that they may have.

The above approach is designed to ensure that the thyroid and adrenal metabolic pathways are well resourced with the important nutrients in order to minimise problems during T3 replacement therapy.

I know of several patients who appeared to have a serious thyroid disorder and then it was discovered a long time later that their issues were primarily due to vitamin and mineral deficiencies. I also know of thyroid patients with adrenal issues that have completely corrected after B vitamins have been introduced (B3 is especially important to the adrenal glands).

I also know of many patients who have begun to take thyroid hormone replacement and then have had significant problems, which appeared to be due to lack of tolerance of the thyroid hormone replacement medication. These problems have often been due to a nutritional deficiency or a combination of several deficiencies including iron, vitamin B12, vitamin D, and folic acid. Deficiencies in magnesium, zinc, copper and selenium can also seriously undermine treatment (a good quality multi-mineral and extra chelated magnesium can address any potential for these latter minerals to be an issue).

Nutritional deficiencies can cripple any thyroid hormone replacement therapy. I understand that many patients, who have been ill for a long time, are desperate to begin thyroid treatment as soon as possible. However, it is imperative that an **equal** effort is placed on clarifying the status of critical nutrients and addressing any issues prior to commencing thyroid hormone replacement. This will save months and possibly years of confusion and problems later. It can often seem as hard to persuade medical professionals to do these tests thoroughly, as it can be to access the necessary thyroid hormone replacement medication. Doing this properly is equally as important as having the correct thyroid hormone replacement.

If any nutritional deficiency is only rectified once someone is already on T3 treatment then there is a risk that the T3 may begin to become far more effective as the deficiency is corrected. Problems with symptoms of tissue over-stimulation may arise. This is another important reason for fully investigating and dealing with any nutritional deficiencies prior to commencing T3 replacement therapy.

Establishing a sound nutritional regime is a commitment for life in my opinion. It is not something that should be viewed as a short-term measure to get thyroid hormone metabolism working. I know I want my T3 to keep me healthy and I want all the necessary processes in my body to continue to work correctly. Therefore, I intend to continue to take my nutritional supplements.

ASSESS ADRENAL STATUS

It is important for a patient's doctor to understand whether cortisol is likely to be a problem once T3 replacement therapy begins. Severely low cortisol might adversely affect glucose levels and the production of cellular energy. There are a number of tests that may be used to do this. A twenty-four hour adrenal saliva test is a highly desirable test as it illustrates cortisol levels over the entire day but a twenty-four hour urinary cortisol test may also be insightful. Depending on the result of any adrenal testing the doctor and the patient may need to discuss various approaches for managing cortisol levels. I have already discussed some of the tests and the options that are typically considered in Chapter 3.

Using T3 replacement offers the possibility of correcting or improving adrenal function in cases of adrenal insufficiency (some patients still refer to this as 'adrenal fatigue'). Clearly, if someone has been diagnosed with Addison's disease or a hypopituitarism problem or any other serious condition for which adrenal hormones must continue to be taken then no T3 dosage is going to make any improvement in the performance of the adrenal glands.

However, in some cases of adrenal insufficiency it may be possible to increase the level of cortisol and other hormones being naturally produced by the careful use of T3. The Circadian T3 Method, which I have briefly outlined in Chapter 16, will be discussed in more detail in the coming chapters.

There are two approaches for using the T3 dosage management process if someone is already on some form of adrenal support medication:

- One approach would be slowly weaning the adrenal support under the supervision of the patient's doctor. If no adrenal hormones are being taken when the T3 dosage management process begins then the T3 dosage may be optimised as much as possible to make full use of the body's natural adrenal hormone production capabilities. This also has the advantage that any adverse effects from adrenal medication will not confuse any problem solving using symptoms and signs.

- The second approach is to leave the adrenal support medication in place and slowly wean this as the Circadian T3 Method is applied during Phase 2 of the dosage management process. Care must be taken to wean the adrenal support enough to allow the adrenal glands to have some demand placed upon them before the Circadian T3 Method is applied. This must be done under the supervision of the patient's doctor.

When the T3 dosage has been optimised as much as possible then any remaining adrenal insufficiency may then be addressed with adrenal support, hopefully at a lower level than would otherwise have been required.

Slowly reducing any adrenal support medication should only be considered as a result of consultation with a qualified and competent medical professional.

Medical advice should be taken regarding changes to any form of medication or supplements including adrenal medication.

INVESTIGATE ANY OTHER SUSPECTED ISSUES PRIOR TO USING T3

In Chapter 5 I discussed a number of problems that might possibly undermine any form of thyroid hormone treatment. These included: environmental toxins, sex hormone issues, gastrointestinal problems and blood sugar balance. If there is any evidence that any of these or any other problems might be relevant and might affect thyroid treatment then it is very important to have them investigated by a doctor or a specialist prior to the start of T3 replacement therapy.

I have already stated my view that T3 is the thyroid hormone of last resort. It is more complex to use and the effort required to arrive at a final working T3 dosage is substantial compared to other forms of thyroid treatment. Therefore, any issues that might be problematic during T3 replacement therapy should be investigated thoroughly before any T3 is administered. This approach may seem slow and tedious but experience has taught me that in this case the tortoise beats the hare every time.

BEGIN REGULAR EXERCISE WHEN ABLE TO

Exercise creates a demand on the entire endocrine system. In particular, it places a demand on the body to increase its metabolic rate, which requires using more thyroid hormone. Muscle also has a higher requirement for thyroid hormone than other tissues. Cardiovascular exercise is very important for our overall health and muscle-toning exercises will also help to improve our fitness. Both cardiovascular exercise and muscle toning will help to create a demand for an increase in metabolic rate.

For patients who have been hypothyroid for a long time, their metabolisms will have slowed down. The consequence of this is that the demand for thyroid hormone will have dropped. Simply providing more thyroid hormone, of any type, is not necessarily enough to see the return of the health that the patient once had. In order to fully recover, the patient will also have to ask their body to work a little harder, to use the T3 that they are prescribed.

If a patient has any medical condition that may be adversely affected by exercise, then they should consult their own doctor prior to starting any new exercise programme. It is worth being aware that exercise depletes iron reserves. Therefore, it is particularly important for a woman, who is pre-menopausal, to have good iron storage if they are exercising.

Any exercise that is done should not be so strenuous or prolonged that it causes exhaustion, injury or any adverse effects. The aim is to start slowly, doing only as much as the individual feels that they can and to build up the level of exercise over time and, in the process, raise the metabolic rate.

However, for those patients, who feel too ill to do any exercise until T3 replacement begins to ease their symptoms, then any exercise regime may need to be delayed until T3 replacement therapy begins to have some positive effects.

CONCLUSION

Each of the steps if omitted or performed poorly, can cost a significant amount of valuable time once T3 replacement therapy begins. In the worst case, not doing one of these steps may result in significant problems during a trial of T3 even to the point of it being discontinued. I had already wasted enough of my life during T4 replacement therapy. I wanted to make sure T3 replacement therapy was a success, so I worked hard on the preparation outlined above.

T3 replacement therapy will not go smoothly if people have not thoroughly addressed these preparatory steps. T3, even more than T4, has the ability to expose nutritional and adrenal issues. If T3 replacement therapy does not progress in a straightforward way then people tend to blame the T3 itself, whereas the real issue is inadequate focus on the essential preparatory steps.

Chapter 20

The Goals of T3 Dosage Management

WHAT IS A T3 DOSAGE?

By the term 'T3 dosage' I mean the total amount of T3 taken each day and the following:

- The number of T3 divided doses taken each day.

- The size of each individual divided dose of T3. Each divided dose of T3 may be of a different size or the same size.

- The precise time that each divided dose of T3 is taken.

THE GOALS OF T3 DOSAGE MANAGEMENT

I developed the following three goals for the T3 dosage management process:

- To find a safe, effective and stable T3 dosage that was the lowest possible dosage of T3, which eradicated symptoms whilst avoiding any tissue over-stimulation.

- To find a T3 dosage that limits, or removes, the need for any adrenal medication or support, if possible.

- The T3 dosage management process needed to be systematic and clear.

Let me now further clarify each of these goals in a little more detail.

Find a safe, effective, stable T3 dosage that is as low as possible

This is the most important goal of T3 dosage management. The words used in this goal are all very important. Let me review each important part of this goal in turn.

Safe: At no time must the T3 dosage cause any tissue over-stimulation. My goal with using T3 replacement therapy has always been to be as cautious and patient as possible, in order to use T3 safely. To do this the process I developed tends to 'creep up' slowly on the ideal T3 dosage.

Tissue over-stimulation by T3 may also be referred to as tissue level thyrotoxicity, or the over-stimulation of the cells by too much thyroid hormone within them. This is not the same as too much thyroid hormone in the bloodstream, as determined by a thyroid blood test, although it may be the same for some people. The types of symptoms and signs that manifest, when there is tissue over-stimulation, will be discussed in more detail later.

My use of T3 replacement therapy has always been very cautious and safe. This emphasis is incorporated within the T3 dosage management process and has meant that I've had no bad experiences.

Effective: The T3 dosage had to be effective in eradicating all of my symptoms associated with hypothyroidism. The result of this is feeling healthy and having energy levels that are normal for one's age.

Stable: It was my aim to be able to continue to take the same T3 dosage each day and only rarely require changes, so that I could get on with my life. My T3 dosage has been stable, apart from occasional alterations every few years due to further thyroid atrophy.

Lowest: My aim was to discover the lowest total T3 dosage, with the lowest individual divided doses, that would still resolve all my symptoms and allow me to regain my health. With this aim built into the T3 dosage management process, I believed that the other parts of this key goal would be more easily achieved. This explicit goal underlined my commitment to the safe use of T3.

Try to limit or remove the need for adrenal medication or support

This was an ideal requirement but not imperative if it wasn't possible. This goal was based on the realisation that the timing and size of the first dose of T3 each day affected my cortisol level. I know of many people who have now used the Circadian T3 Method described in Chapter 16 successfully to reduce or eliminate the need for adrenal support.

I found that simply taking a high enough T3 dosage during the day was no guarantee of adequate adrenal hormone levels. I wanted to ensure that the T3 dosage management process was capable of providing the adrenal glands with enough T3 for them to have every chance to work as well as they were able to.

The T3 dosage management process must make every attempt to explore ways of eliminating or reducing the requirement for adrenal medication by enabling the adrenal glands to produce their vast array of hormones as normally as possible.

By incorporating this goal into the T3 dosage management process in such a way that it had no adverse effect on the primary goal of finding a safe, effective and stable T3 dosage, it offered the possibility of reducing or avoiding the need for any adrenal medication or support. It is my belief that I have managed to do this.

This goal is not achievable if adrenal medication is being taken for Addison's disease, hypopituitarism or any other condition for which adrenal hormones must continue to be provided. Any alteration of any medication including adrenal hormones must always be discussed and done under the guidance of a qualified medical practitioner.

Use a systematic process for T3 dosage management

It was my aim to make explicit the steps that led me to good health. In order to make this as clear as possible, I have structured the T3 dosage management process into three distinct phases:

- Clearing T4 and starting T3 replacement therapy.

- Determining a safe, effective and stable T3 dosage.

- Long-term monitoring of T3 dosage.

Each of the above phases will be dealt with in the next section. I have also defined the assessment approach that I used to determine if my T3 dosage was adequate or not and have documented this at the beginning of the next section.

SECTION 5

T3 DOSAGE MANAGEMENT PROCESS

Chapter 21

Using Symptoms and Signs

The rapid and wide fluctuations of FT3 and the suppressed or fluctuating nature of TSH during T3 replacement therapy make it impractical to use thyroid blood test results to:

- Assess if a T3 dosage is adequate.

- Determine if one or more divided doses are too high or too low.

- Decide upon specific changes to the T3 dosage.

The application of symptoms and signs is a standard approach used by doctors who have experience of using T3 on its own and experienced patients who have been on T3 replacement therapy for a long time. This is the approach I adopted for myself and it has worked extremely well.

MONITORING SYMPTOMS AND SIGNS

Symptoms and signs provide vital clues that can be used to assess whether a dosage change has been effective or detrimental. They have enabled me to decide whether I have needed more T3 in any given dose, whether the dose has been correct, or whether it has been too high and has led to any risk from tissue over-stimulation. Symptoms and signs are also important in the assessment of the timing of divided doses. I was able to determine when the positive effects of each T3 divided dose were declining and only take another divided dose when absolutely necessary.

Doctors use the terms 'symptoms' and 'signs' in a very specific way. A symptom is something that the patient complains about or feels. A sign is a specific observation or measurement that has a more objective value and that someone else can observe or measure. One example is body temperature. If I complained that I was feeling cold and my body temperature reading was below normal, then the sign would be the temperature measurement and the symptom would be my sensitivity to cold.

The main symptoms that I tracked and recorded included: mood; anxiety (including restlessness and irritability); mental ability and clarity; energy level; strength or weakness; digestive symptoms; skin condition; feeling warm or cold and muscle aches or pains.

The main signs that were tracked either by my doctor or by me were: resting heart rate; body temperature; resting blood pressure; weight gain or loss; blood sugar level; adrenal hormone test results; sex hormone test results; checking that the heart was working correctly (no abnormal rhythms or sounds); electrocardiogram (ECG); checking for evidence of bone loss; nutritional deficiencies and thyroid blood test results.

During the early months of T3 dosage management I usually tracked and recorded relevant symptoms and signs every day. If there was a confusing situation then it was not unusual for me to track symptoms and signs hourly, in order to understand the problem. As time went on this became far less frequent. Here are a few more details on the symptoms and signs that I found useful to track:

Symptoms that I tracked:

- Mood – if I was 'down' or depressed, this invariably meant that my T3 dosage was too low.

- Anxiety (including restlessness, hyperactivity or irritability) - if I was anxious, edgy, tense and unable to relax, this usually meant that I had been taking too much T3. This was usually a very reliable indicator.

- Mental ability and clarity – if my T3 was at an appropriate level, I was able to think very clearly and logically. Too little T3 makes clear and quick thinking more difficult and for some people, they can feel as though immersed in a thick, mental fog.

- Energy level – my general energy level and stamina tended to be good if my T3 was at a reasonable level and poor if it was too low. Fatigue during the day and particularly in the evening was typically a good indicator of low T3. Although, if T3 is far too high then any initial hyperactivity can eventually change into fatigue if the hyperactivity is not noticed and acted upon swiftly.

  Low cortisol can also play a role in poor energy levels, so it is important to gather enough diagnostic data in order to determine whether, or not, a low cortisol level is responsible for fatigue rather than too little T3.

- Weakness – if my T3 level was far too low then I would feel weak but I had no symptoms if my T3 level was only mildly low.

- Digestive system – the digestive system rarely lies! If my T3 level was too high I would experience frequent or loose bowel movements. However, if my T3 level was too low I would become constipated. On one occasion only, my T3 level was exceptionally high, because my family doctor had suggested an increase based on a TSH result. This was the one and only time we ever changed my T3 dosage based on a blood test result. I got very constipated and some blood tests were performed that revealed my serum calcium level was slightly elevated. Calcium released into the blood stream can cause constipation, so it is therefore vital to check for an elevated serum calcium level if you have any suspicion that the T3 level may be too high. This only happened to me on one occasion and it was spotted quickly and corrected.

- Skin, hair and nails – changes in the quality of these can provide reliable clues as to whether the T3 dosage is optimised. However, it takes a long time for these changes to become apparent. Therefore, skin, hair and nail quality are only useful indicators after a significant amount of time has passed on a new T3 dosage.

- Heat or cold Sensitivity – usually a good indicator but I tended to use body temperature readings as a sign, when these symptoms arose.

- Muscle aches or pains – I never experienced severe muscle aches and pains. However, I know that many hypothyroid patients do suffer from these symptoms, which may alert them to a low T3 dosage. Occasionally, patients may complain of a feeling of difficulty in swallowing. I have not experienced this either but I have heard that it can be due to thyroid inflammation as a result of insufficient thyroid medication.

Signs that I tracked:

- Resting heart rate – A rapid heart rate, or a feeling that my heart was beating or pounding hard in my chest, usually indicated that an individual T3 divided dose was too high. This is such a useful indicator that I tracked my resting heart rate frequently. This has to be checked when at rest and not within a few hours of exercise.

  Nevertheless, it is important to be aware that heart rate readings can sometimes provide misleading information. Generally, too much T3 can increase the heart rate and this will be something that a patient beginning T3 replacement therapy will need to pay close attention to. Taking too little T3 can also put a strain on the heart and cause an increase in heart rate. Used in isolation the resting heart rate cannot always confirm whether a T3 dosage is too high or too low. It is very important to use the resting heart rate along with other symptoms and signs before making a judgment. I have included some more information on this subject at the end of this chapter.

- Body temperature – I used a basal thermometer to regularly measure my body temperature throughout the day to see how each dose affected my readings. I discovered that if my temperature is around 98.3 - 98.6 degrees Fahrenheit (36.8 - 37.0 degrees Centigrade) then I expect to feel well. If my body temperature was below 98.0 degrees Fahrenheit (36.67 degrees Centigrade) then I suspected my T3 dosage might be too low. If my body temperature was below 97.7 degrees Fahrenheit (36.5 degrees Centigrade) then I was fairly confident that I was under-replaced. There is far more information on the use of body temperature in the next chapter.

Once again, adrenal insufficiency can cloud the picture and cause misleading temperature readings. If the adrenal glands fail to produce enough cortisol then this may have a profound effect on cellular energy production (ATP production by the mitochondria). If this is the case, then low cortisol issues need to be addressed first. The same comment also applies to some essential nutrients like iron, B12, folate and vitamin D.

- Blood pressure (resting) – this was checked regularly, while I was adjusting my T3 dosage. I bought a blood pressure monitor to do this at home and I only took readings when I was resting and relaxed. The upper arm that the BP cuff is on should be aimed away from the body (approximately at right angles to the body) and the arm should be supported on a chair arm or pillow to get an accurate result. I recommend the use of a home BP monitor to any patient who is having their thyroid hormone dosage adjusted.

An individual's blood pressure is expressed as systolic over diastolic blood pressure, for example, 120/80. The systolic blood pressure (the first number) represents the pressure in the arteries as the muscle of the heart contracts and pumps blood into them. The diastolic blood pressure (the second number) represents the pressure in the arteries as the muscle of the heart relaxes following its contraction. The range of systolic blood pressure for most healthy adults falls between 90 and 120 millimetres of mercury (mm Hg). Normal diastolic blood pressure ranges between 60 and 80 mm Hg.

Current guidelines define normal blood pressure range as lower than 120/80. Blood pressures over 130/80 are usually considered high. Low blood pressure (hypotension) is pressure so low it causes symptoms or signs due to the low flow of blood through the arteries and veins. When the flow of blood is too low to deliver enough oxygen and nutrients to vital organs, e.g. brain, heart, and kidneys, the organs do not function normally and may be temporarily or permanently damaged.

A patient's doctor will look primarily at symptoms and signs of low blood flow rather than a specific blood pressure number when considering a diagnosis of low blood pressure. Anyone who has concerns over their blood pressure should consult their doctor who will assess their blood pressure as well as their other presenting symptoms.

- Weight gain or loss – if I was gaining weight, it was likely my T3 level was under-replaced and equally if I was losing weight, it was likely that I was over-medicated. Weight gain or loss is typically a slow process but it is something to look out for, if there is any suspicion that a T3 dosage is not correct.

- Blood sugar – I bought a home blood sugar monitor, as I was aware that poor blood sugar control could produce some of the symptoms associated with hypothyroidism. Blood sugar balance was discussed briefly in Chapter 5. It needs to be remembered that problems with blood sugar metabolism may adversely affect cellular energy production and cause thyroid hormone treatment to fail to produce the desired results. I only tested my blood sugar very occasionally, if I had any concerns, or wanted to rule out unstable blood sugar as a possible cause of symptoms. If a patient had serious concerns about blood sugar metabolism then they should consult their doctor and have the appropriate investigations done, which might include a glucose tolerance test (with or without insulin measurements).

- Pupil dilation test - if I suspected any adrenal insufficiency then this simple test described in Chapter 2 is a useful addition to any laboratory testing that might be required.

- Oximeter reading - to check blood oxygen levels. I have only recently bought one of these devices and so I cannot speak with a lot of experience in its use. However, as described in Chapter 3 these devices offer the possibility of an additional insight into whether iron-deficiency anaemia may be present or not. As such they may become a very valuable tool for thyroid patients.

Signs that my doctor or endocrinologist tracked when required:

- ACTH stimulation test - measures response of adrenal glands in relation to demand. This is sometimes known as a synacthen test.

- Twenty-four hour urinary cortisol test - measures free cortisol and total cortisol output levels - over a twenty-four hour period. The alternative and perhaps better test for cortisol is the twenty-four hour adrenal saliva test. Testing of cortisol levels is immensely useful in the assessment of the correct size and timing of the first daily (circadian) dose of T3. I still tended to make any final decision on the timing of my first divided dose of T3, based on how I felt but this test provided useful information.

- Sex hormone blood tests - to measure my free and total testosterone levels, which are also affected by the timing of the first daily dose of T3. Females should also have other sex hormones tested (oestrogen and progesterone) as well as testosterone.

- Blood pressure (resting) – this was checked whenever I saw my doctor. Luckily, it has never been an issue in my case.

- Listening to the heart for any abnormalities – this is to ensure that the heart isn't under strain from an incorrect T3 dosage.

- ECG - if there is any concern about the heart an ECG should be done immediately. I would also suggest that any patient considering T3 replacement therapy has an ECG done prior to treatment, to ensure there are no previously undiagnosed heart abnormalities. It is also a good idea to repeat the ECG once a stable, safe and effective T3 dosage has been established, or at any time when there are any concerns. A good discussion with a family doctor is advisable, prior to commencing T3 replacement therapy, to get agreement on this and other tests that may be highly useful throughout the T3 dosage management process.

- Serum calcium blood test – if I suspected I might have been taking too much T3 I asked for a serum calcium test. Excess thyroid hormone (T4 or T3) is capable of raising the serum calcium level as a result of bone loss. If serum calcium is elevated hypercalcaemia may be diagnosed. A high level of excess calcium can result in stomach upsets, frequent urination and impaired kidney function. So, it is very important to have a safe T3 dosage.

- Liver and kidney function tests - to ensure that these two organs are working effectively. These were checked occasionally, especially after any significant dosage changes.

- Dexa bone density scan – to be carried out every few years to monitor any bone density changes. Having a Dexa scan every few years is important because this is the only way of comparing the current bone density with previous readings, to determine if any changes have occurred.

- Glucose tolerance test (GTT) - I never asked for one of these but I have included it here for completeness and as a further test beyond the simple blood sugar measurements that may be done at home. In Chapter 5 I discussed the GTT as one mechanism for assessing blood sugar metabolism.

Nutritional deficiencies that my doctor tracked:

- Vitamin D3 – this is characteristically low in hypothyroid patients and easily supplemented.

- Vitamin B12 and folate – a deficiency in vitamin B12 can mimic hypothyroid symptoms and folic acid works synergistically with vitamin B12. These are often found to be deficient in patients suffering from hypothyroidism.

- Iron – hypothyroid patients also often have low iron levels, which should be corrected with iron supplementation. I have already written extensively on the various tests for iron that may be done in Chapter 4. Typically my doctor used serum iron and serum ferritin tests but knowing what I know now before commencing T3 treatment I would have asked for the more comprehensive iron panel: CBC, serum iron, transferrin saturation % and serum ferritin. If there was concern over iron levels and thyroid treatment was not progressing straightforwardly then this more comprehensive iron panel could be re-run as iron stores may be depleted due to the demands of improving metabolic rate.

- Further mineral tests - I have never had this type of testing done but for the case of someone who continues to have issues after everything else has been investigated then this testing may be valuable. For example trace minerals may be tested via twenty-four hour urinary analysis.

Thyroid blood tests that my doctor did occasionally:

- TSH – as a result of my atrophied thyroid gland and my T3 replacement therapy, I expected my TSH level to vary according to when the blood was taken, in relation to my most recent divided dose of T3. I had this test approximately once a year, as it confirmed that no additional pituitary or hypothalamus problem had developed. As already discussed, TSH was not used in any way to determine my T3 dosage. Many people on T3 may find that their TSH is actually suppressed - it depends on the T3 dosage being used and the level of thyroid atrophy.

- Free T3 – the expectation was that my FT3 would be above the reference range, as a result of my T3 replacement therapy, although because of fluctuations in serum concentrations of T3, there was never any guarantee of this.

- Free T4 – this would be likely to be very low, due to the fact that I was no longer taking exogenous T4 and my thyroid gland was progressively failing due to Hashimoto's thyroiditis.

- Autoantibodies – I expected my autoantibody levels (TPOAb, TgAb) to eventually fall. They have in fact already decreased. I will continue to get these tested occasionally, to check that the autoimmune response remains quiescent. In the early stages of my condition, this was a very useful indicator of how vigorously my thyroid was being attacked.

The careful tracking of symptoms and signs is clearly not as easy as doing a simple thyroid blood test. However, it is the only practical way of monitoring T3 replacement therapy.

Over the years, I have learnt to listen to what my body is trying to tell me and I am now very in-tune with the messages it sends me. Whenever I had any doubts about how to interpret my symptoms and signs, I simply made a T3 dosage change and then monitored my symptoms and signs, extremely carefully, following this change.

The use of symptoms and signs does require some time, patience and care, as well as some understanding of how T3 affects the body. This isn't always easy but it does work. It is also a pre-requisite for using the T3 dosage management process that symptoms and signs are rigorously recorded and monitored.

If I had not been prepared to record and monitor my symptoms and signs then there would have been no point attempting to use T3 replacement therapy. At the present time there are no viable laboratory tests that may be used instead of tracking symptoms and signs. Anyone contemplating a trial of T3 replacement therapy has to be prepared to comply with the recording and monitoring of symptoms and signs. This is a discussion that patients must have with their own doctor prior to any decision to use T3 replacement therapy.

ASSESSING CORTISOL LEVELS

I cannot emphasise enough the usefulness of assessing cortisol levels and levels of various nutrients like iron and B12 via laboratory testing. Knowing that a problem exists makes thyroid hormone treatment far more likely to be quick and effective. I will come back to this once again in Chapter 19.

WHEN TO ASSESS SYMPTOMS AND SIGNS?

The T3 dosage management process uses the assessment of symptoms and signs to provide guiding information on the status of the T3 dosage.

I found that it was essential to make recordings of symptoms and signs at different times throughout the day, in order to provide a good overview of the effectiveness of the current T3 dosage. In particular, I began to view the day as a series of time segments, each of which begins with a T3 divided dose. So, when I was very puzzled by some change in symptoms or signs I would collect a range of symptoms and signs data for each time segment in the day. This often helped to clarify how each T3 dose was behaving. Sometimes this necessitated multiple data collections for each time segment.

In particular, I would ensure that I collected data on symptoms and signs **one or two hours after each T3 divided dose** in order to assess how effective that dose had been. I would often also collect data on symptoms and **signs just before the next T3 divided dose was due** and in this way I could assess if the next dose was actually really due or whether the previous T3 dose was still effective. In this way symptoms and signs may used to assess a size or a timing change to an individual T3 divided dose.

The T3 dosage management process makes it clear that it is sensible to adjust only one T3 divided dose at any one time. Any alteration to a T3 divided dose will be either to its size or its timing but not both at the same time.

When a T3 divided dose is being adjusted, by size or timing, symptoms and signs may need to be recorded at regular intervals, often hourly, in between the divided dose being altered and both the preceding and the following divided dose, for all the divided doses throughout the entire day.

It is essential when T3 divided dose changes are being made that adequate time is allowed to collect and analyse symptoms and signs, sometimes recording this information every hour or even half an hour in between divided doses in order to provide information that can be acted upon reliably.

When it is clear that the ideal T3 dosage is being approached then symptoms tend to become far more useful than signs. I used to find that picking my top six symptoms and assigning them a score was very helpful. I could track the progress of these symptoms quite dispassionately as I slowly edged closer to my ideal T3 dosage.

ELEVATED HEART RATE AND T3

I have communicated with several people who have been in the early stages of using T3 and have been having problems with a rapid heart rate. These patients and their own doctors were concerned that it was the T3 that was causing heart rates of 90 - 110 beats per minute.

The way in which these issues have been resolved has been to collect some data before concluding anything. Specifically, there is a simple process to follow:

- It is important to measure the resting heart rate, body temperature and blood pressure just before a dose of T3 is taken.

- Then repeat the measurements every half an hour for several hours afterwards.

- Do not take a further T3 dose when it is normally due until it is clear that either the heart rate has come down to normal or symptoms and signs indicate that the next T3 divided dose is late.

With this heart rate data and the data on body temperature and blood pressure in relation to when the T3 dose was being taken, it may be possible to understand the situation. There are several possibilities that relate to the T3 dosage that may be contributing to the problem:

- The T3 dose prior to the heart rate elevation may be too high.

205

- Two or more T3 divided doses may be being taken too close together, which again results in too much T3.

- A further possibility is that the T3 divided dose is too low. This may seem unlikely but I have seen results from people who have taken these readings that show that, after the T3 dose is taken, the heart rate initially lowers to normal and then rises much later. In this case, it is possible that either the T3 divided dose was not high enough or the intervals between the divided doses were too large. The heart is like other tissues, it requires enough T3 to work normally and if the heart does not have enough T3 then the heart rate can rise until the T3 level becomes extremely low.

- Another very common source of an elevation in heart rate is a nutritional deficiency of iron, B12, folate and vitamin D. Low magnesium may also be problematic and can cause heart rate issues. These underlying issues are very frequently confused with a thyroid replacement dosage issue. Hence the requirement to fully address these issues in the preparation stage prior to T3 replacement therapy. It is significantly less work to thoroughly investigate these prior to using T3 than try to disentangle a confusing array of symptoms during T3 replacement therapy. See Chapter 4 for more details on the relevant nutrients and appropriate testing methods. An electrolyte imbalance (sodium, potassium) may also be problematic and the patient's doctor will need to take this possibility into account.

- The final consideration is that of insufficient cellular energy due or a low level of glucose in the cells. Both of these situations may lead to a poor response, including a rapid heart rate when thyroid hormone is increased. Possible causes include adrenal insufficiency, blood sugar metabolism issues, and deficiencies of important nutrients that the mitochondria use, e.g. vitamin B1 or other mitochondrial issues. The most common of these causes is insufficient glucose reaching the interior of the cells. This is frequently due to low cortisol or blood sugar metabolism problems.

Chapter 3 discusses adrenal insufficiency in some detail and the possible investigation and treatment approaches. In the case of low cortisol, the mechanism that is responsible for the elevated heart rate may be due to low blood glucose because of the low cortisol. This will tend to create low cellular levels of glucose. When thyroid hormones are raised then this can quickly result in a depletion of glucose, ATP and a consequent rise in adrenaline in response to this and the elevated heart rate and even an increase in blood pressure or flushing of the skin (often the face).

Chapter 5 briefly discusses blood sugar balance and touches on the possibilities of dietary issues and the relevance of both cortisol and insulin. If an imbalance in blood sugar levels is suspected then it is important to take proper medical advice in the process of investigating this.

If low cortisol levels are the cause of the elevated heart rate then patient's using T3 may sometimes gain some benefit from the use of the Circadian T3 Method, first mentioned in Chapter 16 and to be discussed in more detail in the coming chapters. If this method fails then some form of adrenal support may well be required for a short time or indefinitely depending on the severity of the problem. These options should be considered during discussions between the patient and their personal physician.

For any patient with heart rate elevation then the key to understanding the situation is to take frequent heart rate measurements and then to discuss the results with their own doctor. The patient's doctor may also listen to the patient's heart, take a blood pressure reading and perform an ECG to rule out any heart abnormalities.

If the most likely cause is a T3 dosage issue then the test may be repeated after an increase or decrease or a timing change to a specific dose of T3. The data usually reveals the reality of the situation. Sometimes a change to the T3 dosage is required to compare the results and gather more information.

Other common causes of heart rate elevations when on T3 replacement include nutritional deficiencies, adrenal issues and blood sugar imbalances. Some people give up using T3 because they don't realise that they have other problems that are being exposed by the use of the T3 thyroid hormone.

AVOIDING COMPLEX PROBLEMS BEFORE STARTING TO USE T3 IS EASIER THAN SOLVING THEM DURING T3 REPLACEMENT

I have become completely convinced that it is far easier to put the initial effort in before using T3 in order to **avoid** getting into complex and confusing problem solving that involves issues like elevated heart rate. When T3 replacement is being used it is not possible to use simple thyroid blood tests to assess the T3 dosage. Consequently, it can become extremely difficult to work out if a problem like a raised heart rate is related to the T3 dosage or a low level of some nutrient or low cortisol. **The solution is simple and that is to eliminate as many of the other possibilities prior to using the T3.** Hence the preparatory steps described in Chapter 19 are critical to this process and I do not consider them to be optional or just 'nice to have'.

Chapter 22

Taking Body Temperature Readings

I want to discuss taking body temperature readings, because this is such a useful sign that can help determine whether a T3 dosage is too high or too low. There are also several pitfalls that need to be avoided when taking body temperature readings that I need to point out.

The great American physician, Dr. Broda Barnes, emphasised the importance of taking temperature readings for thyroid patients. Most of Dr. Barnes's work was carried out between the 1930s and 1980s. He first described his Basal Temperature test to the rest of the world, in 1942 via a publication. Basal, in this context, means when the patient is completely at rest.

Basal was a term that many doctors were familiar with at the time, due to the prevalence of the basal metabolic rate (BMR) test, which was a complex test, used at the time to measure metabolic rate in order to determine appropriate levels of thyroid medication. The BMR test measured oxygen consumption and heat output for a patient who was completely at rest. The BMR was used because it was known that metabolic rate is below normal when a patient's thyroid gland was failing. By measuring BMR it was possible to not only diagnose thyroid disease quite accurately but also the doctor could determine when the correct amount of replacement thyroid hormone was being provided.

Dr. Barnes noticed a very close correlation between BMR test results and the measurement of body temperature when the patient was at rest and he communicated his results and belief that the basal temperature test was very valuable. Clearly, Dr. Barnes did not believe that measuring body temperature, when a patient is at rest, can be used on its own to determine if a patient is hypothyroid or not. He did believe that body temperature is highly valuable when used alongside a multiplicity of other symptoms and signs.

Basal temperature refers to a resting body temperature, measured away from food, drink and exercise. Using this method it is possible to get an assessment of core body temperature without the influence of any energy released from exercise, food or drink. It is one method of measuring the effect of thyroid hormone on our metabolism. In the absence of any useful thyroid blood tests, the basal temperature test can be quite helpful. Women of childbearing age must be aware of the influence that female hormonal fluctuations can have on basal temperature readings. This can complicate matters somewhat and Dr. Barnes suggested that women's basal temperature readings are more accurate if they are taken on days two to five of each new cycle.

HOW TO TAKE BODY TEMPERATURE MEASUREMENTS

The body temperature is usually taken by placing the thermometer under the tongue for at least three minutes. An alternative method, which has to be with a mercury thermometer, not a digital one, is to place the thermometer under your armpit for at least ten minutes.

If the temperature is taken under the tongue, then a normal body temperature is 97.7 - 99.0 degrees Fahrenheit (36.5 - 37.2 degrees Centigrade). An under-the-armpit normal body temperature is 97.8 - 98.2 degrees Fahrenheit (36.6 - 36.8 degrees Centigrade).

For the rest of this chapter, I will only refer to a body temperature that is taken with a thermometer placed under the tongue, because I believe that it is the least time consuming and most convenient method.

Hypothyroid patients tend to have lower than normal body temperatures that often fall 1.5 - 3.0 degrees below normal on the Fahrenheit scale. However, any body temperature below 97.7 degrees Fahrenheit (36.5 degrees Centigrade) might suggest the presence of hypothyroidism.

Several body temperature readings should be taken over a period of days, ideally at the same time each day, in order to develop a clearer picture of how body temperature is varying.

When to take body temperature when using T3

Dr. Barnes suggested that the most realistic basal temperature reading is obtained by taking body temperature readings when a patient first wakes up in bed in the morning. However, with T3 replacement therapy, the fluctuating level of T3 means that body temperature also fluctuates to some extent. I prefer to take body temperature readings during the morning or afternoon, based on my view that T3 is at a more healthy level in my body during these hours of the day. I believe body temperature when I first wake up is misleading.

However, I feel that body temperature readings are a big asset and help me to monitor my treatment, especially when used in conjunction with other symptoms and signs.

Using a liquid basal thermometer

I prefer to use liquid filled basal thermometers, rather than the digital ones. Personally, I use an oral body temperature reading, rather than placing the thermometer under my armpit, because I find it to be a much more convenient way of taking my temperature. I am fully aware that oral temperature readings may be susceptible to fluctuations due to infections. If I have a cold or a virus I don't take any readings.

Prior to taking my temperature, I shake down the thermometer so that it reads well below 95 degrees Fahrenheit (35.0 degrees Centigrade). I then keep the thermometer under my tongue, with my lips closed, for a full three minutes to ensure an accurate reading.

Some things can adversely affect body temperature readings

There are some things that can affect the result of taking body temperature via a thermometer under the tongue:

- Any exercise within the previous two hours can increase body temperature.

- Any mild activity within the previous fifteen minutes can also increase body temperature, so reclining or sitting in a room that is comfortably heated, for at least fifteen minutes before taking a temperature reading is important.

- Eating or drinking anything during the prior fifteen minutes can affect the result, because it changes the temperature in the mouth.

- Taking a shower or a bath during the hour before can temporarily lower temperature readings.

- A cold or virus can affect the body temperature - avoid taking temperature readings if a virus or other illness is suspected.

Interpreting the results

If my body temperature readings were consistently below 98.0 degrees Fahrenheit (36.67 degrees Centigrade) then I suspected that my T3 dosage was too low. This is a little higher than the 97.7 degrees Fahrenheit (36.5 degrees Centigrade), which Dr. Barnes suggested but this is what I personally found.

Temperature readings consistently above 98.6 degrees Fahrenheit (37.0 degrees Centigrade) led me to suspect that my T3 had been over-replaced.

Certainly, if my body temperature was lower than 97.7 degrees Fahrenheit (36.5 degrees Centigrade) then I strongly suspected that I was under-replaced.

In the early stages of establishing an optimum T3 replacement dosage, I took multiple temperature measurements throughout the day, in order to see how each dose affected my temperature. Whenever I got confused about whether a T3 divided dose was too high or too low I would take body temperature readings every half an hour, just before taking the divided dose of T3 and for several hours afterwards. I'd also assess other symptoms and signs at the same time as the body temperature readings.

I have discovered that if my temperature is around 98.3 - 98.6 degrees Fahrenheit (36.83 - 37.0 degrees Centigrade) I am usually on a reasonable T3 dosage.

I never exclusively relied on body temperature readings, instead, I used them alongside the other symptoms and signs that I tracked. There will inevitably be individual variations, because we don't all have the same body temperature. However, at the very least, any general trend of changing body temperature will provide useful information.

For Women of Childbearing Age

When a woman ovulates her body temperature will rise naturally by a small amount. Often this increase is only between 0.2 and 0.4 degrees Fahrenheit (0.1 to 0.2 degrees Centigrade). The detection of this small rise in body temperature is how some couples that are finding it difficult to conceive identify the time of ovulation, i.e. the prime time to get pregnant. A day or two before menstruation, body temperature normally returns to normal.

This type of natural body temperature fluctuation for a woman who has a fairly normal monthly menstrual cycle needs to be taken into account when symptoms and signs are being used to understand the effectiveness of a T3 dosage. At certain times of the month it might be easy for a woman to believe that she needs to modify her T3 dosage if body temperature alone is being used to make decisions.

To make matters a little more complex, some women have reported to me that during certain phases of their menstrual cycle they have found that they appear to require a little more T3 each day, e.g. 5 to 10 micrograms extra per day. I have been told that the extreme hormonal fluctuations after ovulation appear to interfere with the action of T3 in some manner. One lady identifies the point of ovulation, via the temperature increase and other indicators, then increases her T3 dosage to avoid any 'hypo' symptoms that she experiences after ovulation. She then waits until her body temperature returns to a more normal level, one to two days before she menstruates, then reduces her T3 dosage to the normal level.

These fluctuations and the way that they affect women may vary from person to person depending on their own hormonal balance. Not every woman may find that their T3 is affected by fluctuations in sex hormones and women who are perimenopausal may have entirely different experiences. Consequently, without adequate research it is difficult to draw any general conclusions.

However, it is clear that body temperature alone may be misleading for women of childbearing age and in some cases more subtle T3 dosage management may be required.

Chapter 23

Recognising a T3 Dosage That is Too High

I have already outlined the symptoms and signs that I tracked as part of the process of T3 dosage management. One of my main goals was to ensure that any dosage changes were always safe. Consequently, I wanted to place extra emphasis on identifying if a T3 dosage was too high. A T3 dosage that is too high incurs a risk of tissue over-stimulation by thyroid hormone, otherwise known as thyrotoxicosis.

It was clear that thyroid blood test results were not going to provide any useful indication of whether my T3 dosage was too high. To further ensure that safety was always in the front of my mind, I developed a specific list of symptoms and signs that summarised the indicators of tissue over-stimulation by thyroid hormone, which could be reviewed if I had any suspicion that my T3 dosage might be too high.

Common symptoms of tissue over-stimulation by thyroid hormone include:

- Anxiety or nervousness or sensation of inner tension - this has always been my first indication that one of my divided doses may be a little excessive.

- Loose bowels or frequent bowel movements - this has also been a fairly early indicator for me.

- Feeling hot or increased perspiration.

- Weight loss, despite increased appetite - clearly this won't be noticed immediately and hopefully, the T3 dosage will have been reduced, well before this occurs.

- Fatigue - worsening with increasing dosage of T3. It would be typical to have fatigue prior to starting T3 replacement therapy. What is being looked for here is an increasing level of fatigue, in the presence of one, or more, of the other symptoms and signs of tissue over-stimulation

Common signs of tissue over-stimulation by thyroid hormone include:

- Hyperactivity - as if someone had drunk too many cups of coffee.

- Heart palpitations - faster than normal heart rate, unpleasant sensations, more forceful beating of the heart, irregular heart beat. I have never had any irregular heart behaviour but, if a T3 divided dose has been too high, then it may have raised my heart rate, by a small but noticeable amount, for two to four hours. This has been a rare occurrence, because I increase T3 divided doses in very small amounts. I have already mentioned that a faster heart rate than normal can be caused by too little T3 as well as too much. It can also be caused by nutritional deficiencies of iron, vitamin B12, folate and vitamin D, adrenal insufficiency (low cortisol) or blood sugar metabolism problems. This particular sign may require quite careful analysis, along with other symptoms and signs, before any conclusion may be drawn over the T3 dosage.

- Raised body temperature - above 98.6 degrees Fahrenheit (37.0 degrees Centigrade).

- Systolic hypertension - slightly raised systolic blood pressure (the first, of the two blood pressure numbers).

Less common signs of more excessive tissue over-stimulation by thyroid hormone, which would only be likely to occur if the above symptoms or signs had not been recognised, or had been ignored, include:

- Arrhythmia - heartbeats that are too slow, fast, early or irregular.

- Tachycardia - are rapid arrhythmias, greater than 100 beats per minute.

- Fibrillations - irregular heart rhythm.

- Warm, moist, and smooth skin.

- Lid lag (von Graefe's sign) - when a patient tracks an object downward with their eyes, the eyelid fails to follow the downward moving iris.

- Staring eyes due to eyelid retraction (not to be confused with exophthalmos due to Graves' disease).

- Tremor or trembling - often of the hands.

- Muscle weakness.

In extreme and very rare cases, excess thyroid hormone can lead to a thyrotoxic crisis known as *a thyroid storm*. A thyrotoxic crisis can cause a sudden increase in body temperature (to over 104 degrees Fahrenheit, 40 degrees Celsius); heart abnormalities; vomiting; diarrhoea; dehydration, coma and even in some cases, death.

When the T3 dosage management process is followed carefully, it is extremely unlikely for any unusual, or adverse, effects to go unnoticed, long enough, for any serious symptoms or signs of thyrotoxicosis to occur.

I used a patient and cautious approach, during T3 dosage management, with only small, 2.5 microgram, or 5 microgram, increases in any single T3 divided dose, at any given time. Due to this approach, with safety foremost in my thoughts, I only ever experienced mild symptoms of excess T3, which were easily detected and corrected. If any symptoms or signs of tissue over-stimulation by T3 are detected, then the T3 dosage should be reduced immediately - typically to the dosage prior to the last increase that appeared to create the problem.

If my heart rate and body temperature are normal, no adverse symptoms or signs are present and I feel well, then I am extremely unlikely to be taking too much T3. However, symptoms and signs do need to be recorded and monitored. If I had not done this, I would not have been able to use the T3 dosage management process and T3 replacement therapy would not have been a viable option.

ELEVATED HEART RATE AND T3

I have included a small section entirely on this topic at the end of Chapter 21, in which I have listed some investigation possibilities that I have personally found to be valuable.

A SPECIAL CASE OF A T3 DOSAGE THAT IS TOO HIGH

In circumstances where one or more essential resources, e.g. nutrients or cortisol, are in scarce supply in the body, a too high divided dose of T3 may cause the rapid usage of the available resources and result in symptoms rather more like hypothyroidism than tissue over-stimulation. A frequent example is if cortisol is low and individual T3 doses are increased too quickly. In this case body temperature may fall rather than rise. This may often be avoided by lowering the peak levels of T3 within the tissues by the use of less T3 within each divided dose. Sometimes this might be accompanied by the addition of a further T3 dose so that enough T3 is provided but the scarce resource is not fully used up at any one time.

This is a special case of recognising a divided T3 dose that is too high but it needs to be borne in mind, as it may appear rather counterintuitive to lower a T3 dose when what is hoped for is an improvement in symptoms and signs.

Chapter 24

Phase 1: Clearing T4

By the time I was prescribed T3 thyroid hormone, it was very clear to me that T4 was nothing more than a hindrance. Consequently, in this first phase of the T3 dosage management process, I had to stop using T4 completely and, very carefully, begin to use T3 replacement therapy.

Why have this phase of clearing T4 at all prior to using T3? Why didn't I just stop using T4 and immediately start using T3? My concern was that any T3 taken could potentially cause the existing circulating T4 to be processed far more effectively, as a result of the T3 starting to raise my metabolic rate. This could potentially cause a rapid onset of severe symptoms of hyperthyroidism. With high levels of T4 still in my body, this created an unpredictable and possibly dangerous situation.

I felt that extreme caution and patience was required, to allow the T4 to clear, before I used anything other than small amounts of T3. I knew that one of the consequences of this was that my symptoms of hypothyroidism would remain, or might worsen, during this period. However, it was only around eight weeks to wait to allow most of the T4 to clear and I had been ill for so long I felt it was worth being cautious. The safe use of T3 was a clear goal that I had established and I was going to stick to it.

Remember, at this point I had already addressed my nutrition and was on a supplement regime. I had also begun a limited exercise regime.

ADRENAL STATUS AND THE USE OF ANY ADRENAL HORMONE MEDICATION

I had also assessed my adrenal status. One of the main problems that people experience when trying to use T3 is that the symptoms may be confusing and there may be a number of possible causes for these symptoms. I believed that the T3 dosage management process would be simpler to run if I were not taking adrenal hormones. Clearly, if I had been taking adrenal hormones and my doctor believed that my health would suffer if I attempted to wean these prior to applying the T3 dosage management process then I would have continued to use adrenal support at this stage.

However, if my doctor felt it was acceptable then I may have attempted to slowly wean the adrenal medication prior to applying the T3 dosage management process. If reducing the use of all adrenal hormones was not possible then it may have been possible to slowly wean them during Phase 2 of the T3 dosage management process.

Any patient with Addison's disease or other severe disorder that requires the taking of adrenal medication, in order to avoid life-threatening consequences, **must** continue with adrenal medication.

It is important that any changes to any medication or supplement are done under the **supervision of the patient's doctor.**

PHASE 1 PROCESS
This is the process I used:

STEP ONE - stop T4, wait, start with two divided doses of T3
- I stopped taking any T4 medication.

- I waited as long as I could before starting to take any T3, in order to let as much T4 clear as possible before introducing T3.

- The symptoms of hypothyroidism got progressively worse. When the symptoms were too difficult to cope with I began taking some T3.

My first T3 dosage consisted of 10 micrograms at 9:00 am and 10 micrograms at 4:00 pm. I knew that this initial dosage of T3 was going to be completely inadequate but it was important to ensure that there were no bad reactions to the medication. I remained on this low dose for several days, until my symptoms and signs indicated that I definitely required more T3 and I was confident that there were no symptoms of tissue over-stimulation.

STEP TWO - switch to four divided doses of T3
- I then switched to a T3 dosage that consisted of four divided doses of T3 per day, taken at: 8:00 am, 11:00 am, 2:00 pm and 5:00 pm.

I used four divided doses of T3 per day, as a starting point, to ensure that no single divided dose created a peak tissue level of T3 that caused any indication of tissue over-stimulation. If I had felt that three divided doses were more appropriate then I would have used 8:00 am, 11:00 am or 12 noon and 5: 00 pm.

- My new T3 dosage was: 10 micrograms at 8:00 am, 5 micrograms at 11:00 am, 5 micrograms at 2:00 pm and 5 micrograms at 5:00 pm, which provided a total of 25 micrograms of T3.

I had to break up a UK 20-microgram T3 tablet into halves and quarters to achieve this. This T3 dosage was also completely inadequate. This was expected but starting very cautiously was important. I have rarely found that 5 micrograms of T3 in a single dose was adequate but this was just a safe starting dosage.

- I began recording relevant symptoms and signs, in order to provide an accurate record of my T3 treatment and to help me solve any problems that arose. I recorded the date, the exact T3 dosage I was taking and the relevant symptoms/signs every day. In particular, symptoms and signs were recorded in between each T3 divided dose.

STEP THREE - increase T3 dosage only enough to cope during T4 clearance

- I increased one of the T3 doses by 2½ or 5 micrograms, every three to fourteen days, in order to make my symptoms more tolerable, whilst the T4 was clearing.

Initially, I concentrated on the first T3 dose of the day, until the symptoms were not as severe. My goal in this phase was **not** to eradicate my symptoms but to avoid being too uncomfortable.

I then did the same with the next divided dose of T3 and so on. I kept the timing of the individual divided doses the same, as I felt that it was not worth spending too much time fine-tuning it until the T4 had cleared at the end of the phase.

- I stayed in this phase of the dosage management process for eight weeks, which was enough time for the T4 to stabilise to the level produced by my own thyroid gland. Using only enough T3, taken in four divided doses, avoided the worst of the symptoms of hypothyroidism.

I did expect to continue to have symptoms of hypothyroidism during this phase. This was because I realised there was almost no possibility of identifying an adequate T3 dosage until the T4 had cleared. I only sought to raise my T3 dosage in order to overcome the symptoms that I simply did not want to cope with. It was also desirable to remain on a T3 dosage that was likely to be quite a lot lower than my final T3 dosage, in order to provide the next phase with the best starting conditions.

OBSERVATIONS ON FIRST PHASE OF T3 DOSAGE MANAGEMENT

The intent of this phase is simply to allow the T4 to clear. In order to do this some T3 replacement does need to be started to avoid causing even worse symptoms of hypothyroidism.

I tried to use two divided doses to begin with. However, I rapidly discovered that two divided doses required too much T3 in each dose and I had some symptoms of tissue over-stimulation. My heart rate was very slightly raised and my heart felt as if it was beating too hard. By using four divided doses this problem was removed completely. The number of divided doses may be fine-tuned during the next phase of the T3 dosage management process.

I did have a few minor adverse symptoms during this phase. I had a slight headache, which I refer to as my 'thyroxine headache'. I had a slight heart rate increase at times. I also found that the beneficial effects of T3 did not appear to last for very long to begin with. However, as the T4 cleared all of these effects disappeared and I was able to slowly increase my T3 dosage.

A T3 dosage of around 30 - 35 micrograms of T3 per day was all that was required to get me through the first six to eight week period, while I was waiting for the T4 to clear. Other people may need significantly more or less T3. However, I definitely did not feel fully well on this T3 dosage and I knew that I would require more T3. I was simply not prepared to take any chances. I knew that it was more important to do this correctly and safely, than to do it quickly.

It is important to remember that not all the T4 will clear during this phase of the T3 dosage management process. The exogenous T4 medication that a thyroid patient has been taking will clear. However, as long as a thyroid patient has some healthy thyroid tissue remaining and has a TSH that is not suppressed by T3 thyroid medication then some T4 will continue to be produced by the patient's own thyroid gland. A great deal of T4 will clear during this phase (possibly most of it) and as the T3 dosage is increased the patient's TSH will begin to be lowered, thus reducing any endogenous thyroid hormone production. During Phase 2 of the T3 dosage management process, as the ideal T3 dosage is carefully determined, more of the patient's own T4 (and consequently more reverse T3) will be cleared.

T3 was going to work!

By the end of this phase I had already concluded that T3 was actually going to work. I did have some symptoms of hypothyroidism remaining but I felt much better - far more like my old self. It was a wonderful feeling to realise that I had at last found a treatment that could allow me to be healthy once more.

Chapter 25

Phase 2: Determining a Safe,
Effective and Stable T3 Dosage

After eight weeks had passed, the majority of the synthetic T4 had cleared from my system. I turned my attention to the task of attempting to find a safe, effective and stable T3 replacement dosage - the second phase of the T3 dosage management process.

With most of the synthetic T4 cleared, a lot of things could be different. I was open-minded about whether I would require one, two, three or more divided doses. Some patients live perfectly happily on a single T3 dose per day and other patients require up to six T3 doses per day. I also knew that three to five divided doses were very commonly used.

When I began this phase, I thought about two approaches for setting the sizes of each T3 dose:

- **A level-dose strategy,** with each divided dose being the same size. I believed that it would be simpler to arrive at a T3 dosage like this but it would not be optimal. If I had wanted to use a level-dose strategy, then I would have changed all the T3 divided doses at the same time and restricted the size of each change to, perhaps, 2.5 micrograms. I really believe that this approach is far from ideal and I would never use it.

- **A tailored-dose strategy,** with each divided dose potentially being of a different size and located at the ideal time. I believed that the process of determining a T3 dosage that was tailored, although more complex, was more likely to be optimal. I felt, that it might allow me to discover the minimum number of divided doses that I could use and still feel well. This is clearly the best approach and the T3 dosage management process is based on this.

I decided to use a tailored-dose strategy. I have divided the process I used into a series of steps in order to help communicate it more clearly. I have included two versions:

- Detailed Phase 2 Process - this describes the complete process.

- Simplified Phase 2 Process - this is included immediately following the Phase 2 Process. This provides an overview of the Phase 2 process.

DETAILED PHASE 2 PROCESS

STEP ONE - assess starting T3 dosage

I was still taking four doses of T3 per day, at the following times: 8:00 am, 11:00 am, 2:00 pm and 5:00 pm.

I assessed my symptoms and signs, including body temperature, heart rate and blood pressure, throughout the day following the first T3 divided dose. I picked a day when I was going to be in the house and not highly active. I then recorded symptoms and signs every hour from the point I took the first T3 dose right through the day and evening.

This established an accurate record of body temperature, heart rate, blood pressure and other symptoms, which helped to assess the effectiveness of each T3 divided dose. I also wanted to be sure that the symptoms and signs showed evidence that the effectiveness of each T3 divided dose was declining prior to taking the T3 divided dose that followed it.

STEP TWO - adjust size of first T3 divided dose and times of subsequent doses

I slowly and carefully adjusted the size of the first T3 divided dose, to try and improve my symptoms and signs. My first dose of T3 was still being taken at 8:00 am. This first T3 divided dose needed to act as a 'platform' for the other doses. If my first T3 dose corrected my symptoms and signs, then I felt that it would be possible to maintain this state, with the subsequent T3 divided doses.

The process I used, to adjust the size of the first T3 divided dose, was:

a. I assessed my symptoms and signs, including body temperature, heart rate and blood pressure, to determine whether the first T3 divided dose was effective.

I made sure that I assessed symptoms and signs each hour that followed taking the T3 divided dose, collecting data right up until the next divided dose was taken. My goal was to have a sustained period, of at least a few hours, following the T3 dose, during which I felt totally well, with no tissue over-stimulation.

b. I then made a decision, on whether a change to the size of the divided dose, was necessary:

- Based on my symptoms and signs, if I clearly had no improvement at all, or my symptoms and signs indicated that I was still definitely hypothyroid, during the hours that followed taking the divided dose, then I knew that the divided dose was still far too low. In this case, the divided dose was **increased by 5 micrograms.**

- If my symptoms and signs indicated I still had some degree of hypothyroidism during the hours that followed taking the divided dose but it was less severe than it had been, then I knew I should be more cautious in the size of any further divided dose changes. In this case, the divided dose was **increased by only 2.5 micrograms,** to avoid overshooting the optimum dose. When I was close to the final dose size, I felt that 2.5 micrograms was the largest change that I could afford to make. 2.5 micrograms, is only one eighth, of a UK 20 microgram T3 tablet and is quite hard to split accurately. Changing a divided dose by more than this, when very close to the correct dose, would be foolhardy.

• Based on my symptoms and signs, if I appeared to have too much T3 in the divided dose, or symptoms of tissue over-stimulation in the hours that followed taking it, then the divided dose was **decreased by 2.5 or 5 micrograms,** depending on the scale of the problem.

• If there was any evidence of a very adverse change in heart rate, blood pressure, or any other symptoms or signs of tissue over-stimulation during the hours that followed taking the divided dose, then I immediately **reversed** the T3 dosage back to a previous T3 dosage that I knew had none of these problems.

• If I felt healthy and my symptoms and signs suggested that I was adequately replaced with T3 during the hours that followed taking this divided dose, then **no further change was required** to this divided dose.

c. Based on my symptoms and signs, I decided whether the time that I was taking the following T3 divided dose was correct or not.

It was important to have evidence that the T3 divided dose was 'running out of steam' and a further T3 divided dose was necessary before actually taking it. This was achieved by assessing symptoms and signs every hour, or even half an hour, when the next T3 divided dose was due. However, I did not actually take the next divided dose until I was sure that it was required. It is essential to only take T3 divided doses when the body requires them. The taking of the following T3 divided dose should be delayed until enough information is collected to be sure that an appropriate time can be identified to take it.

So for instance, if I was adjusting the **size** of my first T3 dose, which was being taken at, say 8:00 am, then I would not take my second T3 dose until I was confident that it was needed. For example, if by 11:30 am I began to feel slightly tired, with a lower body temperature and I was sure that the symptoms and signs indicated my T3 was low at this point, I would take my second T3 dose immediately (11:30 am). However, thereafter I would take my second T3 dose either half an hour or one hour earlier to avoid ever feeling any symptoms of low thyroid levels. Consequently, I would adjust the time of my second T3 dose to 10:30

am or 11:00 am, so that I felt healthy throughout the first and second dose periods without any 'dip' in symptoms or signs.

If the time of the T3 divided dose that follows the first one is altered, then the subsequent T3 divided doses should have their timings adjusted so as to maintain the intervals between them for the moment (until each of them is adjusted in turn).

d.   After each single alteration of the first T3 divided dose size and any subsequent timing adjustments had been made, I then waited between **three and fourteen days,** to allow this T3 dosage change to take effect, before any further changes were made. Whether this was three days or longer depended on whether the effect of the dosage change had stabilised. If changes in my symptoms or signs were still occurring then I waited for up to fourteen days. There was little point in making further changes, until symptoms and signs had completely adjusted.

e.   I repeated stages 'a' to 'd', until the first T3 divided dose appeared to be optimised in size and the timings of the subsequent T3 divided doses that followed it were also adjusted. In particular, the time that the second T3 divided dose would have been accurately adjusted. Then I proceeded to step three.

STEP THREE - adjust sizes of second through last T3 divided doses and the times of subsequent doses

At this point I had established a reasonable size for the first T3 divided dose. I had also adjusted the timing of the second T3 divided dose and made the same timing adjustments to the subsequent T3 divided doses.

I simply applied the same process outlined in step two to adjust the size of the second T3 divided dose and the timings of the subsequent divided doses. I used symptoms and signs to assess the size of the second T3 divided dose and to determine when the third T3 divided dose should be taken.

Using this process, it is possible, one by one, to adjust the size of each of the T3 divided doses and to adjust the time to take the following T3 divided doses. Remember it is essential to only take each T3 divided dose when symptoms and signs indicate that it is required.

By taking only sufficient T3 to feel well and only taking a T3 divided dose when it is absolutely required is it possible to avoid any tissue over-stimulation by thyroid hormone.

STEP FOUR - assess removal or addition of a T3 divided dose

After the previous step was complete then three possibilities will occur regarding the timing of the last T3 divided dose:

- Symptoms and signs may indicate that there is enough T3 to feel healthy for the rest of the day. In this case, **nothing further is required** and step five may be performed.

- The last T3 dose may now be too late in the evening and causing issues with symptoms and signs during the evening or night, which may include difficulties in getting to sleep. In this case, it is important to consider **removing** this last T3 divided dose completely.

- The last T3 dose may now be earlier than it was and may not be sufficient to ensure that symptoms and signs remain healthy throughout the rest of the day. In this case, it is important to consider **adding** a new divided dose at an appropriate time after the current last dose of T3. Any additional T3 divided dose will have to have its size and timing adjusted.

STEP FIVE - optimise T3 dosage as much as possible

I repeated steps two, three and four as many times as I needed to all the T3 divided doses (from the first to the last).

This is necessary for several reasons. Firstly, the assessment of individual divided dose sizes and timings may not be completely ideal. Secondly, as each divided dose is adjusted in size or timing it may have an overall impact on the body that makes it necessary to fine-tune the other T3 divided doses.

This process is fundamentally iterative and needs to be repeated a number of times until no T3 divided dose requires changing in size or timing. The T3 dosage must be optimised as much as possible before proceeding to the next step.

STEP SIX - gather more information through laboratory tests

I now asked my doctor to test for the following: a test for low cortisol (twenty-four hour adrenal saliva test or twenty-four hour urinary cortisol), TSH, FT4 and FT3. Other tests that could be done at this stage are: total and free testosterone (sex hormones for males), oestrogen and progesterone (sex hormones for females).

The reasons behind these tests were:

- Twenty-four hour adrenal saliva or twenty-four hour urinary cortisol: This was a useful test at this point. I wanted to assess how my adrenals were responding and whether I needed to make any T3 dosage adjustment, in order to help my adrenals produce more cortisol. I relied primarily on how I was feeling and what my symptoms were when making any final decision over whether I had adrenal insufficiency or not.

- TSH: This was not used to determine how much T3 I should be taking. I just wanted to monitor my TSH to ensure that nothing highly unusual was occurring that could suggest a pituitary problem.

- FT3: This was also not used to determine my T3 dosage. However, if the symptoms and signs suggested that I was under-replaced and my FT3 levels were not at the top of the laboratory reference range, then this may have helped to confirm these suspicions, even though I knew that the FT3 level was subject to fluctuations.

- FT4: I expected my FT4 level to be very low, as the only T4 left in my system would, perhaps, be a small amount, produced by any residual thyroid function. This result would be interesting if it was higher than expected, which would alert me to potential endocrine issues, or if it had dropped significantly, alerting me to my failing thyroid gland.

- Testosterone and free testosterone (oestrogen and progesterone for women, although I have done no specific research relating to how T3 might affect oestrogen and progesterone): potentially these may be adjusted also, via moving the first divided dose of T3 into the main cortisol production window. It is low cortisol that is the main focus of this step. Therefore, it is not essential to test for sex hormones unless there is a specific concern.

Further evidence that may also suggest low cortisol levels also include a body temperature that does not rise in response to T3 and a rapid heart rate. These signs may be indicative of other conditions but I have already discussed the way in which cortisol may affect the body in other chapters including Chapter 3, Chapter 5 and Chapter 16.

If my symptoms and signs, including the cortisol test result, indicated that cortisol levels were healthy then I would have skipped step seven and proceeded directly to step eight.

My cortisol was low so I proceeded to step seven.

STEP SEVEN - apply the Circadian T3 Method (CT3M) and then finalise sizes and times of subsequent doses
This step is optional and should **not** be performed if:
- Symptoms and signs and any cortisol testing suggest that cortisol levels are already normal.
- If the adrenal glands will not respond directly to the availability of more T3. Conditions that might mean the adrenal glands cannot respond include Addison's disease and hypopituitarism. Although the CT3M will not do any harm - it just wouldn't help.
- In either of these circumstances I would have taken my first dose no earlier than 8:00 am (the time that I woke up from sleep).

It is desirable to encourage the adrenal glands to work as normally as they are able to. This step is aimed at trying to improve the performance of the adrenal glands as much as possible by providing them with the T3 they need to do their job in producing hormones like cortisol and aldosterone.

I did not apply the Circadian T3 Method and adjust the timing of the first dose of T3, until my total daily T3 dosage was close to being optimised. **If I had been aware that my adrenal hormone levels were far from optimal then I would have applied Step Six and Step Seven and used the Circadian T3 Method a lot earlier and before my T3 dosage was optimal.** The decision to apply Steps six and seven earlier would need to be made on an individual basis and based on many symptoms and signs and the actual progress of T3 replacement therapy.

The references to the 4:00 am to 8:00 am main cortisol production window in Step Seven assume that someone wakes up around 8:00 am in the morning. For someone who wakes up later or earlier then these times need to be adjusted. The Circadian T3 Method was described in Chapter 16. This is how I used it in detail to adjust the timing of the first T3 dose of the day:

- Symptoms and the cortisol testing results were reviewed. If these results suggested the need for more adrenal output, then I moved my first T3 dose of the day back into the main cortisol production window, to 6:30 am initially - a <u>move back by one and a half hours</u>.

- I waited to see if this resulted in any improvements in symptoms and signs. Particular attention should be paid to blood pressure as improved adrenal function can raise blood pressure. It was important to be patient at this stage, because cortisol levels can take several weeks to fully adjust, even though some benefits may be detectable within days. I found that my cortisol levels did not stabilise until about six weeks had passed. I did not wait for six weeks in between each timing change but I did allow several days and then longer when I was fine-tuning. This stage of the T3 dosage management process can take a while.

- During the preparation stage for the T3 dosage management process my doctor and I would have needed to make a decision about whether I should wean down any adrenal support prior to starting. **If the decision had been taken to leave me on adrenal support during this process, then it may have been possible to gradually wean down the adrenal support during this Step Seven (applying the Circadian T3 Method) with my doctor's approval.** For this to have worked properly then there would need to be some weaning of the adrenal support in advance of any first T3 dose change to ensure that the adrenal glands had demand placed upon them via pituitary ACTH. This weaning may take a long time and must be **done slowly**. In some cases it may take six to twelve months or longer to fully wean adrenal medication. In a few cases complete weaning may never be possible.

- If I had been on any adrenal medication such as hydrocortisone or adrenal glandulars then I would **not** have taken any of these with my first (circadian) dose of T3, because adrenal medication would tend to suppress the natural production of adrenal hormones.

- The timing of the first T3 dose of the day continued to be adjusted, by taking it half an hour earlier, gradually getting closer to 4:00 am. I monitored symptoms and signs throughout this process and took care not to make too early a judgement because of the time it takes for the adrenals to adjust. A change of **half an hour** can significantly change cortisol levels.

- If, **after adjusting the timing of the first dose**, between the hours of 4:00 am and 8:00 am, I failed to notice any satisfactory improvements, I may have **increased the size of the first dose of T3 (or decreased it if I thought it was too high)**. In this case, I may have **moved the time of the first dose forward** (possibly as far as one and a half hours before getting up - 6:30 am) to avoid causing the adrenals to produce too much cortisol. The process of **adjusting the first dose timing** would then be repeated.

- The typical range of the T3 required to successfully apply the CT3M is between 10 and 30 micrograms, with 15 to 25 micrograms being more common.

- If necessary, I made timing and possibly size adjustments to all the other T3 doses, i.e. I used the process outlined in the previous steps as many times as I needed to. Changing levels of other hormones, like cortisol, may affect the way T3 acts and so, it is important to fine-tune the T3 dosage, in order to meet the goal of it being safe, effective and stable. In particular it is likely that all the other T3 divided doses may become more effective at this point as natural levels of adrenal hormones may be produced with the consequent positive effect on ATP production.

- When I felt that my T3 dosage was optimised, I went back to my family doctor and requested another cortisol test (and optionally a sex hormone blood test). It is very important to actually assess cortisol levels through a laboratory test and not attempt to guess whether the cortisol output is adequate or not simply based on symptoms alone. Symptomatic assessment of cortisol levels can be very misleading. If aldosterone had also been a concern then this would have needed testing.

- I repeated this step until my T3 dosage was stable.

- If adjusting the first T3 divided dose cannot adequately regulate cortisol then I would have needed to work with my doctor to consider some form of adrenal support.

- I was able to fine-tune my first T3 dose of the day and I managed to establish adequate levels of cortisol without the need for any additional medication. Once I had established a working T3 dosage, cortisol testing was repeated to determine if I still had cortisol insufficiency.

STEP EIGHT - fine-tune the T3 dosage

Several repetitions of steps two through seven may be needed. Eventually, when I felt that my T3 dosage had stabilised, I moved into the long-term monitoring phase - Phase Three.

STEP NINE - optionally add some T4 back in to tolerance

As discussed in Chapter 11, T3 may be safely and effectively used as a long-term thyroid hormone replacement. I have seen no compelling evidence that the T4 thyroid hormone needs to be present in the body. Future research may change my opinion on this but for the moment this appears to be the case. The important thing to remember is that thyroid patients who resort to using T3 replacement therapy have usually remained very ill whilst on T4 based treatments. Consequently, using T3 replacement is the only option for some patients to fully regain their health.

This step is only included here for completeness as I can see no compelling reason to use T4 at all. However, for any readers who would not feel comfortable without using some small amount of T4 then this process Step Nine has been specifically included to provide this option.

This process step is **optional,** as some thyroid patients simply cannot tolerate any T4:

- Once the T3 dosage has been determined it is possible to add T4 back and find out how much can be tolerated.

- I would not suggest doing this until the T3 dosage has been completely fine-tuned, which in many cases will take many months and possibly even a year. There is no point adding in T4 and creating another variable until the T3 dosage is very stable.

- Start dose of T4 would be of the order of 12.5 micrograms (to be discussed with the patient's doctor).

- Every 6-8 weeks add 12.5 micrograms to this daily dose.

- Check symptoms and signs and determine how much T4, if any, can be tolerated.

- There may be a need to re-tune the T3 dosage.

SIMPLIFIED PHASE 2 PROCESS

- **Step One** - Assess Starting T3 Dosage. Starting T3 dosage was being taken at: 8:00 am, 11:00 am, 2:00 pm and 5:00 pm. Assess symptoms and signs.

- **Step Two** - Adjust size of first T3 divided dose and times of subsequent doses.
  Determine whether to increase, decrease or leave the first divided dose unchanged. Use small dose size changes. After the first T3 divided dose has been changed then accurately adjust the time that immediately subsequent T3 divided dose (second dose) is being taken. Then make similar timing changes to the T3 divided doses that follow (third to last doses). T3 divided doses may be taken earlier, later or left unchanged. The correct timing of T3 doses is just as important as their sizes if you want to ensure that T3 is being used effectively and safely.

- **Step Three** - Adjust sizes of second through last T3 divided doses and the times of subsequent doses. Use the method outlined in step two and apply it to each of the other T3 divided doses (second to the last).

- **Step Four** - Assess removal or addition of a T3 divided dose.
  As a result of timing changes in the previous steps there may now be too many or too few divided doses. Add or remove one if necessary.

- **Step Five** - Optimise T3 dosage as much as possible.
  Repeat steps two to four as many times as necessary. Note: if it is clear that low cortisol or poor adrenal function is impacting T3 replacement therapy then Steps Six and Seven could be applied earlier in the process and before the T3 dosage is close to ideal.

- **Step Six** - Gather more information through laboratory tests.
  Need to decide if cortisol is low. If cortisol is low then do step seven. If cortisol is healthy, or this step is not possible then proceed to step eight.

- **Step Seven** - Apply the Circadian T3 Method to attempt to regulate cortisol and other adrenal hormones. This is followed by fine-tuning the timing and sizes of T3 divided doses. For a patient on adrenal medication then the weaning of this may be possible during this step. If this cannot regulate adrenal hormones then some adrenal support may be required.

- **Step Eight** - Fine-tune the T3 dosage. Repeat steps two to seven as many times as necessary to yield a safe, effective and stable T3 dosage.

- **Step Nine** - Optionally add some T4 back in to tolerance. This step is definitely not required but is present for those that believe they may get some benefit from adding a small amount of T4 back in. This should not be attempted until the T3 dosage has been completely fine-tuned and has been stable for a long time (several months at least).

OBSERVATIONS ON SECOND PHASE OF T3 DOSAGE MANAGEMENT

I have quite a few observations and I will group them into some relevant areas.

Tracking Symptoms and Signs

It is imperative that any indications of tissue over-stimulation are detected quickly. In the absence of useful blood test results, symptoms and signs have to be tracked carefully and frequently during this phase. Sometimes, this might involve tracking these multiple times during the day.

By tracking body temperature, heart rate, blood pressure and symptoms regularly and only adjusting one divided dose at a time by a small amount, this protected me from any significant adverse effects. If I did raise a T3 divided dose by too much, then it was quite obvious that this had happened, because I was monitoring symptoms and signs, which included heart rate, blood pressure, body temperature and any appearance of anxiety, stress or hyperactivity.

It can be very valuable to track symptoms and signs every hour following a divided dose of T3. In particular, recording of these one or two hours following a T3 dose and also when the next T3 dose is due to be taken will allow the assessment of whether a T3 dose has been effective and when it begins to 'run out of steam'. This will enable the following dose of T3 to only be taken when the effectiveness of the prior dose is declining. In this way each divided dose of T3 will not be taken before it is required (which can cause problems).

So, by tracking symptoms and signs carefully it is possible to not only assess the size of the divided dose that is being focused on but it also allows the review of the timing of the following divided dose. It is by having this level of information that the timing of T3 divided doses may be adjusted to their optimal timings. **The intent is to only take a T3 divided dose when it is needed and not before. This is the way to achieve the minimum amount of T3 for good health with no T3 divided dose causing any symptoms or signs of tissue over-stimulation.** If the following dose timing is adjusted then any further divided dose timings should also be adjusted to maintain the current intervals between subsequent doses. If, as a result of this process the subsequent doses are being taken later in time then it is possible that the last divided dose may be omitted completely, if it is determined that it is too late to take it. **In this way the numbers of divided doses may be reduced during this phase.** Of course, if the divided doses need to be taken closer together then this may necessitate taking one or more additional divided doses rather than a reduction.

If time is limited then recording symptoms and signs mid-way between each T3 divided dose may often be adequate. For a thorough assessment, which will certainly be needed when fine-tuning of T3 dosage is in progress, hourly recordings are far more useful at revealing the effectiveness of T3 divided doses and how long this effect is sustained for.

Symptoms and signs need to be reviewed as a whole in order to understand what is happening. I found that it was important to look for indications of when a T3 divided dose was starting to be less effective and that another T3 divided dose was due. Temperature will often lower a little. Heart rate may be more difficult to read. Heart rate may change but sometimes heart rate rises due to the strain on the heart of operating with too little T3 but some people heart rate will lower a little when another T3 dose is due. Blood pressure needs to be tracked as a matter of safety but it is unusual for BP alone to provide a subtle indication of a dose being due. The use of symptoms is as important as the signs. It is subtle process. Once I had 'tuned-in' to my body I found this to be quite an easy process, although it did take a little practice.

Divided Doses

When making a change to a divided dose, I tried to **alter only one divided dose at a time**, in order to keep things simple and avoid any confusion. Therefore, when making changes **I would only change the amount of T3 I took in an individual dose or the time I took it**. This approach enabled me to clearly understand what was happening.

I experimented by only taking one or two doses of T3 per day but was not able to tolerate a large enough dose of T3 to make either work. Everyone is different and one or two divided doses may work for some people. However, I was able to reduce my number of divided doses from four to three during this phase of the T3 dosage management process.

The longest interval without taking any T3 precedes the first T3 divided dose. Consequently, the first T3 divided dose is less affected by previous doses of T3 than any other T3 divided dose. The first T3 divided dose must to a certain extent 'stand alone' and be capable of normalising the metabolism. This is why I often state that my first T3 divided dose has to provide a 'kick-start' at the beginning of the day.

It is essential to only take just enough T3 in any divided dose. However, **the adjustment of the time that each T3 divided dose is taken is as important as the titration of the divided dose size. Taking divided doses of T3 at the latest point possible following the preceding T3 divided dose is crucial to avoid tissue over-stimulation.** The focus on identifying the best T3 divided dose timing is just as critical part of this process.

When fine-tuning is being done small changes in T3 dose size will be required to achieve an ideal T3 dosage. **This will require the use of 5-microgram and 2.5-microgram T3 dose size changes.**

Adrenal Function

I can't stress enough how useful it was to optimise my cortisol level, by applying the Circadian T3 Method. As simple as changing the timing of my first dose of T3 and placing it within the main cortisol production window sounds, it took me nearly three years to realise that this was possible.

Low levels of cortisol can reduce the effectiveness of T3 as a result of limiting cellular energy production. However, it is also important for our health not to have too much cortisol. Therefore, it is very important to only consider taking the first T3 divided dose within the main cortisol production window if there is sound evidence that cortisol levels are low.

It is critical to be aware that some people cannot manage without taking their adrenal hormones. For people with Addison's disease or other conditions that dramatically affect the capability of the adrenal glands there is simply no option but to take adrenal hormones. Hypopituitarism is another condition for which adrenal hormones have to be taken.

It is also important to realise how many hormones the adrenal glands produce. Far more hormones are produced than just cortisol, DHEA, adrenaline and aldosterone. So many hormones are produced by the adrenal glands and the optimal way to achieve good health is to encourage the adrenal glands to work normally rather than compensate for them by taking adrenal hormones. **The Circadian T3 Method can promote better function of the adrenal glands and help to produce more cortisol, aldosterone and the many other adrenal hormones. The CT3M is not just about improved cortisol production.** Many patients I have spoken to that have applied the Circadian T3 Method have improved their adrenal function and have addressed low cortisol and low aldosterone symptoms. In many cases this amazingly simple Circadian T3 Method has allowed patients to <u>slowly</u> wean themselves from the use of adrenal medications under the guidance of their doctor.

There are many articles available on the Internet that discuss the merits of providing low levels of adrenal hormones for a short while during thyroid hormone treatment. These articles invariably state that this should only be done for a short period of time and then, once the thyroid hormone treatment is working, the adrenal hormones should slowly be reduced then stopped. However, many patients appear to still be on adrenal hormones after several years have passed by. I suspect that in at least some of these cases the adrenal insufficiency is due to hypothyroidism and that adequate T3 to the adrenal glands when they are working at their hardest may be of value (the Circadian T3 Method).

If I had been on adrenal hormones when I began to apply the Circadian T3 Method and my doctor had advised me not to wean them before applying the CT3M then, with my doctor's approval, I may have tried to **slowly wean** (reduce) these adrenal hormones during Step 7, when the Circadian T3 Method was applied. At the very least it may have been possible to reduce the amount of adrenal support that I required. In this case then some reduction of adrenal support might have needed to be done at various times when the Circadian T3 Method was being applied in order to ensure that enough demand was being placed on the adrenal glands. It is possible that the weaning of adrenal hormones may take many months for thyroid patients who have been using these for a long time. In some cases it may take six to twelve months or longer for adrenal function to return to an adequate level for all the adrenal medication to be safely removed. In some cases complete weaning may not be possible. Thyroid patients should work closely with their own doctor during the weaning process.

Once a decision has been taken to move the first T3 divided dose within the main cortisol production window, I found it critical to do this with extreme care. After the initial move of the first T3 divided dose to 6:30 am (one and half hours before I got up on a morning) then movements of half an hour at the most should only be used when a change is made. After any timing change, it is important to allow at least several days and ideally a week or more to elapse to fully understand if a change is effective or not prior to any further change.

The effect of more adrenal hormones being produced may be to increase the apparent potency of the T3, however, this is probably just as a result of more cellular energy being produced. It may require the reduction in the size of T3 divided doses or timing changes to avoid tissue over-stimulation.

It is very important to use a twenty-four hour adrenal saliva test or a twenty-four hour urinary cortisol laboratory test to gain an informative and accurate assessment of cortisol levels during the process of using the Circadian T3 Method. This is because it is very easy to be misled by symptoms alone and an inappropriate first T3 divided dose may be selected. A laboratory test of cortisol will take much of the guesswork out of this process and potentially save a considerable amount of time and stress.

If I had still had some adrenal insufficiency after having adjusted my first T3 dose then I may have needed to use of some form of adrenal support at this stage. Fortunately, I did not require any adrenal support at all.

I am not against the use of any form of appropriate adrenal support when it is essential to provide it. **If at any time during the T3 dosage management process it becomes obvious that the entire process is being undermined because of low cortisol levels then clearly the patient and their doctor should consider the use of adrenal support.**

First T3 Divided Dose Titration Options in the Circadian T3 Method

I have already discussed this in Chapter 16 but it is worth mentioning again. If a patient's doctor decides that the Circadian T3 Method should be tried then there are a number of things to consider.

Patients who have had good experiences using the Circadian T3 Method have kindly provided much of this information to me and I thank them for this.

The Phase 2 Process provides an overall framework. However, life can be a little more confusing and complex. Sometimes, symptoms of adrenal insufficiency may be present when the first T3 divided dose is too early, too late, too low or too high. For some people the first T3 divided dose needs to be perfectly titrated in order to avoid symptoms of adrenal insufficiency.

This is especially true for those people who have been severely hypothyroid for a long time and have weakened adrenal glands.

Being very systematic and carefully exploring all the possible options with the first T3 divided dose is very important. Adjusting the timing of the first T3 divided dose through the entire main cortisol production window may be required. If this is done then several days will need to be allowed to elapse after each change in order to evaluate it. A timing change of half an hour or one hour to the first T3 dose may be sufficient in some cases to alleviate symptoms of adrenal insufficiency but sometimes the symptoms may not go away until the first T3 dose has been moved by a few hours within the main cortisol production window.

If, after all timing options have been explored, symptoms of adrenal insufficiency are still present then these timing options may need to be explored once again with either a higher or lower first T3 divided dose.

Many patients simply need a higher first T3 divided dose in order to improve. However, it is also clear from feedback that some people simply cannot cope with too much T3 in the first divided dose and they do better with a reduction in the size of the first T3 dose.

Typical dose sizes for this circadian T3 dose are between 15 and 25 micrograms of T3 but some people do well with only 10 micrograms and some require more than 25 micrograms. It is important that no adrenal hormones are taken with the circadian dose in order to allow the adrenal glands to have the best opportunity to produce their hormones naturally.

As I have stated elsewhere, some people simply cannot resolve their adrenal issues with T3 alone and have to use some form of adrenal support. However, it does appear that the Circadian T3 Method is helpful in reducing the need for this in some people.

Patience

The full effect of T3, may take many days and even weeks to occur. Enough time must be allowed after a T3 divided dose change before any further changes are made. Patience is very important. If changes are made too quickly, while there is still some underlying adjustment occurring, this will result in extreme confusion. A slow, methodical and systematic process is required and symptoms and signs need to be carefully monitored and logged. If the situation still remains confusing, then some laboratory tests should be carried out, in order to gather more data.

Within the cells of the body, there are a myriad of chemical processes that have to adjust to any new thyroid hormone dosage. When thyroid hormone levels change, the entities responsible for these processes may have to adjust their own scale of operation, in order to cope. This is a chemical and biological adjustment and it may not be instantaneous. A simple example illustrates this. One of my referenced texts explains how thyroid hormones are responsible for increasing the number and activity of the mitochondria within the cells. One of the consequences of hypothyroidism is that the number and activity of the mitochondria diminishes.[1]

Even when a correct T3 replacement dosage has been determined, it may take some time before the mitochondria recover. I believe it's important to continue to do regular exercise, to eat well and to take adequate nutritional supplements. Regaining full health may take some time, after a prolonged period of hypothyroidism. It may have taken a long time to get ill and it may take some time to get well again.

Detective Work

Inevitably, there have been times when confusing symptoms have occurred. I found that it was important to remain calm and objective in these situations and carefully consider what might be causing the problem. The fastest way to resolve issues is to plan a logical approach to dosage adjustments and to systematically try out different T3 dosages, in order to find the optimum strategy.

The biologically active T3 thyroid hormone has a profound effect on many other hormones and systems in the body. Confusing symptoms can arise, as a result of an incorrect T3 dosage that is affecting one or more other hormones. Understanding how the endocrine hormones work and what their effects might be, if they are too high or too low, will help in understanding situations like this. So, doing some studying is a very worthwhile exercise.

Some problems might not be straightforward. This may sometimes take days to work out and a lot of experiments may have to be done in order to understand what is actually going on. Whenever I struggled to make sense of symptoms or signs, it was better to put my dosage back to a previously more stable dosage.

As I approached my optimum daily dosage, the changes to my regime became far less frequent. Any remaining dose adjustments needed to be very small. A typical change at this stage might have only involved adding or reducing a dose by one eighth of a 20-microgram T3 tablet (2.5 micrograms).

Patience is essential to using T3 effectively and, more often than not, it is actually the fastest way to determine a safe, effective and stable T3 dosage. With the T3 thyroid hormone it is important to be the tortoise not the hare.

Timescales

It took me around three years to arrive at the T3 dosage that fully restored my health but most of this time was wasted because I had not realised I could regulate cortisol using T3. If I had known about that at the start then I would have expected to have taken between three and six months to reach a fine-tuned T3 dosage but only two to three months to feel quite healthy. These latter estimates appear to be reasonably consistent with the experience of other people and are certainly not longer than it takes with T4. However, the T3 dosage management process requires a great deal of work in order to deliver good results.

T3 Dosage Management and Patients who have had Thyroid Cancer

Patients who have had their thyroids removed after thyroid cancer and are placed on thyroid hormone replacement must take the advice of their own medical professionals where dosage management is concerned.

Once the thyroid cancer has been treated as effectively as it can be (often by surgery and/or radioactive iodine) then thyroid hormone replacement commences. This treatment will usually start with T4 and the patient's doctor will be trying to keep the TSH as suppressed as can be tolerated by the patient, with most doctors trying to get the TSH well below 1.0. I am told that most doctors treating thyroid cancer patients prefer to see TSH values as low as 0.1 or less if the patient has tolerated the thyroid hormone well. The idea behind this is that by totally suppressing TSH this will reduce the possibility of stimulating any cancer cells, should any unfortunately remain.

Occasionally, a thyroid cancer patient does not do well on T4 or T4/T3 and may require T3 replacement. Consequently, the T3 dosage management process described in this book may not be ideally suited to the requirement to fully suppress TSH.

It is very important for any thyroid cancer patient who is prescribed T3 treatment that they work closely with their doctor. The T3 dosage management process defined in this book is designed to find the absolute minimum amount of T3 that is required to be effective. The consequence of this is that for some people this may not result in a suppressed TSH (as this is not a goal of the process). Consequently, a patient recovering from thyroid cancer should work with their doctor to ensure that they are doing everything that is necessary to ensure that their health is as good as it can possibly be. This may mean ignoring elements of this T3 dosage management process in order to comply with medical advice regarding the optimal recovery from thyroid cancer. Clearly, TSH will be a driving factor in adjusting the T3 dosage for a patient who has had thyroid cancer.

Chapter 26

Phase 3: Long-Term Monitoring

Once a safe, effective and stable T3 dosage has been established, it will occasionally need to be changed. Our need for thyroid hormone sometimes changes over time. Patients that require thyroid hormone replacement need to make adjustments to cope with these changing needs, because their own thyroid glands can no longer do this for them automatically. I have Hashimoto's thyroiditis and I fully expected some further deterioration of my thyroid gland, which would potentially need a T3 dosage change.

I have been in this long-tem monitoring phase for well over ten years now. The T3 dosage that I established rarely requires adjustment and I have never had any nasty surprises whilst being on this treatment. In the past two years, as my thyroid gland has almost stopped producing any T4, I have had to adjust my T3 dosage a little more frequently.

PHASE 3 PROCESS

This process is simple and may be communicated with a few simple guidelines.

ONLY MAKE VERY SMALL CHANGES

If I have any cause to modify my T3 dosage during this phase then I use the process defined in the previous chapter. However, any changes now are only very small and occur infrequently. This applies to the number of T3 divided doses, individual divided dose sizes as well as timing changes.

Any dose size adjustments are limited to 2.5 micrograms and timing adjustments to plus or minus 30 minutes.

I allow plenty of time after a change to assess it, prior to any further adjustment - a minimum of two weeks is fairly typical, unless the change was obviously bad, in which case, I just reverse it.

As the optimal T3 dosage is approached, small T3 dosage changes can have a significant effect after several weeks have passed as the dosage change can affect various physiological systems and take some time to fully occur. Consequently, even an increase of 2.5 micrograms per day may take a month or two to fully evaluate when the T3 dosage is close to being ideal.

CONTINUE TO USE SYMPTOMS AND SIGNS

Throughout this long-term monitoring phase I have continued to assess symptoms and signs, as a means of determining whether the T3 dosage I was taking was still ideal. However, as time went on I found that I became far more aware of how my body was responding and it became increasingly straightforward to monitor the symptoms and signs that I have described. I have become 'tuned-in' to how my system is behaving and I am now highly sensitive to any changes in how I am feeling. This has made the on-going assessment of symptoms and signs incredibly easy to do. It has become intuitive.

During this phase if there were a downturn in how I felt, I would re-start recording my T3 dosage, symptoms and signs. The recording of all of this information has been extraordinarily useful and I have gone back and reviewed all of my records on several occasions.

The laboratory tests that my doctor does occasionally have already been listed but I always ensure that I ask my family doctor to check my heart and blood pressure from time to time.

It is also important for thyroid patients, regardless of the type of thyroid hormone replacement they are using, to have a bone density scan every few years, to ensure that no bone loss is occurring. If there were any noticeable bone loss, then action would need to be taken to prevent the situation from worsening.

I have no heart or bone loss issues as far as I am aware. I do continue to have my thyroid blood tests done occasionally, which includes having my thyroid autoantibodies checked. The autoantibodies show whether the autoimmune response remains quiescent and the FT4 level provides an indication of how much thyroid function I have remaining. These are useful because they provide an indication of whether my T3 dosage is likely to remain stable. Thyroid blood tests remain unhelpful in providing any insight into what T3 dosage I should be using.

I have also never had any problems with low cortisol or adrenal issues since using a divided dose of T3 in the main cortisol production window. Clearly, my adrenal glands were healthy and just required the right environment to function correctly.

KEEP DOING EXERCISE AND MAINTAIN NUTRITIONAL REGIME

I continued to do regular exercise and have increased this as time has gone by, even though I am now older. It is important to do some form of regular exercise, as failing to exercise may make thyroid replacement therapy less effective.

I have also maintained a supplementation regime, which I feel has helped to avoid any nutrient deficiencies, which may have compromised the T3 replacement therapy.

ADDING IN SOME T4

As soon as I saw that my autoantibody levels had dropped in 2006, I attempted to try T4 replacement once again, just in case this change in circumstances had made any difference to the effectiveness of T4. Unfortunately, T4 replacement continues to quickly produce the symptoms of hypothyroidism.

However, it is now clear that my thyroid gland is producing almost no T4. A recent very low FT4 result of 0.3 pmol/L (reference range 9.0–25 pmol/L) suggests that my thyroid gland is almost completely dead now.

This prompted me once more recently to try to see if a small amount of T4 produced any benefit. I now appear to be able to tolerate 12.5 micrograms of T4 quite easily and have the option to take this daily if I feel that it is beneficial (which I do not as yet). Whether this change in tolerance is due to the fact that my Hashimoto's autoantibodies have now fallen to zero or the fact that my own thyroid gland is producing less T4 of its own I do not know.

The T3 dosage management process allows for the optional addition of T4 to tolerance once the ideal T3 dosage has been determined. The variation in the type and severity of cellular level problems with thyroid hormone between individual patients may mean that some patients will be able to add some T4 back to their overall regime without any difficulty.

DIVIDED DOSES

Over the years, as my thyroid has atrophied, occasional changes have been made to my T3 dosage. In the past several years, each T3 divided dose appears to have a slightly longer lasting effect. Consequently, the intervals between each divided dose has increased slightly. I have had to use symptoms and signs to determine that my T3 divided doses were actually sustaining me for a longer period of time. This experience emphasises the importance of knowing whether an individual's thyroid condition is autoimmune or not, i.e. whether on-going deterioration of the thyroid gland should be expected.

T3 DOSAGE WILL NOT REMAIN THE SAME OVER THE YEARS

Once I had my T3 dosage finalised it did not remain completely stable. How could it? The human body has different needs at different times in your life. As I have got older several changes have occurred. I have become healthier as I have completely recovered from the damage that was done by so many years of hypothyroidism. I have also fine-tuned my vitamin and mineral supplements and this has helped me significantly.

As I complete this book I am in the process of re-evaluating the various times that I take my T3 divided doses, as each divided dose that I take appears to remain effective for longer than in the past. I am not sure whether improved adrenal health, nutritional improvements or lower thyroid autoantibodies may have contributed to the apparent extended effect of the T3.

Any adjustments I make will only be to one divided dose at a time with adequate time allowed for a systematic assessment of symptoms and signs. Any timing change of my first T3 divided dose will of course be no more than a half an hour at any one time, as even this small adjustment can have a profound impact on the level of adrenal hormones produced. I have discovered that I need less in my first T3 divided dose and at a slightly later time. The most likely reason for this is that my adrenal health is now better than it was in the past.

Chapter 27

Conclusions on T3 Dosage Management

I was slow to take responsibility for my own health and slow to recognise that I needed to limit the time that was slipping away from me, due to incorrectly treated hypothyroidism. Eventually, I realised that I had to make the decision to ignore the advice of the endocrinologists and to choose T3 replacement therapy instead of the recommended T4 treatment. I was just too slow in recognising this.

Meeting with much resistance and fed false information about how inappropriate T3 replacement therapy was, I was repeatedly told that my problems were not related to thyroid hormones and that T3 was either a waste of time, unavailable or dangerous.

All of the above required me to trust my own instincts, which some may deem a brave or even foolish step. However, this decision eventually paid off, as I succeeded in finding a path to recovery.

Eventually, I found a doctor who did believe my problems were due to thyroid hormones and allowed me to try using T3 replacement therapy. Shortly after this I was also fortunate in finding a family doctor and endocrinologist who were both supportive and empathetic. Despite the fact that both my family doctor and my endocrinologist did not really offer insight into the practicalities of using T3, they did a great job of listening to me and providing specific help, when it was required. They encouraged me to adjust my medication based on the symptoms and signs, which I have described. My endocrinologist also filled in some gaps in my knowledge, which I found extremely helpful. Without their support using T3 replacement therapy would have been a much more difficult task.

However, I have had to search a large number of sources of information and then digest these in order to develop the process that enabled me to manage my T3 dosage. In doing this I have realised just how critical the right vitamins and minerals are to the support of the cellular processes that enable thyroid hormones to work correctly. I have also been forced by necessity to understand the many problems that I encountered and then develop creative solutions to these in order to regain my health. The majority of this learning is embedded in the T3 dosage management process.

The T3 dosage management process is an organised and systematic process. I followed it and determined an effective, safe and stable T3 dosage. I am living proof that it can be made to work.

I still view T3 replacement therapy as a treatment that should only be attempted after all the other thyroid hormone treatments have failed to resolve a patient's symptoms. The T3 dosage management process is inherently more complex than the equivalent for T4.

I have presented the following:

- A set of lessons relevant to T3 replacement therapy that I have learned over many years.

- Some information on the preparation that I did prior to using T3. This preparation is **critical** to the success of T3 replacement therapy.

- The goals I established for the T3 dosage management process.

- The T3 dosage management process that I used, including the use of symptoms and signs.

I hope that I have conveyed the practical methods that explain how I used T3 to recover from hypothyroidism.

In addition, I hope that any doctor who is contemplating a trial of T3 for a patient will consider the content presented within these pages. Fully appreciating the practical aspects of using the T3 thyroid hormone can make the difference between the success and failure of T3 replacement therapy.

I now believe that the T3 dosage management process I have presented in 'Recovering with T3' is best in class in that it appears to work extremely well, whilst ensuring that the T3 dosage that is produced as a result is the lowest possible and creates no issues with tissue over-stimulation.

It is also clear that the Circadian T3 Method that is part of this T3 dosage management process is an extremely potent tool whether used with pure T3 or with natural desiccated thyroid. The CT3M appears to be a highly valuable tool that may be used to promote better adrenal function in thyroid patients who have sluggish adrenal glands.

For more information on the effectiveness of the Circadian T3 Method and the T3 dosage management process as documented by thyroid patients the reader should visit the Recovering with T3 website, which is listed in Appendix B at the end of this book.

SECTION 6

UNDERSTANDING WHY T4 FAILED

Chapter 28

Why Did T4 Fail and T3 Succeed?

This is a question that I have asked myself many times. There was such a dramatic difference between my poor response to T4 replacement therapy and the success of T3 that I fully expected to be able to find out what was causing the failure of T4. Unfortunately, none of the doctors I saw could provide any explanations of why T4 failed to resolve my symptoms.

It is only in the past seven or eight years that I have realised how many people are in a similar situation to myself. I used to think that my problems were unusual and that I might never get an answer to this question. As long as I thought that the failure of T4 replacement therapy was rare, I was prepared to forget this question and accept that I would never get close to an answer. However, since it became obvious to me that this is quite a common problem and having communicated with many other patients who have been forced to use T3 replacement therapy, I have not been able to ignore the question of 'why?'

What were the reasons for T4 failing, so miserably, to remove my symptoms? Why did T3 work when T4 failed to?

I have read a great deal on this topic, finding a vast, variety of information by delving into various research publications. It is clear that medical research has only just begun to understand the problem but a good start has been made. There have been some individual studies that shine some light on certain types of problems that can occur but other potential problems have not been researched as much and remain in the shadows.

From what is known through current research, one thing is very clear, there are many different possible reasons that T4 replacement therapy fails for some patients and they can all result in the symptoms of hypothyroidism, regardless of how perfect thyroid blood test results appear to be.

I would love to be able to present a comprehensive summary of all the relevant research but that would be a book in its own right and not one that I would feel competent to contribute to. This is too large an area of research, too complex and too little advanced at present, for me to do anything other than touch on some possibilities. This chapter, therefore, is a summary of my own musings on the problem that had such a large impact on my life. These thoughts have been informed by medical research but I will save any specific referral to relevant medical research until the next chapter.

IMPAIRED CELLULAR RESPONSE TO THYROID HORMONE

Can I give a name to the reason why T4 failed to correct my symptoms of hypothyroidism? No, I can't - not a single name anyway, because there are many classes of potential problems that can occur within our cells. Each of these classes can impair the action of thyroid hormones. I prefer to use 'impaired cellular response to thyroid hormone' to describe my problem with T4 replacement therapy.

The expression 'impaired cellular response to thyroid hormone' makes it clear that the issue occurs within the cells and stops thyroid hormone creating a normal response, i.e. it leaves the patient with symptoms associated with hypothyroidism. 'Impaired cellular response to thyroid hormone' implies no assumptions about any particular reason for the impairment. Therefore, it is an ideal description to use, because it covers a range of possible causes of thyroid hormone failure.

Many research papers and textbooks use the term 'partial tissue resistance' to refer to the same problem.[1] However, a number of other descriptions are also used: partial tissue resistance to thyroid hormone, partial peripheral cellular resistance to thyroid hormone, peripheral resistance syndrome, euthyroid hypometabolism, or type 2 hypothyroidism.[1, 2, 3] The word 'partial' is important in 'partial peripheral tissue resistance', because other forms of resistance are usually more severe and are often associated with genetic defects that are present from birth.[4]

The expression 'tissue resistance to thyroid hormone' has been adopted by some researchers to refer, almost exclusively, to defects in the genetic makeup of cells that affect the thyroid receptors in the cell nuclei. This is a very narrow use of the term 'tissue resistance' and other researchers have sought to use the term to include a broader range of issues within the cells.

I would use any existing terminology, if it covered a wide range of potential cellular issues and if there was general agreement on what it meant. Neither am I especially keen on the term 'type 2 hypothyroidism', because it tends to imply that it is not as severe a condition as hypothyroidism, in much the same way that type 2 diabetes is often less severe than type 1 diabetes. In the case of hypothyroidism, many patients with impaired cellular response to thyroid hormone, can have extreme symptoms of hypothyroidism - it is not a less severe condition than hypothyroidism due to a failing thyroid gland.

I will continue to use the term 'impaired cellular response to thyroid hormone'. It is a little wordy but relatively unambiguous and it perfectly describes my view on why T4 replacement therapy failed to make me well. With this terminology in mind, I believe that it was the impaired cellular response to thyroid hormone that caused T4 replacement therapy to fail to relieve my symptoms. For some reason either insufficient T3 was reaching its intra-cellular targets, or T3 was failing to regulate cell function correctly when it got there.

FURTHER CLUES ABOUT MY OWN THYROID HORMONE PROBLEM

Let me start with my medical history. As a child I had urticaria (hives) for several years. It began for no apparent reason and then, around seven years later, stopped almost as quickly. I was placed on high levels of anti-histamines for several years to control the urticaria. Most cases are triggered by an allergic reaction and only last a few weeks. The longer-term cases, like mine, are thought to have an autoimmune involvement. It appears that even at age eleven, I already had the potential for some autoimmune issues.

At around twenty years of age I had a bad case of glandular fever, which is also known as mononucleosis, or Epstein-Barr virus. Interestingly, there are doctors who believe that long after the symptoms have disappeared, the virus may still be lodged within the cells of the thyroid gland, causing long-term damage to the thyroid itself.[5]

However, during my twenties I was processing thyroid hormones extremely well. When I was at university I would do regular five-mile runs at a decent pace. I played tennis. I was active and was very slim. My own thyroid hormones must have been working correctly within the tissues of my body at this stage, even after the glandular fever. Very active throughout my twenties, I was healthy right up until a year prior to the diagnosis of Hashimoto's thyroiditis. Only once the autoimmune thyroid problem occurred did my health deteriorate.

T3 replacement therapy was the only solution that overcame the problems and removed the symptoms associated with hypothyroidism.

When I developed Hashimoto's thyroiditis something happened that caused me to develop impaired cellular response to thyroid hormone. I am also confident that this problem includes both my own natural T4 and synthetic T4.

I asked a couple of the endocrinologists I saw, during the early years on synthetic T4, whether I might have developed a problem that resulted in less T3 reaching my cells than I had prior to developing hypothyroidism. I was consistently told that this was not possible and that the only circumstances when this can occur are when a patient is critically ill, or starving. I have subsequently found various texts that confirm that starvation and serious illness may result in less T3 being produced.[6, 7] Clearly, these circumstances were not applicable to me. I received no other answers or explanations.

I have experimented with high levels of synthetic T4 replacement as well as natural thyroid replacement and neither solution has resolved my symptoms, or made me feel well. T3 is the only thyroid replacement therapy that works for me. I discounted a poor conversion rate of T4 to T3 as being a possible cause of my problems with T4, which is a widely discussed idea amongst some thyroid patients. I already knew that any temporary degraded T4 to T3 conversion, due to stress or elevated cortisol levels, only lasts a few weeks. This is well documented and I have already cited references in this regard. In addition, I investigated a variety of combinations of T4 and T3 and I realised that no modest impairment of T4 conversion to T3 could explain my symptoms.

I also believe that I had no issues with cortisol, insulin, glucose or any other essential nutrient, like selenium, iron, B12 or folic acid. I have done such a thorough job of assessing all of these potential issues and have such a good nutritional regime that these potential issues are not relevant to my problems with T4.

During T4 replacement therapy my FT4 and FT3 were high enough that any problem had to be occurring at a cellular level. At times I had taken such high levels of synthetic T4 and natural thyroid that it was very clear that no T4 replacement therapy was ever going to make me well.

Due to the fact that it is possible for me to feel well on T3 alone, I have discounted the possibility that I had a hypothalamic or pituitary problem. My problem is not due to central hypothyroidism, because increasingly high dosages of T4 should have been able to resolve all my symptoms and I wouldn't have expected such dramatic benefits from T3.

The other major clue that I now possess, due to a nearly extinct thyroid gland, is that my issue is unlikely to be due to reverse T3. I now have almost no T4 left in my body. Yet even in this situation a number of other 'blocking chemicals' are capable of interfering with my T3 medication and may cause the symptoms of hypothyroidism if they are taken in too high a dosage. These include: hydrocortisone, DHEA, alcohol, certain prescription drugs like some antibiotics. Even if I take more T3 when any of these blocking chemicals are taken it makes little difference.

My problem is linked to how thyroid hormone is handled within my cells and T3 fully overcomes whatever the issue is as long as no other blocking chemical is present. I have completely concluded that my thyroid hormone problem is due to the impaired cellular response to thyroid hormone. It only remains to have this confirmed by a laboratory test that is yet to be invented and to identify the specific class of problem that is causing it.

MUSINGS ON IMPAIRED CELLULAR RESPONSE TO THYROID HORMONE

Impaired cellular response to thyroid hormone causes either insufficient amounts of T3 to reach its intra-cellular targets, or the incorrect regulation of cell function when T3 does reach them. Based on everything I have read, it appears that there are classes of problems that can cause impaired cellular response to thyroid hormone. Some of the possible classes of problems are:

- A problem with the transport of FT4 or FT3 into the cells. Unbound T4 and T3 were thought, until recently, to passively diffuse through the walls of cells. It has been recently discovered that transporter proteins are involved in the movement of both FT4 and FT3 across cell membranes and into cells. Consequently, one cause of impaired cellular response to thyroid hormone might be due to a problem with one or more transporter proteins or associated mechanisms.

- Damage to any of the numerous enzymes involved in the cellular processing of thyroid hormones, including the deiodinase enzymes.

- Interference to thyroid hormone progress within the cells. Hormones, amines, immune system chemicals, or other compounds, might interfere with how thyroid hormone accesses the cells, progresses within the cells, or binds to the intra-cellular targets.

- Problems with the nuclear thyroid hormone receptors. Poor binding to the T3 thyroid receptors in the cell nuclei can be caused by mutations to one or more genes that affect the thyroid hormone receptors. It is possible that other mechanisms might degrade the binding of thyroid hormone to the thyroid hormone receptors.

- Problems with the mitochondria. Damage, disease or malfunction of the cells' mitochondria or T3 mitochondrial receptors might lead to normal levels of thyroid hormone not enabling healthy levels of mitochondrial activity within cells.

- Post-receptor effector mechanism problems that affect the effectiveness of T3 once it has bound to the T3 thyroid receptors on the genes in the cell nuclei.

- Autoantibodies to hormones or hormone receptors.

- A problem with the cellular processing of thyroid hormones, due to low or missing co-factors, or some other chemical, or toxin causing interference etc.

- ... and there will be more problems that are found, as this area is researched over the coming years.

I have long suspected that immune system chemicals might be responsible for interfering with the progress of thyroid hormones in my cells and the eventual binding of T3 to the mitochondrial and nuclear thyroid receptors (third item on the above list). I have this 'pet theory' for a few reasons. Firstly, all my health issues appear to have an immune system connection. Secondly, my impaired cellular response to thyroid hormone began after the onset of Hashimoto's thyroiditis. Thirdly, I have found some research evidence that supports the idea that some immune system chemicals can impair thyroid hormones within the cells.

Unfortunately, there is no way of investigating this further, because no laboratory tests are currently available to enable this.

IMPLICATIONS OF IMPAIRED CELLULAR RESPONSE TO THYROID HORMONE

It's not sufficient to have adequate FT4 and FT3 levels in the bloodstream. Regardless of blood levels, T3 actually needs to enter the cells efficiently, successfully reach its intra-cellular targets and become effective at regulating cell function. T3 needs to do this in the presence of optimal levels of cortisol, insulin, glucose and relevant enzymes and nutrients. T3 needs to do all of this, within cells that are producing enough chemical energy and are working correctly.

I can now easily imagine how I could remain with the symptoms of hypothyroidism, while my FT4 and FT3 levels appeared to be perfectly adequate. If a patient has impaired cellular response to thyroid hormone, then it is likely that many doctors will conclude that the patient's symptoms are not associated with thyroid hormone issues. I can now understand why my thyroid blood test results were unhelpful and why I struggled to work out why my T4 treatment was failing.

The only way that a correct diagnosis can currently be made, for a patient with this type of issue, is to consider the patient's symptoms, as well as his or her detailed medical history. Even after that, a trial of a different hormone replacement method, like T4/T3, or T3, would be needed to confirm the diagnosis.

WHY DID T3 WORK?

By taking T3 there is no need for the body to convert any T4, as T3 is already biologically active. Taking the biologically active thyroid hormone T3 increases the probability of avoiding some of the potential obstacles. Taking T3 results in a rapid increase in bloodstream levels followed by cellular levels of the hormone. It is this singular nature of T3 that makes it so ideal for overcoming impaired cellular response to thyroid hormone. Increasing the daily dosage of T3 is the equivalent of 'carpet bombing' the cells. Using T3 replacement therapy, it is possible to saturate the tissues with the biologically active thyroid hormone and attempt to overcome any impaired cellular response to thyroid hormone. I believe that it is the pure T3 form that is particularly helpful in overcoming impaired cellular response to thyroid hormone. I doubt that slow release T3 would be as effective for many of those people who require a full replacement dosage of T3.

Even if there is a severe problem, it may still be possible to find a T3 dosage that will work successfully by using much larger, individual doses of T3 that provide the right amount of T3 to its intra-cellular targets. Even if this results in a fully suppressed TSH and an elevated FT3 level, a patient might still feel well and display no evidence of tissue over-stimulation. As far as the patient's cells are concerned, they will behave perfectly normally, with just the right amount of T3 becoming effective there. This might require bloodstream levels and possibly cellular levels of T3 to be exceptionally high in order to achieve this.

Using the car analogy again - if all other thyroid hormone replacement therapies have failed, then using T3 is the equivalent of putting the best quality, high-octane fuel into a car engine that is struggling to generate enough energy. The best way to do this is to completely drain the fuel tank of the current lower octane fuel and to then fill up the tank with the more superior fuel that enables the car to become roadworthy again. The driver then needs to learn how to use the accelerator in the most efficient way, to deliver the right amount of fuel, to make the engine run perfectly.

In many cases, patients' symptoms may be resolved using high enough dosages of natural thyroid, or a synthetic T4/T3 combination. However, if the impaired cellular response to thyroid hormone is severe enough, a pure T3 replacement therapy may be required. Only a small proportion of patients are likely to require T3 replacement therapy. However, for those patients, the use of T3 may be the only way for them to become well again.

CONCLUSIONS ON THE FAILURE OF T4 AND THE SUCCESS OF T3

I have many concerns, the largest among them being that even though many years have passed since I began using T3 replacement therapy, very little appears to have changed in the way patients are being treated. There are still too many patients who continue to have severe symptoms of hypothyroidism and yet have normal blood levels of TSH, FT4 and FT3. I believe that impaired cellular response to thyroid hormone may be at the root of many of these cases. I also believe that a great many people may be suffering from undiagnosed nutrient deficiencies that can completely disrupt correct thyroid hormone metabolism.

Impaired cellular response to thyroid hormone requires a radically different diagnostic and treatment approach. There is medical research being carried out that will hopefully one day provide more comprehensive diagnostic tests and solutions. Of course, if more focused research could be funded, then patients may greatly benefit from this.

However, thyroid patients need this problem to be acknowledged now. They also require better diagnostic and treatment practices to be established as soon as possible

A CAUTIONARY NOTE ON VERY HIGH DOSES OF T4 BASED THERAPIES

I have stated earlier in this chapter that higher doses of synthetic T4/T3 or natural thyroid may often resolve a patient's symptoms. I want to briefly express some concerns that I have about high dosages of any T4 based medication. Any hormone, if taken in excess, may be said to be at a supraphysiological dosage. If a T4 based thyroid medication is increased then eventually, at some point, the level of conversion of T4 to T3 will reach its theoretical minimum conversion rate (because the conversion rate is influenced by TSH as already mentioned). This conversion rate will not reduce even as the supraphysiological dosage of the T4 based medication is further increased.

If the supraphysiological dosage of the T4 based medication continues to be increased then the FT4 and FT3 levels in the bloodstream are both likely to rise. Eventually, even the more resistant symptoms and signs may improve (providing that the cause of the impaired cellular response to thyroid hormone is not severe) but some symptoms and signs may not be at a healthy level because of the far from natural effects of this strategy. Blood pressure and heart rate may rise. There could be a wide range of adverse physiological effects. These may even include mood swings as a result of the effect on the brain and central nervous system of the supraphysiological dosage. I believe that these adverse effects may possibly be associated with the clearance of excess thyroid hormone that is being forced upon the body. It would require a scientific study to truly understand this.

I have seen these effects first hand from an experiment I performed on myself several years ago. Noticing that my thyroid autoantibodies had dropped to near zero, I wanted to explore T4 replacement therapy once more. For several months I placed myself on T4 medication to determine whether it would now work. The T4 proved to be as unpleasant as it had been in the past but I decided to explore higher dosage ranges than before. I eventually reached 300 micrograms of T4 per day. My FT4 and FT3 levels were both higher than the top of the reference ranges and my body temperature normalised. The FT3 level on this T4 dosage was virtually the same as being on T3 replacement therapy. However, my blood pressure rose alarmingly and I became mentally unstable and felt suicidal. I would never do this again but it was a valuable learning exercise and not one I would suggest anyone else ever tries.

When people tell me that it is possible to get well by simply increasing natural thyroid, T4/T3 or just T4 then I want to know whether there are any symptoms or signs of a supraphysiological dosage present. If all is normal and healthy then this is wonderful - really it is wonderful! However, if there is evidence of adverse symptoms then there is a need to be very, very wary. I've been there and it can be extremely dangerous and may risk long-term cardiovascular damage amongst other problems.

Chapter 29

A Sprinkling of Research on T4 Failure/T3 Success

As I have already stated, I am not able to provide a comprehensive summary of all the relevant medical research, regarding impaired cellular response to thyroid hormone. It would not be possible for me to do justice to the large body of research that has been done so far, in one or two chapters of a book. I will simply try to select some relevant medical research studies that illustrate the range of potential problems that can cause impaired cellular response to thyroid hormone and hope that by the time the reader has finished this chapter it will be clear that:

Impaired cellular response to thyroid hormone is a very real issue.

- Impaired cellular response to thyroid hormone can be undetectable through thyroid blood tests and it can cause T4 replacement therapy to fail to resolve a patient's symptoms.

- T3 replacement therapy may have genuine value in helping some patients that still continue to have severe symptoms of hypothyroidism on T4 replacement therapy.

I will now try to select some research, which I believe supports and illustrates the existence of impaired cellular response to thyroid hormone.

DISCREPANCIES BETWEEEN SERUM AND TISSUE LEVELS OF THYROID HORMONE

There are three different studies, which I would like to highlight.

TSH does not correlate to physical functioning and ability

In one study, the authors present evidence that suggests that TSH may be viewed as a poor tool on its own, in the assessment of progress during the treatment of thyroid disease. A number of doctors are starting to realise that TSH results can be highly misleading.[1] The referenced study investigated the links between TSH, T4, free T4, T3, TBG and rT3 (reverse T3) and various aspects of physical functioning and ability.

The study showed that TSH and FT4 levels are poor indicators of tissue thyroid levels. In particular, the results showed that for a large percentage of patients, the level of TSH (and FT4) in the bloodstream is not useful in determining whether a person is euthyroid in the tissues, i.e. whether the cells of the body are receiving an adequate supply of thyroid hormones.

It is vital to remember that in order to feel well a person must have normal levels of thyroid hormones in the cells and these hormones must be effective once they are inside the cells. Having normal levels of thyroid hormones in the bloodstream cannot guarantee that a person will feel well, regardless of whether the TSH, FT4 and FT3 levels are within the laboratory reference range.

In addition to the above, the referenced study showed that FT4 levels had a negative correlation with tissue thyroid levels, i.e. higher FT4 levels were associated with decreased peripheral conversion of T4, low FT3 levels and high rT3 levels in the cells. The study demonstrated that the higher the rT3 level in the bloodstream, the worse the physical performance scores were.

The study also showed that increased FT4, rT3 levels and decreased FT3 levels in the bloodstream are associated with hypothyroidism at the tissue level, inevitably leading to diminished physical functioning. The study suggests that the FT3/rT3 ratio may be a potentially useful indicator of tissue levels of thyroid hormone. This is an idea that has the support of some doctors in the USA. This implies that FT3/rT3 may be a more useful marker of actual thyroid levels than TSH for some patients. However, the FT3/rT3 ratio may not detect all cases of tissue level thyroid hormone deficiencies.

This finding is very interesting because it highlights the value of using FT4, FT3 and rT3 along with patients' symptoms to assess actual thyroid hormone activity. This is a finding that is very similar to that reached in two papers that I have already referenced in Chapter 12.[Chapter 12: 2, 3] There appears to be sufficient evidence to suggest that substantially more research is required in this area, which may lead to a different approach to assessing thyroid hormone levels for many patients - an approach which may not use TSH in the significant way that it is used at the present time.

This study also adds to the evidence that suggests that simply prescribing T4 on its own may not be enough to achieve adequate thyroid hormones in the cells of the body. It also highlights how a normal TSH reading cannot be used as confirmation that cells have adequate thyroid hormone. According to some doctors, TSH levels can be even more misleading if a patient is suffering from any other systemic illnesses or condition, including: diabetes, heart disease, hypertension, systemic inflammation, asthma, CFS, fibromyalgia, rheumatoid arthritis, lupus, insulin resistance, obesity and chronic stress.

There are two further research studies that add further weight to the potential discrepancy between bloodstream levels and cellular levels of thyroid hormones.

TSH, FT4 and FT3 blood test results may not reflect tissue levels of T3

In two related studies, the researchers present evidence that indicates that the standard treatment with T4 replacement therapy (using synthetic T4) may not correct cellular levels of T3 thyroid hormone.[2, 3]

T4 replacement is the first and often the only thyroid replacement that many doctors and endocrinologists will prescribe. This is based on a widely held assumption that the body will convert the required amount of T4 into the biologically active thyroid hormone T3. Based on this assumption, many doctors and endocrinologists believe that laboratory tests, predominantly the TSH test, will enable the T4 dosage to be adjusted accordingly, which in turn will result in adequate tissue levels of thyroid hormones. This assumption had never been directly tested, until the two studies referenced above were published. Both of these studies involved the use of rats rather than human subjects, because it required the dissection of various tissues and the measurement of thyroid hormones within those tissues.

The first of the two studies investigated whether, or not, T4 replacement therapy results in adequate T3 levels in different tissues of the body. TSH, FT4 and FT3 levels in the bloodstream and ten different tissue levels of T4 and T3 were measured, after synthetic T4 had been infused for twelve to thirteen days. In other words, ten different areas of the body were measured, to see how much T3 and T4 they actually contained, in comparison to blood levels of TSH, FT4 and FT3, after the rats had been given a T4-only preparation for twelve to thirteen days.

The second of the two studies compared the TSH, FT4 and FT3 levels in the bloodstream and thirteen different tissues levels of T4 and T3. These comparisons were made with infused T4 and then they were repeated with an infusion of a combination of T4 and T3.

The studies showed that even when normal levels of TSH and FT4 were achieved in the bloodstream, **only very few tissues** had normal T3 readings. The pituitary gland was one of the few tissue samples to display normal levels of T3, which would explain the normal TSH level. However, the vast majority of tissues were still deficient in T3, despite the normal blood test results of FT3.

These studies provide scientific evidence that suggests that the current thyroid function blood tests of TSH, FT4 and FT3 fail to reflect low levels of T3 in the tissues of the body. These results suggest that some patients can continue to experience symptoms of hypothyroidism despite normal laboratory test results.

T4 may not be able to create healthy levels of T3 in the tissues for some patients

The two studies also suggest that it is impossible for hypothyroid patients to achieve normal tissue levels of T3 by taking T4 only preparations, unless supra-physiological dosages of T4 are given. The authors of these studies concluded that T4 replacement therapy should no longer be considered an adequate treatment for people suffering from hypothyroidism.

The pituitary gland tissues may more easily maintain healthy T3 levels

What is perhaps more significant, is that the **second of the pair of studies** showed that the cells in the pituitary gland were able to maintain adequate levels of T3 when T4 was provided, despite the rest of the body having less than adequate levels of T3. This is important, as the pituitary gland is responsible for producing TSH, which many doctors rely on as the sole indicator of a patient's thyroid hormone status. If the pituitary gland can maintain optimum levels of T3, when the rest of the body can't, it is again easy to see how TSH results could be misleading. Under normal conditions, it was shown that the pituitary would have 7 to 60 times the concentration of T3 compared to other tissues of the body. However, when overall thyroid hormone levels drop, the pituitary was shown to have 40 to 650 times the concentration of T3 compared to the other tissues. Thus, it was shown that the pituitary gland is unique in its ability to concentrate T3, even when thyroid hormone levels are low. This does not appear to occur in other tissues - the TSH can provide a highly inaccurate picture of overall thyroid hormone levels.

No surprise T4 does not work for some patients

Doctors who are aware of all of the above studies have commented that it is no surprise that many patients on T4 preparations continue to suffer with symptoms associated with hypothyroidism, despite being told their levels are within the laboratory reference range. However, the majority of doctors still haven't adopted this viewpoint, which is very unfortunate for suffering thyroid patients around the world.

PROBLEMS WITH TRANSPORT OF THYROID HORMONES INTO THE CELLS

Thirty or forty years ago, medical researchers believed thyroid hormones just passed into cells via passive diffusion. It is now clear that this is not the case and that various transporter proteins are involved in the movement of FT4 and FT3 into cells.

Because proteins are required and therefore have to be made in the first place, this creates an additional point of failure for thyroid hormones within our cells. Mutations in one of these transporter proteins, known as the MCT8 transporter, have been identified in male patients, which gives rise to severe psychomotor retardation, in a condition known as Allan-Herndon-Dudley Syndrome (AHDS).[4] This is a form of tissue resistance to thyroid hormone or impaired cellular response to thyroid hormone.

The research on transporter proteins and possible problems that may be associated with them is still at a very early stage and more problems may be identified.

DAMAGE TO ENZYMES INVOLVED IN THYROID HORMONE METABOLISM

A recent study in the UK highlights a potential genetic defect that affects critical enzymes involved in the processing of thyroid hormone within the tissues. This problem cannot be detected by TSH, FT4 or FT3 thyroid blood tests, yet may prevent patients from feeling well on T4 replacement therapy.[6]

The study analysed over six hundred hypothyroid patients treated with T4 and combined T4 and T3 replacement therapies and looked at whether genetic defects might lead to problems with the deiodinase enzymes responsible for processing thyroid hormones, including the conversion of T4 into T3. This was the largest and most comprehensive study to date, involving hypothyroid patients treated with T4 and combinations of T4 and T3.

Defective gene linked to poor health on T4, patients on T4/T3 healthier

This study concluded that some patients only achieve an improved sense of well being when taking a combination of T4 and T3. The results identified that a commonly impaired gene (DIO2), is associated with a poor sense of patient health when on T4 replacement. The impaired gene is associated with problems with one of the deiodinase enzymes involved in the conversion of T4 to T3. However, this impairment is undetectable in blood tests, as the problems occur entirely within the cells of the body. Patients on a combined T4/T3 replacement fared considerably better, despite possessing the same genetic defect.

The results of the study have encouraged some inspired doctors to make public statements emphasising that the medical profession should take patients far more seriously, if they claim that they do not feel well on T4 replacement therapy. This is particularly worrying because these patients may possess normal thyroid blood test results, despite the fact that hypothyroid symptoms may persist. One doctor even stated that patients in these circumstances should be asking for a combined T4/T3 treatment option, because it is likely that T4, on its own, is unable to replenish the reduced intra-cellular levels of T3.

There is no reason to believe that this is the only cause of defects in, or diminished levels of, critical enzymes involved in thyroid hormone metabolism within our cells.

INTERFERENCE TO THYROID HORMONE PROGRESS WITHIN CELLS

In the previous chapter, I suggested that one possible cause of impaired cellular response to thyroid hormone, might be that other hormones, amines, immune system chemicals or other compounds interfere with how thyroid hormones access cells and then progress towards the intra-cellular targets within them. I am highly suspicious that immune system chemicals, possibly inflammatory cytokines, may have been responsible for the failure of T4 replacement therapy to resolve my symptoms.

Recently, I consulted an immunologist, as I was experiencing various gastro-intestinal symptoms that now appear to be linked to a high level of the immune system chemical histamine. I had severe urticaria when I was young. Urticaria is known in some cases to be associated with autoimmune thyroid disease.[6] Patients with urticaria have an increased frequency of Hashimoto's thyroiditis. According to the immunologist, some cases of urticaria are caused by autoantibodies. He also told me that people, who have had urticaria, are twice as likely to develop autoimmune thyroid disease, compared to the rest of the population, although I do not know how accurate this statistic is. It is not clear what the exact reasons are for the relationship between urticaria and Hashimoto's thyroiditis but it is suspected that there is a link that involves one, or more, damaged or defective genes.

Low levels of thyroid hormones are associated with an increase in the release of chemicals from mast cells including histamine.[7] This illustrates the potential connection between low levels of thyroid hormones and the development of sensitivities and allergies.

My gastro-intestinal issue is caused by histamine being released in the upper part of my digestive system. According to my immunologist this is almost certainly caused because of internal urticaria (rather than IBS or food allergies). Luckily, I was already following an appropriate treatment regime, which included antihistamines and high levels of vitamin C.[8] This recent problem with internal urticaria is another instance of immune system related problems that I appear to be prone to.

Cytokines from immune system linked to conversion of T4 to T3 in tissues

Over recent years of reading published medical research, I have become aware of the existence of immune system chemicals called cytokines. Cytokines are a collection of proteins released by cells that have a specific effect on the interactions between cells, on communications between cells or on the behaviour of cells. The cytokines includes the interleukins, lymphokines and cell signal molecules, such as tumour necrosis factor and the interferons, which trigger inflammation and respond to infections. Various studies exist that indicate that various cytokines may be capable of inhibiting the conversion of T4 to T3 in the tissues.[9, 10, 11, 12] In other words, it is possible that some of the chemicals from my compromised immune system may have been responsible for the failure of T4 replacement therapy to return me to good health. It is even possible that various immune system chemicals began adversely affecting me when I first developed urticaria as a child.

This class of issue takes effect entirely within the cells of the body and is therefore undetectable by thyroid blood tests, although the symptoms may be very apparent..

Cytokines may be linked to Hashimoto's thyroiditis

Recently, I read a book in which the author suggests that cytokines are often present as a direct result of Hashimoto's thyroiditis, due to the fact that it is an autoimmune disease.[13] The book suggests that cytokines are responsible for partially blocking access to the nuclear thyroid receptors.[14, 15, 16, 17] This idea fits well with the idea of chemically induced impaired cellular response to thyroid hormone. The author highlights the frequent association between low vitamin D levels and hypothyroidism and discusses the important role that supplementing with vitamin D3 may have in calming the immune system (discussed in Chapter 4).

The following are examples of further studies that suggest potentially important relationships between cytokines and impaired cellular response to thyroid hormone.

Elevated levels of the cytokines IL-6, tumour necrosis factor-alpha, and interferon-alpha have been reported to have a strong association with the reduced T3 and increased rT3 found under stressful conditions.[18, 19] Administration of IL-6 to healthy subjects results in decreased T3 and increased rT3 levels, with TSH levels slightly suppressed.

Other chemicals may also be found that interfere with thyroid hormones within cells

Another example of a naturally occurring chemical in the body, that may be relevant to intra-cellular problems affecting thyroid hormones, is the recent discovery of a particular amine. [20] This amine may be significant for people who have a low metabolic rate. The referenced study investigated 3-Iodothyronamine (T1AM). T1AM is a derivative of T4, which is created by decarboxylation and deiodination. The study revealed that T1AM is capable of inducing a hypometabolic state. This is just one example that illustrates that we still have a great deal more to learn about the biochemical problems that may lead to a low metabolism.

Far more research is required

The research in the area of cytokines and other immune system related compounds has a long way to go, before a full understanding is reached. However, I believe that more relationships between the actions of the immune system and impaired cellular response to thyroid hormone will be found.

PROBLEMS WITH THE NUCLEAR THYROID HORMONE RECEPTORS

Over recent years tissue resistance to thyroid hormone has come to be regarded, by some medical researchers, as a class of problems that lead to poor levels of binding of thyroid hormone within the cell nuclei. Other researchers still prefer to use this term to discuss the broader failure of thyroid hormone within the cells that I have described as the impaired cellular response to thyroid hormone.

Tissue resistance to thyroid hormone

Tissue resistance to thyroid hormone or thyroid hormone resistance syndrome was identified in 1967.[21] Because of subsequent identification of gene mutations the term 'resistance to thyroid hormone' became frequently associated with defects of the thyroid receptors.[22, 23, 24]

Tissue resistance to thyroid hormone is frequently defined to be one of three types:

- General resistance to thyroid hormone, where the pituitary and the peripheral tissues are resistant.[25]

- Pituitary resistance to thyroid hormone, where it is only the pituitary gland, which is resistant.[26]

- Peripheral resistance to thyroid hormone. This is sometimes also known as partial tissue resistance, partial cellular resistance to thyroid hormone or even type 2 hypothyroidism (because it is analogous to type 2 diabetes).

Genetic Defects in the thyroid receptors linked to general and pituitary resistance

Patients with general, or pituitary, resistance to thyroid hormone may be detected relatively easily via laboratory tests. Both general and pituitary resistance are often associated with defects in the c-erbA-beta gene on chromosome 3. The c-erbA-beta gene, codes for the main thyroid hormone receptor, in the cell nucleus and a defect results in a thyroid receptor, which does not bind as easily to thyroid hormone, i.e. this receptor has a lower affinity than it should have to thyroid hormone. Many different types of mutations to the c-erbA-beta gene have been discovered so far. However, a defect in the thyroid receptors are only one of several possible causes.[27] Over the years since the identification of mutant thyroid receptors, many patients with these types of genetic defect have been studied. Whilst some have quite severe clinical features, some have very mild features and others have none.

Causes of peripheral resistance to thyroid hormone less clear

In peripheral resistance to thyroid hormone, the pituitary gland responds normally to thyroid hormone but the other tissues may be in varying states of hypometabolism, i.e. they may be starved of thyroid hormone at the cellular level. Patients with peripheral tissue resistance are far harder to identify, because their thyroid blood test results may appear normal. When they are identified, the treatment is typically to provide high dosages of T3 in order to provide a high enough level of thyroid hormone to regulate the thyroid receptors and overcome the resistance.[28] By providing T3 at a high enough dose, the symptoms of peripheral tissue resistance may be resolved in many cases.

The causes of peripheral tissue resistance are far less clear than those of general and pituitary resistance. Partial peripheral resistance is an even more subtle variety of peripheral resistance, in which the degree of resistance to thyroid hormone may be varied, with respect to different tissue types within the body, making this even more difficult to detect through laboratory testing.

More medical research needed

One of the most well known medical researchers in this area has written a useful history of tissue resistance to thyroid hormone.[29] The research on this topic is still only in its relative infancy, after the work on the human genome presented the researchers with more opportunities to investigate the operation of thyroid hormone within the cells of our bodies.

Could some form of thyroid hormone resistance be relevant to me? I don't know. What I do know is that the medical research in this area will continue for many years. It has already provided an explanation for the symptoms of many patients. My suspicion is that a wider array of problems will be identified, regarding thyroid receptors and other causes of low binding affinity, between thyroid hormones and thyroid receptors. I suspect that some of these problems may give rise to mild symptoms and others will cause more severe symptoms.

MITOCHONDRIAL PROBLEMS

I have already mentioned the mitochondria. The majority of the energy needs of the human body are met by the action of the mitochondria. Each human cell has one mitochondrion, which is a tiny organelle. When thyroid hormone levels increase, the action of thyroid hormone at the cell nuclei generates more mitochondrial proteins that in turn cause the mitochondria to produce more energy. If the cells of our bodies require more energy, then this must be forthcoming from the mitochondria. Apart from thyroid hormone and several co-factors, one of the main chemicals that the mitochondria require in order to produce chemical energy (ATP) is glucose. Hence, the correct functioning of our blood sugar metabolism is essential for the mitochondria to function optimally.

Consequently, the presence of low thyroid hormones, low cellular glucose levels or some other condition that impacts the mitochondria, may result in too little cellular energy being produced. Therefore, both thyroid disease and problems with the mitochondria can produce similar symptoms.

There may turn out to be many different classes of mitochondrial problems, including missing or low enzymes, co-factors or essential nutrients, blood sugar metabolism problems, damage or disease of the mitochondria and damage to the mitochondrial thyroid hormone receptors. If there is a problem with the mitochondria, then the effect of thyroid hormone within the cells will be seriously impaired. Hence, this is such a critical area for more research.

Many co-factors are necessary for correct mitochondrial function, these include: L-carnitine, coenzyme Q-10, NADH, B complex vitamins, lipoic acid, magnesium and various other nutrients. One study clearly illustrates the links between mitochondrial malfunction and diseases that have similar symptoms to low levels of thyroid hormone.[30]

This is another burgeoning area of research.

POST-RECEPTOR EFFECTOR MECHANISM PROBLEMS

It has been proposed that deterioration in the effectiveness of thyroid hormones within the cells might sometimes be caused by problems that occur after the T3 hormone has bound to the thyroid receptors. The actions that occur after the binding of thyroid hormone to the thyroid receptors are known collectively as the post-receptor effector mechanism.

Some researchers have suggested that impaired cellular response to thyroid hormone might occur due to a post-receptor effector mechanism defect.[31, 32]

AUTOANTIBODIES TO THYROID HORMONES

Autoantibodies to T4 and T3 have been found in the serum of some patients with autoimmune thyroid disease.[33, 34, 35] These autoantibodies are rarely measured and their value has not been evaluated but they are thought to disrupt the balance between thyroid hormones and their binding proteins.[36, 37]

There have also been articles that have speculated about the existence of naturally occurring autoantibodies to mitochondrial and nuclear thyroid receptors.

More medical research is required in this area to identify the full range of relevant autoantibodies and their effect and relevance to impaired cellular response to thyroid hormone.

PROBLEMS WITH LOW OR MISSING CO-FACTORS, CHEMICAL OR TOXIN INTERFERENCE

It is clear that the symptoms associated with hypothyroidism can exist in the presence of normal thyroid blood test results, if an important nutritional deficiency exists. I am not going to spend more time discussing the impact that a nutritional deficiency can have on the impaired cellular response to thyroid hormone. I have already discussed vitamins and minerals and a great deal of information is readily available on this subject from multiple sources. However, it is worth mentioning the contribution that some toxins can have on the impaired cellular response to thyroid hormone.

Dioxins and PCBs can bind to transthyretin and perhaps to nuclear thyroid receptors, thus competitively inhibiting T3 binding.[38] Other toxins that are known in animals to produce decreased serum levels of T4 and increased rT3 include: chlorinated paraffins, polychlorinated biphenyl, hexachlorobenzene, 3-methylcholanthrene, 3,3',4,4'-tetrachlorobiphenyl, 2,3,7,8-tetrachloro-p-dioxin and clofibrate.[39]

Drugs that reduce T3 and increase rT3 include: dexamethasone, propylthiourcil, iopanic acid (radiographic contrast agent), amiodarone and propranalol.

CONCLUSIONS ON T4 FAILURE AND T3 SUCCESS

The above classes of problems, that can cause impaired cellular response to thyroid hormone, have been chosen somewhat arbitrarily in order to allow me to more easily discuss them. There are many other ways of categorising the type of failures I have just discussed. I leave it to the medical researchers, to create a common language for the various problems that can impair the cellular response to thyroid hormone. Having a common language for the overall problem of impaired cellular response to thyroid hormone, which identifies various class problems that give rise to it, would be an advantage for researchers, doctors and patients.

This research is still only in its early stages

The above summary of various types of problem, are as my chapter title suggested, just a sprinkling of a few elements of relevant medical research. However, even given the body of research that is available on this topic, it feels to me as if we are still only in the very early stages of understanding. In most of the above areas, the research is only just beginning to uncover parts of the whole story. Medical research does not yet have a complete understanding of the cellular action of thyroid hormone and, as a consequence, all the potential failures that can cause symptoms for patients are far from understood. As for having laboratory tests available to family doctors and endocrinologists, that can detect all of these problems, well, we can only dream of such things at the present time.

I am confident that I have impaired cellular response to thyroid hormone

I have managed to come to terms with all of this now. To a certain extent, I am 'at peace with it'. After developing Hashimoto's thyroiditis, T4 replacement therapy failed to correct my symptoms. I tried to use treatments containing synthetic T4 and T3, which also failed to restore me to good health. In addition, I also tried using natural thyroid preparations in conjunction with additional T3 but this also failed. I have supplemented with all the nutrients that are relevant to thyroid hormone metabolism, which made no difference to the effectiveness of T4. On T3 replacement therapy I feel healthy, my body temperature is normal, my pulse rate and blood pressure are normal, my energy is good and my weight is normal. I am now operating reasonably normally at a cellular level, regardless of my serum levels of thyroid hormones - which look far from normal. I have read and understood enough medical research to know that T3 replacement therapy solution is a perfectly reasonable treatment for me.

The only treatment that worked and continues to work for me is T3 replacement therapy. I expect that I will never find out in my lifetime what caused my particular brand of impaired cellular response to thyroid hormone. This prediction is based on my understanding of how much medical research is really left to do.

Thyroid blood tests are misleading for patients with impaired cellular response to thyroid hormone

I know that far too much emphasis and trust is still being placed on thyroid blood test results. Clearly, for many patients, thyroid blood test results provide an excellent insight into tissue levels of thyroid hormone. However, for those patients who respond poorly to T4 replacement therapy, thyroid blood test results provide no genuine insight during treatment. I have tried to explain some of the reasons behind the unreliability of thyroid blood test results, including some relevant research in this chapter, yet many doctors still remain slaves to clinical pathology.

If a patient fails to respond symptomatically to T4 replacement therapy, the only current reliable measures of whether the tissues are receiving enough T3 are how the patient actually feels and what their remaining symptoms actually are. Unfortunately, many doctors ignore patients' hypothyroid symptoms once their blood test results fall within the laboratory reference range. As previously discussed, there are many vital clues as to whether a patient is hypothyroid at the tissue level. Patients' symptoms, appearance and body temperature can provide major clues but very few doctors focus on these basic and insightful measures. The presence of frequent infections, allergies, myxoedema and muscle weakness are other valuable diagnostic clues that are often ignored, or are relegated to a position of less significance than laboratory test results.

Reverse T3

It should be implicitly clear from this chapter that I believe that there are many different ways in which the human body can sometimes fail and not respond well to T4 based therapies. Some of these failure modes may result in elevated rT3 levels whilst others may not.

Reverse T3 may be a useful adjunct laboratory test to perform for some people and I am convinced by various research studies and by the experience of some doctors and patients that in some cases T3/rT3 ratio may be a valuable diagnostic tool and may even be used to titrate thyroid hormone replacement in some people. What I am less convinced about is the application of T3/rT3 ratio in all cases of impaired cellular response to thyroid hormone. When rT3 is a problem then I believe that it is a resulting artifact of the underlying cause of the impaired cellular response to thyroid hormone and not the fundamental issue in its own right.

My personal view is that in those patients that exhibit this, an elevated rT3 or a low T3/rT3 ratio is the fallout or consequence of the underlying issue. However, I believe that some forms of impaired cellular response to thyroid hormone may not exhibit an alteration in rT3 or T3/rT3 ratio.

Consequently, my own opinion at the present time is that rT3 or T3/rT3 ratio cannot be relied upon as a diagnostic tool in all cases of impaired cellular response to thyroid hormone. In particular, I would be concerned if rT3 or T3/rT3 ratio were being relied upon on its own to determine the suitability of a patient for T3 replacement therapy or for the subsequent dosage management using T3.

Having said all the above my view is that if someone has an unusually high level of rT3 then this may obviously be a problem as reverse T3 will slow down the metabolism. So, looking at rT3, along with other laboratory test results can be highly valuable.

Once a decision has been taken by a doctor and patient that it is time for the patient to have a trial of T3 replacement therapy then the decision has been taken that T4 based medication should no longer be the predominant thyroid hormone being used. After this decision there is little point having any real interest in reverse T3 as correct titration of T3 thyroid hormone can only be done well using symptoms and signs at the present time.

Consequently, I believe the only real scenarios where rT3 may have some use are in treatments that are predominantly T4 based, i.e. with T4, T4/T3 or natural desiccated thyroid replacement therapies. I believe that in predominantly T4 based treatments rT3 may be useful in a lot of cases but in some patients the value of rT3 may be irrelevant to the real problem that the patient has or rT3 may appear normal and yet the patient may still have problems with the T4 thyroid hormone.

More research is needed into treatments aimed at calming down the immune system in Hashimoto's Thyroiditis Patients

I have already mentioned that some doctors believe that by keeping the TSH very low or suppressed this may help to reduce the autoantibody response in some Hashimoto's patients. In Chapter 4 I also briefly mention that some doctors have had success at calming the immune system through the use of vitamin D3. Many patients and doctors are also convinced that eliminating gluten-based foods from the diet can also benefit some thyroid patients, especially patients with Hashimoto's thyroiditis. Some doctors also believe that eliminating dairy products and other immune system stimulating foods or additives may also be valuable.

It is not possible to discuss the topic of calming down the immune system without mentioning a medication known as low dose naltrexone (LDN). Naltrexone is an opioid antagonist that has been used and approved to treat opioid addiction and alcohol addiction - at high doses.

When naltrexone is taken in low doses it is known as low dose naltrexone or LDN. LDN has been shown by researchers to work in a different way to naltexone. LDN is believed to stimulate the production of more endorphins, which modulate the immune system and re-balance any excessive immune system responses through its effect on opioid receptors. It is claimed that any side effects of LDN are minor. LDN is only used with a starting dose of 1.5 milligrams, rising to 4.5 milligrams at the most as compared with the much higher dosage usage of naltrexone. Although, extensive clinical trials have not been done specifically on LDN there is extensive information available on the safety of the much higher dosage naltexone, which is an approved medication.

Low dose naltrexone (LDN) is currently being used to treat some autoimmune diseases including rheumatoid arthritis, multiple sclerosis and Crohn's disease. These applications as far as I know are not FDA approved uses of LDN but some successes are being claimed. Other autoimmune conditions may also benefit from LDN treatment. Interestingly, LDN is thought to reduce the production of pro-inflammatory cytokines and this one more reason why I have included this brief review of LDN here. Research teams are continuing to investigate the potentially very important benefits that LDN is alleged to bring.

I have communicated with many patients who have Hashimoto's thyroiditis and they have told me that LDN has made their Hashimoto's autoantibodies drop to zero and has relieved many of their symptoms including fibromyalgia. Some claim that LDN has eliminated their fibromyalgia or brain fog. It is also claimed that LDN promotes healing and reduces sensitivity to gluten and casein as well as reducing or stopping autoimmune reactions.

If LDN fulfils the potential that some people believe it has and has no significant side effects then it might be the silver bullet that many Hashimoto's thyroid patients have been hoping for. However, it is important to be absolutely clear that full clinical trials resulting in approval to use LDN for autoimmune thyroid conditions or other autoimmune conditions have not been done yet. Campaigners are in the process of trying to get approval for these trials. Extensive trials have been done for naltrexone but the low dose naltrexone works in a different way and may require more specific trials.

There is extensive information regarding LDN on the Internet and via patient based forums.

LDN should be the subject of further research, even though many thyroid patients and patients with other conditions are already using it and are claiming extremely good results.

Thyroid patients, who are not healthy on T4, need better care

It is encouraging that research is still being conducted into why T4 fails for some patients. The fact that a growing number of studies are exposing the potential unreliability of the current thyroid function blood tests, for some patients, means that there is the possibility, that listening closely to how patients actually feel may finally become important again.

I have now outlined some of the reasons why I believe T4 failed to resolve my symptoms and why T3 succeeded in doing so. I hope I have been able to provide some insights into why a substantial number of thyroid patients fail to regain their health using synthetic T4 replacement therapy.

I believe that it is now possible to understand why some patients feel better on one of the following thyroid hormone replacement therapies:

- Natural thyroid (because it contains T3).

- Synthetic T4 / T3 combinations (because of the extra T3).

- Pure T3 (this can provide a sufficient level of T3 to overcome severe resistance issues).

When it comes to thyroid problems, I do not believe that there is a 'one size fits all' solution. Some patients may require a natural thyroid preparation or a combination of synthetic T4 and T3 in order to regain their health. A few may do better using pure T3. Some other patients may simply get well once they are given all the important vitamins and minerals that the thyroid and adrenal hormone pathways require to work correctly. For those patients who have failed to regain their health with T4 replacement therapy, it is often impossible to initially determine which treatment option is going to be the most successful. Trial and error is usually the only way to do this. However, I believe it is important to trial all the T4 based treatments prior to trying T3 replacement therapy. Despite the fact that T3 has the fewest biochemical barriers to overcome, I feel that it is by far the most difficult thyroid hormone replacement therapy to use, in terms of dosage management.

Those doctors, who are more open-minded, are utilising the latest research findings and are adopting new treatment protocols are having good success in treating patients who have suffered for many years on ineffective T4 replacement therapy. Unfortunately, far too few of these physicians exist at the moment. Consequently, many patients are missing out on adequate thyroid treatment.

I strongly believe that the wider range of thyroid treatments need to become available, so that patients who are continuing to suffer with the symptoms of hypothyroidism whilst on T4 replacement therapy, stand a chance of recovering.

Furthermore, I believe doctors and endocrinologists need to start listening to thyroid patients who tell them that they still feel unwell. The focus of diagnosis and treatment in particular, needs to place a higher emphasis on how patients feel and what their symptoms are, rather than relying far too heavily on blood test results, which may repeatedly fail to provide a clear picture for some patients.

SECTION 7

RECOMMENDATIONS & FINAL THOUGHTS

Chapter 30

Suggestions for
Doctors and Researchers

I cannot complete this without making some suggestions, aimed at all doctors involved in the diagnosis or treatment of thyroid disease or in any relevant medical research. I believe that the current situation, where so many thyroid patients continue to feel unwell on T4 replacement therapy, will not improve until family doctors and endocrinologists recognise that this is occurring and begin to handle these situations differently.

Some patients manage to overcome the lack of adequate available treatment by self-medication. I am not an advocate of this 'do it yourself' thyroid treatment.

Substantial change, for the benefit of all unfortunate patients, who have some level of impaired cellular response to thyroid hormone, has to arrive through changes brought about by the medical profession. In this penultimate chapter, I will try to communicate a few suggestions that I think would have significant benefits for thyroid patients like me.

HOW DOCTORS MEASURE THEIR SUCCESS

I have discussed this earlier but feel that it is really significant. As long as family doctors and endocrinologists are satisfied that they have successfully treated the hypothyroid patient, by focusing so much on thyroid blood test results, then no substantial change for the better will occur. In particular, it should no longer be acceptable to believe that thyroid replacement treatment has been a success just because thyroid blood test results are 'normal'.

People in all professions re-orient themselves and work differently depending on the measures that are used to determine whether they are successful or not. In my previous professional life I was measured using various criteria, which included whether a certain new technology worked according to its design specification and also whether it was produced in time for a customer to use. Doing one of these on its own but not the other would have been deemed a failure.

At present a doctor can feel satisfied if the thyroid blood test results are normalised according to certain criteria. Whilst thyroid blood test results may be a subset of the measures being used, they are not sufficient on their own. Doctors need to begin to measure the progress of the treatment in terms of improvements in symptoms and other useful signs that actually reflect how the patient feels. In the absence of better measures of tissue levels of thyroid hormones this is the best we can do at present but it is useful and it does reflect the action of thyroid hormones within the cells.

Changing how the success of thyroid hormone replacement is measured, to explicitly include what a patient most cares about, is a profoundly important change and it will radically alter the focus of treatment. I believe that this needs to be incorporated into medical training. I also believe that over time, it will improve the quality of care and treatments offered to thyroid patients. If T4 replacement therapy fails, then the close tracking of symptoms and signs will enable the patient and the doctor to have a common understanding that this has occurred. The doctor will feel at a deeper level that the treatment has not been successful. These measures will become part of how the doctor assesses his or her own ability to treat patients. It is a potent tool.

It is too easy at present, for some doctors to 'wash their hands' of the patient who has not responded to T4 replacement and offer reasons such as 'it is a psychological problem' or 'it must be some other disease that is causing these symptoms'. This has to stop, unless there are *exceptionally* good reasons to believe one of these hypotheses.

If T4 replacement therapy fails for a specific patient, then thyroid blood tests will be of reduced value in further treatments offered. In this case, continuing the use of symptoms and signs will be very critical, until medical researchers deliver usable methods of measuring the degree of successful activity of thyroid hormone within a patient's tissues.

I am sure that the provision and use of a simple symptoms/signs tracking tool would be relatively easy. Output from such a tool could quite easily be incorporated within on-line patient record systems. This is not rocket science by any means - it is just common sense.

If there is to be improvement in the quality of care of thyroid patients who do not respond well to T4 replacement therapy, then this is an essential step.

MEDICAL RESEARCH

Medical research is of course absolutely critical in this area. Medical research will ultimately provide clear and irrefutable solutions to all the issues that I have raised but we are a long way away from this at the present time. In the years ahead, medical research needs to be resourced and focused. If this is done well then the lives of thyroid patients all around the world will improve.

I have a few suggestions that I would like medical researchers and the people in control of research funding to consider. I know that there may be all kinds of opinion, inertia, organisational issues and difficulties involved in making any of this happen. However, I believe ultimately that this type of research needs to happen. My suggestions for research areas are:

- Continuing research aimed at thoroughly understanding the action and metabolism of thyroid hormones within our cells.

- More research aimed specifically at understanding all the possible causes of impaired cellular response to thyroid hormone. Any problems that hinder the progress of thyroid hormone, or make it less than effective at its targets within the cells, need to be studied. Researchers that are focused on the causes of failure of T4 replacement therapy need to ensure that when they begin to look at human subjects, that at appropriate times, they study a genuine population of people who are known to not respond symptomatically to T4. We exist - use us. We need to know that the medical researchers understand the problems that brought us to use T4/T3 or pure T3 in the first place.

- Research that leads to new diagnostic markers that can identify the presence of the problems that cause the impaired cellular response to thyroid hormone.

- Whilst there are no current laboratory tests to detect the causes of impaired cellular response to thyroid hormone we must rely on the assessment of the patient's symptoms and signs to provide insight into the successful action of thyroid hormones within the cells. Therefore, I would like to see at least one new laboratory test developed, that could be used to truly assess the level of biologically active T3 hormone, that is actually reaching the important intra-cellular targets and is actively contributing to the regulation of cell function. It is not sufficient to have adequate levels of T3 in the bloodstream. It is not even sufficient to have a healthy level of T3 within the cells. We need to have some graded measure of how much T3 is actually reaching the mitochondria and cell nuclei and being effective there. I have no idea if it will be possible to develop a test like this within the next ten years. However, we desperately require some interim laboratory test that can help medical professionals understand why T4 replacement therapy is failing so many patients.

- There needs to be improved communication of relevant medical research results to those doctors responsible for setting the standard of diagnostic and treatment methods for thyroid disease. I would like to see more medical researchers, who are practising doctors, involved in determining current medical practices regarding thyroid disease treatment. These improvements need to be rapidly passed on to all doctors and medical schools.

- If new diagnostic tests can be made available, it would be sensible to consider applying these diagnostic tests to patients with other conditions like ME, chronic fatigue syndrome or fibromyalgia. It may be likely that a proportion of these patients also have some degree of impaired cellular response to thyroid hormone, even though they may not have any obvious thyroid disease as determined by standard thyroid blood tests.

Properly funded, focused and coordinated medical research could revolutionise the way in which thyroid hormone disorders are diagnosed and treated.

ALL THE THYROID REPLACEMENT THERAPIES

There is not a single doubt in my mind that synthetic T4, natural thyroid, combinations of T4/T3 as well as pure T3 should all be available treatment options that family doctors and endocrinologists can use, rather than just the widely prescribed T4 replacement therapy.

Imagine that someone asked a professional gardener to look after their large home and provided the gardener with a lawn mower, trowel, spade, fork and clippers for trimming small shrubs. These tools are gleaming new and of the finest quality. Unfortunately, the gardener then discovers that at the rear of the house there are several large, overgrown hedges that require re-shaping. The gardener requires a professional quality electric hedge-trimmer, as none of his other tools are appropriate. The owner of the house is angry and complains that he has already provided the gardener with perfectly adequate tools for the job and he points to the clippers that the gardener is holding. The owner is so angry that the gardener goes back to work and begins to attempt to trim the hedges with the small clippers. The clippers make no impression on the hedges and the gardener eventually gives up.

T4/T3 and T3 replacement therapies need to be available to doctors as treatment options that may be used in the right circumstances, just as the gardener above requires a suitable power tool.

Some training or educational information would also need to be made available to cover topics such as the impaired cellular response to thyroid hormone and the failure of T4 replacement therapy. Training or educational information would need to be made available for T4/T3, natural thyroid and T3 thyroid hormone replacement therapies.

Doctors that do employ T3 replacement therapy need to begin adopting a wider range of divided doses of T3, with the awareness that three to five divided doses of T3 have been found to be effective by a large number of patients successfully using T3. Total daily dosages in the range of 40-60 micrograms of T3 are not going to be sufficient to resolve the symptoms of some patients, who may require 70 or 80 micrograms of T3 or more in some cases.

In the case of a combined T4/T3, or pure T3 treatment, any patient requiring one of these treatments has already failed to become well on T4 replacement therapy. Consequently, conventional treatment practices are not going to be successful. Some doctors who have good success rates with managing T4/T3 replacement find it useful to focus more on the patient's symptoms and signs, in combination with using FT4/FT3 levels. This is probably due to their awareness of the unreliability of TSH, as an indicator of tissue levels of thyroid hormones.

In the case of T3 replacement therapy, the type of approach outlined in this book will be required, which has virtually no reliance on thyroid blood tests to assess treatment progress. This may require more training or specialist support.

These changes should **not** be tied to and paced by further discoveries in the area of medical research. Thyroid patients cannot wait for more research to occur.

NUTRIENT TESTING AND SUPPLEMENTATION

I have communicated with too many thyroid patients over the past several years to not include some comment here about vitamin and mineral deficiencies. I have learned that far too frequently some nutrient that is critical to thyroid hormone metabolism has been too low. In some cases this state of affairs has continued for many years and the patient has continued to experience severe symptoms associated with hypothyroidism even though various thyroid hormone treatment approaches have been tried. In a few cases the appropriate tests had been performed but the patient's doctor had just not realised that a desperately low level of some nutrient may have actually been critical.

Many doctors appear to consider that investigating nutritional deficiencies and supplementing with a wide range of vitamins and minerals is some form of alternative medicine. If more doctors were aware of the essential need for these nutrients in the processing of thyroid and adrenal hormones and within the mitochondria then perhaps there would be more attention on this area. I also have concerns over some of the laboratory reference ranges for nutrients that appear to be applied to all categories of patient in a uniform manner.

I would like to see more thorough testing of important vitamins and minerals incorporated into the protocol for diagnosing and treating thyroid patients. If an important nutrient is found to have a tested value that is just within the laboratory reference range then this should not be ignored. People with already compromised thyroid hormone metabolisms require very healthy levels of nutrients and better guidelines need to be in place for doctors who do this type of testing for thyroid patients. Perhaps a specific set of nutrient tests and more helpful laboratory ranges could be developed specifically for patients with compromised thyroid hormone metabolism.

I also believe that it is right and proper for thyroid patients to be encouraged to use a broad range of vitamin and supplements to maximise their chances of correct thyroid hormone activity. I do not know whether it would be practical for this to be available via the UK NHS but provision of good supplementation and a healthy diet appears to be an important factor in the ultimate recovery of some people. I know that this approach has helped me significantly.

There is sound science behind the need to test for nutrient deficiencies and to ensure that key nutrients are provided at healthy levels. Many thyroid patients would benefit from thyroid diagnosis and treatment protocols that have been updated to include a far more robust and proactive approach to nutrients that are critical to thyroid hormone metabolism.

MEDICAL SCHOOLS

At the present, medical school training does not adequately cover the potential failure of T4 replacement therapy to correct a thyroid hormone problem. This needs to be addressed.

The use of the various thyroid hormone replacement therapies needs to be introduced into medical training as soon as possible This will allow doctors to have all the tools they need to treat all thyroid patients, not just a large number of them. Universities and medical schools should incorporate the updated thyroid treatment protocols into their teaching, so that the next generation of doctors are aware of all the treatment options available.

PHARMACEUTICAL COMPANIES HAVE A ROLE

Pharmaceutical companies need to make liothyronine sodium (T3) tablets available in smaller tablets than the 20 micrograms currently available in the UK.

A patient using T3 replacement therapy often has to split a T3 tablet in order to produce a 5-microgram, 7.5-microgram, 10-microgram, 12.5-microgram, 15-microgram and 17.5-microgram T3 divided dose. The availability of 2.5-microgram and 5-microgram T3 tablets would be an enormous help, as it would avoid the need to have to split a T3 tablet into eighths (2.5 micrograms). If 5-microgram and 10-microgram T3 tablets were also available, then no tablet splitting would be required at all, just the ability to do simple maths. I have not spoken to anyone yet who has needed to break tablets into smaller sizes than 2.5 micrograms. I believe that almost all patients using T3 replacement therapy would benefit from being able to increment individual T3 doses by 2.5 micrograms.

INTERIM SOLUTIONS

What happens to thyroid patients who remain unwell on T4 replacement therapy at the moment? These thyroid patients require some interim solutions to be put in place. One example of an interim solution would be to train a number of endocrinologists or family doctors to specialise in dealing specifically with patients who fail to respond to T4 replacement therapy. These doctors would need to become adept in using alternative ways of detecting thyroid conditions, apart from simply using blood tests, for example placing more emphasis on symptoms and signs.

Treatments offered would need to include natural thyroid, synthetic T4 and T3 in combination as well as pure T3 for the more difficult cases. T3 replacement therapy in particular requires far more intensive patient support during the initial dosage management phase than T4 replacement therapy.

There may be doctors or politicians who would deem this interim solution too expensive. However, I believe that the long-term savings that could be made, by restoring thyroid patients to full health, would easily cover these costs. A considerable number of thyroid patients find that they are unable to work due to continued ill health and have to survive on State Benefits. Restoration of good health would enable these patients to return to work. This would remove their dependence on State support and allow them to make a positive contribution once more. Apart from the on-going expenses associated with dealing with patients who do not feel well on

T4 treatment, there are the further costs that will be incurred if some of these patients go on to develop other diseases as a result of prolonged hypothyroidism, e.g. cardiovascular diseases, diabetes etc. Any short-term costs should be regarded as an investment that will be recouped over time.

BASELINE THYROID TESTING

Mindful of my own thyroid problems and with the knowledge that at least one other family member was diagnosed with a thyroid issue and another may have had thyroid disease, I suggested to my two sons that they had a complete set of thyroid blood tests done before leaving home and going to university. They are both well and are fully grown adults now. I thought that it was advisable for my sons to have the knowledge of their thyroid hormone levels, especially FT4 and FT3, when they were adults and in good health. Armed with this information, should any future thyroid problems arise, then it could take some of the guesswork away from diagnosis and treatment, as both of my sons will already have a fair idea of the levels of FT4 and FT3 that enable them to feel healthy. Much to her credit, our family doctor was supportive of these laboratory tests.

Given that it is sometimes difficult to diagnose thyroid disease and it can certainly be difficult to treat in some cases, then this approach may be something that the medical profession might want to consider for families with thyroid problems in their medical history. A simple baseline test for offspring once they have become young healthy adults may save a considerable amount of time, money and stress later on.

NEED FOR CHANGE

Thyroid patients desperately need a more comprehensive treatment protocol available, so that other treatments may be attempted, in those cases where T4 replacement therapy fails to resolve symptoms. The above suggestions for enhancements to the treatment for hypothyroidism are not made lightly. I have been considering this area for many years and have communicated with many thyroid patients who have had similar problems to myself.

The only way to have a significant impact on the lives of thyroid patients is to make changes from within the current system and have more doctors and endocrinologists treat the very real problem of impaired cellular response to thyroid hormone. This will hopefully reduce or eliminate the need that some patients feel to go outside of the medical system and self-medicate.

In the long-term, medical research needs to deliver a comprehensive solution to all the practical diagnosis and treatment issues associated with impaired cellular response to thyroid hormone. In the short-term, some focused medical research needs to happen, to provide better interim diagnostic and treatment tools that can aid doctors in their handling of cases where T4 replacement therapy does not adequately resolve a patient's symptoms.

It is very important that adequately funded and focused medical research occurs and is encouraged and monitored. This research is vital for those thyroid patients who feel that they have been abandoned and condemned to live with the symptoms of hypothyroidism for the rest of their lives.

Chapter 31

Final Comments

I am a thyroid patient who failed to recover on any form of T4 treatment. I eventually discovered that T3 replacement therapy successfully eliminated all my symptoms and allowed me to recover my health. T3 continues to work well for me.

Thankfully, I refused to accept the many misinterpretations of my symptoms and of my thyroid blood test results, given to me in the early years of my illness.

I was repeatedly told that my symptoms had nothing to do with my thyroid hormones and that I would simply have to learn to live with the situation. One endocrinologist diagnosed me with ME and suggested that I join a support group. I was also told that my symptoms were psychological in origin and one doctor warned me that if I wanted any further help from him I would have to agree to a trial of the anti-depressant, Prozac.

The responses I received from doctors during those early years are very similar to the stories I have heard from so many other thyroid patients who fail to recover on T4 replacement therapy. Worryingly, one doctor even told me that medicine cannot be considered a proper science and that I couldn't expect to find explanations for everything.

Virtually none of the doctors I saw showed any interest in the data I had carefully collected, including my temperature and the array of symptoms that are so representative of hypothyroidism. Some endocrinologists told me that measurements like my low body temperature were irrelevant.

The only data that appeared to be important to the doctors that I sought help from, in those early years, were thyroid blood test results. These doctors were satisfied and content when my thyroid blood test results fell into the laboratory reference ranges. Their job was done. They could pat themselves on the back and take my payment if it was a private consultation.

As far as these doctors were concerned, any problems I was left with were either not related to thyroid hormones, or were issues I was going to have to live with. The fact that my work and family life were being destroyed at the time, by the effect of these symptoms and that these symptoms exactly mapped onto the symptoms of hypothyroidism, didn't make any of these doctors want to take ownership for getting my health problems resolved.

A great deal of what I was told during those early years, by supposed experts, was absolute rubbish!

Unfortunately, there are still patients being told the same sort of misleading information, in the face of failing T4 replacement therapy. I feel deeply frustrated by the stories that I hear about every week on Internet forums dedicated to thyroid disease. I know that there are perfectly good alternative thyroid replacement therapies available that are likely to be more effective than T4 replacement therapy and that ought to be available to those patients who continue to feel unwell on T4. I want to be clear and state that if T4 replacement therapy is working well for a patient and successfully eliminating all of their symptoms, then it is clearly a good treatment for that particular patient.

I was recently told a story by a thyroid patient who completely recovered many years ago as a direct result of using the T3 thyroid hormone and is now healthy and has retrained in a highly regarded and intellectually challenging profession. Prior to treatment with T3 replacement therapy this person had clear symptoms of hypothyroidism, was completely unable to work and function normally, even though thyroid blood tests were within the laboratory ranges. Various 'diagnoses' were suggested by different doctors, which included chronic fatigue syndrome. It was not 'chronic fatigue'. It was impaired cellular response to thyroid hormone. This patient has been taking quite a high dosage of T3 for the past ten years, has no symptoms of tissue over-stimulation by thyroid hormone and feels completely normal. I have met this person and can testify that this individual appears to be in the absolute best of health. This patient's doctor apparently now wants to withdraw the T3 medication that has been prescribed for many years and has told the patient that the use of T3 is just 'a simple lifestyle choice, which is likely to cause avoidable long term health problems'. This was a selection of words that was actually committed to paper in a letter to another doctor! There is a need for some re-education of those doctors that display this type of ignorance, arrogance, lack of ability to think beyond inadequate thyroid disease training and lack of empathy. Significant change is required if patients are to get the treatment and support that they require.

I wish to see better care become available for those patients who aren't recovering using T4. Nutrient deficiencies do need to be considered and dealt with in a more intelligent, thorough and comprehensive manner than is currently being done. Patients, whose nutrient levels are healthy but still fail to recover using T4 replacement therapy, may have impaired cellular response to thyroid hormone and may require a higher level of T3 within their cells in order to recover. This may frequently be achieved through a T4/T3 based treatment or through the use of T3. Contrary to popular belief, T4 isn't the only thyroid hormone replacement available and some people may feel better on one of the other treatment options. Many patients do fully recover once they are prescribed one of the other thyroid replacement therapies - I communicate with these people quite often. This is not a fairy tale - it is reality.

I believe that it is also possible that some proportion of patients who have been diagnosed with ME, chronic fatigue syndrome, fibromyalgia or other conditions that are related to low metabolic rate, may also have impaired cellular response to thyroid hormone. A deficiency in T3 at the tissue level will not necessarily show up in routine thyroid function blood tests, which implies that there may be no obvious blood test markers of thyroid disease for a subset of these patients.

KEY FACTORS IN MY RECOVERY

To summarise, the following points enabled me to fully understand my thyroid problem and recover my health through T3 replacement therapy:

- I considered my medical history.

- I carefully logged my symptoms and signs, in order to fully understand how they changed over time and with different dosages of thyroid hormone. I kept detailed records of all the medication I took and how it affected me. Gathering data is essential in order to understand the patterns associated with the illness. It also provides a documented record to share with doctors.

- I kept records of all my blood tests and familiarised myself with the laboratory reference ranges.

- I learned as much as I could about thyroid hormones and how they work. Knowledge does empower you and with this disease, at this moment in time, it is very important.

- I took responsibility for my own health and did not simply accept everything and every opinion I was told. I wish I had taken responsibility for my own health a lot sooner, as I now recognise that time disappears all too quickly with thyroid disease.

- I tried to keep up to date with current research on my condition as knowledge definitely defeats fear! I didn't do this thoroughly but I made sure I spent some time on this every few months.

- I found competent medical professionals that I could work with. I actively sought for these doctors. This was one of my most important goals. I found a doctor who was experienced in prescribing natural thyroid and combinations of T4/T3 and fortunately he allowed me to go on a trial of T3 replacement. I was lucky to find an open-minded family doctor who supported me superbly. I was referred to a brilliant and far more open-minded endocrinologist, who I could really talk to. Working with competent doctors makes a huge difference. It enabled me to have some confidence about a consultation, rather than be apprehensive that I was about to have another confrontation.

- I was extremely determined and never gave up looking for a solution. I refused to accept that I would have to live with the symptoms that T4 treatment failed to resolve. I rejected the all-too-easy diagnosis of ME, which I felt in my case was an admission of defeat by one endocrinologist. I remained active and assertive in trying to find a workable solution to my problems.

Most of these points are largely associated with a change of attitude. This mind-set change was a critical part of my recovery. I began to take responsibility for getting my thyroid problem resolved and was unwilling to accept the close-minded and unhelpful approach of some of the doctors who attempted to treat me during the first six or seven years of my illness. I believe that until excellent diagnostic and treatment practices regarding impaired cellular response to thyroid hormone are prevalent, then this type of positive, proactive state of mind by the patient may be an important part of the recovery process.

UK THYROID TREATMENT APPEARS TO BE LAGGING BEHIND

In the UK particularly, there seems to be a reluctance to adopt any of the emerging new research findings and to apply them to the clinical treatment of thyroid disease. There is also a continuing refusal to believe that T4 replacement therapy simply isn't working for some patients. Many doctors adhere to rigid methods based on thyroid blood test results during treatment, even when T3 thyroid hormone forms a part of the treatment. This is in spite of research findings that suggest that thyroid blood test results may be misleading for some patients.

Over the past eight or ten years, I have communicated with hundreds of thyroid patients from all over the world including the UK, the USA, some other European countries and Australia. Many patients in these other countries are being taken far more seriously when they complain that T4 isn't effectively eliminating their symptoms. Patients in the USA are finding it easier to locate doctors who will provide them with alternative thyroid treatments, including natural thyroid preparations and combinations of T4 and T3 therapies. In fact, the UK is well known, amongst sufferers in other countries, for providing very limited treatment options for thyroid patients.

In the UK, a few doctors have dared to place more emphasis on patients' symptoms and signs rather than blood test results and TSH levels. Some of these doctors have also offered their patients alternative thyroid treatments to T4 replacement therapy. A few of these enlightened doctors have been forced to cease practising medicine, simply because they refused to be slaves to the rigid and inadequate guidelines laid down by the UK endocrinological community on the treatment of thyroid conditions. The refusal of many UK doctors to prescribe anything other than T4 means that many thyroid patients have a limited chance of ever recovering, because there aren't many resources to turn to. Thyroid patients in the UK are having an extremely difficult time - perhaps even harder now than when I was struggling twenty years ago.

Patients, who are aware of any of the recent research concerning thyroid disease, or those who hear of other patients recovering using alternative thyroid treatments, are likely to become extremely frustrated that other treatment options are not being made available.

Let me make it quite clear that I do believe that thyroid patients all over the world require significant improvements in thyroid diagnosis and treatment and they need far more easy access to doctors who are capable of helping them. I just believe that here in the UK the medical profession has been particularly slow to make improvements in the areas that this book is focused on.

T4/T3 AND T3 REPLACEMENT THERAPY ARE GREATLY UNDER-UTILISED

It is very unfortunate that the T3 thyroid hormone is often overlooked, misunderstood and even slightly feared by some patients and doctors. There are so many negative myths surrounding T3 and many people continue to be doubtful of using T3 as a proper thyroid hormone replacement therapy, despite mounting evidence of its success in certain patients. I believe T3 should be used far more frequently than it is today, as it would help many thyroid patients recover as I did. It is surprising to me that T3 is used so infrequently as a therapeutic tool. T3 should be a mainstream thyroid replacement hormone, alongside natural thyroid and synthetic T4.

I recently read an article in a newspaper that was generally positive about the potential use of T3 as a treatment. However, the response from an endocrinologist who was interviewed was to point out that the rapid way in which T3 reaches high peak levels is a risk for heart problems and bone loss. This view that I hear so often completely misunderstands two things. Firstly, the rapid absorption and high peak levels of T3 are what makes it so incredibly useful in addressing impaired cellular response to thyroid hormone. Secondly, there are perfectly good ways of managing a T3 dosage to ensure that there are no instances of tissue over-stimulation by T3.

The unique properties of pure T3 make it possible to help people like me regain their lives. T3 should be a drug that doctors are delighted that they have available rather than one that so many view with fear and distrust.

When you consider what thyroid disease does to peoples' lives when it is incorrectly treated, then it is simply a tragedy that T3 replacement therapy and the T4/T3 therapies are not available to all doctors, as basic tools at their disposal. The devastating effect that incorrectly treated hypothyroidism can have on the lives of other people around the patient, needs to be considered. The emotional, relationship, work and financial consequences can be extremely high.

For me, the effect of using T3 was like throwing a switch. Within weeks of using T3 I had my life back, although I had a lot of lessons to learn about its use. I am quite a careful and cautious person. I would not have continued to use T3 if I thought for one minute that there was anything unsafe about it.

THYROID DISEASE MAY OCUR MORE FREQUENTLY

It is possible that over time far more patients will require T3 in order to overcome their impaired cellular response to thyroid hormone. This is not just because many patients already exist that would be healthier on T3 replacement than any other treatment.

I believe that, albeit very slowly, contaminants in our air, food and water supplies are having an insidious effect on our immune systems. Our diet and modern life is also having a stressful effect on our bodies. Modern medicine has enabled us to live longer lives. Therefore, any genetic defects that we may possess are no longer being weeded out, whereas even as little as one hundred years ago the same genetic defects may have shortened lives to the point that defective genes were not passed to another generation.

I believe that as our immune systems are gradually more compromised then more people will develop thyroid problems and a higher proportion of thyroid patients will find that only T3 resolves their symptoms. I derive no pleasure from this viewpoint because I see it as a sad situation for the human race. I just believe that it is the most likely scenario.

Therefore, it is imperative that the T3 and T4/T3 replacement therapies are fully embraced by the medical profession as soon as possible so that the increasing numbers of patients who require them can be cared for correctly.

FINALLY

For any patient, about to embark on a trial of T3 replacement therapy, when all other thyroid treatments have failed, I wish you good luck. With the support of a well informed and intelligent doctor and armed with patience and caution, there is every reason to assume that T3 replacement therapy can be made to work both effectively and safely and help you to recover, just as I managed to.

Now it's time for the endocrinologists who govern the diagnosis and treatment methods for thyroid patients, to begin to make long overdue changes that incorporate all the available thyroid hormone therapies that already exist and work well for so many people.

It is also the time for the thyroid researchers to come to our rescue and do the good work that will finally bring about the necessary understanding, new laboratory tests and breakthroughs that we so desperately need.

I believe that it is in the long-term interest of both the medical profession and thyroid patients that more positive partnerships are established to share knowledge, ideas and recipes for success in the treatment of patients who do not feel well on T4 replacement therapy. It is essential that the medical profession utilise all successful diagnostic and treatment methods when necessary to help people recover from thyroid disease. I really am hoping that we may soon enter an era of more partnership and cooperation with medical professionals, as I firmly believe that this is the only sensible way forward. I for one would be happy to contribute to this in whatever form was necessary.

It is a fact that some thyroid patients simply cannot recover through the use of T4 replacement therapy. It is unfortunate that at the present time in the world of thyroid disease, this still appears to be the elephant in the room!

SECTION 8

APPENDICES

Appendix A

Books for Further Reading

Dr. John C. Lowe: *The Metabolic Treatment of Fibromyalgia.* Boulder, McDowell Publishing Company, 2000. ISBN 0-914609-02-05.

Dr. Gina Honeyman-Lowe and Dr. John C. Lowe: *Your Guide to Metabolic Health.* Boulder, McDowell Health-Science Books, 2003. ISBN 0-974123-0-3.

Dr. Barry Durrant-Peatfield: *Your Thyroid and how to keep it healthy.* London, Hammersmith Press Ltd. Second Edition, 2006. ISBN 978-1-905140-10-7.

Mark Starr, M.D.: *Hypothyroidism Type 2: The Epidemic.* Columbia, Mark Starr Trust, 2010. ISBN 978-0-9752624-0-5.

Janie A. Bowthorpe, M.Ed.: *Stop The Thyroid Madness. A Patient Revolution Against Decades of Inferior Thyroid Treatment.* Colorado, Laughing Grape Publishing, 2008. ISBN 978-0615-477121.

Datis Kharrazian: *Why Do I Still Have Thyroid Symptoms? When My Lab Tests Are Normal.* New York, Morgan James Publishing, 2010. ISBN 978-1-60037-670-2.

James L. Wilson N.D., D.C., Ph.D.: *Adrenal Fatigue. The 21st Century Stress Syndrome.* USA, Smart Publications, 2001. ISBN 1-890572-15-2.

Steve Hickey Ph.D. and Andrew W. Saul Ph.D.: *Vitamin C: The Real Story.* Basic Health Publications Inc., 2008. ISBN 978-1-59120-223-3.

Dr. Steve Hickey & Dr Hilary Roberts: *Ascorbate The Science of Vitamin C,* 2004. ISBN 1-4116-0724-4.

Patrick Holford: *The Optimum Nutrition Bible.* Judy Piatkus (Publishers) Ltd., 1998. ISBN 0-7499-1748-2.

Midred S. Seelig, M.D., MPH, Andrea Rosanoff, PhD.: The Magnesium Factor. Avery, 2003. ISBN 1-58333-156-5.

Two Excellent Endocrinology Books (for those who wish to dig deeper):

Lewis E. Braverman and Robert D. Utiger: *Werner and Ingbar's The Thyroid: A Fundamental and Clinical Text.* Lippincott Williams & Wilkins, 2005. ISBN 978-0781750479

K.L. Becker (Editor), John P. Bilezikian (Editor), William J. Bremner (Editor), Wellington Hung (Editor), C.Ronald Kahn (Editor): *Principles and Practice of Endocrinology and Metabolism.* Lippincott Williams and Wilkins, 2001. ISBN 978-0781717502.

Appendix B

Useful Websites

Recovering With T3
Website: http://recoveringwitht3.com or http://rwt3.com
- The purpose of recoveringwitht3.com is to provide information for people who are trying to recover from hypothyroidism using the T3 thyroid hormone. It includes a section on T3 Success Stories that have been submitted by thyroid patients from around the world. Many of these provide evidence of the effectiveness of the T3 dosage management process and the Circadian T3 Method (CT3M or T3CM).

Recovering with T3 Facebook Page
Website: http://www.facebook.com/recoveringwitht3
- Provides information regarding new updates to the Recovering with T3 website and additional information for people trying to recover from hypothyroidism using the T3 thyroid hormone.

Thyroid Patient Advocacy
Website: http://www.tpa-uk.org.uk/
- This is a UK based (but international) independent, user-led, organisation established to ensure that all thyroid disease sufferers are given a correct diagnosis and receive effective treatment. TPA believes that all patients should have access to all relevant tests and treatment, including synthetic or natural T3. Thyroid Patient Advocacy is registered as a UK Charitable Trust.

Thyroid UK
Website: http://www.thyroiduk.org
- This is a thyroid website aimed at providing information and resources to promote effective diagnosis and appropriate treatment for people with thyroid disorders in the UK. Thyroid UK is registered as a charitable company.

DrLowe.com
Website: http://www.drlowe.com
- The purpose is to provide an abundant source of information solidly based on science and logic and of practical value to patients and clinicians who deal with hypothyroidism, thyroid hormone resistance and fibromyalgia.

Thyroid Science

Website: http://www.ThyroidScience.com

- This is an open-access journal for truth in thyroid science and thyroid clinical practice.

Stop The Thyroid Madness Website

Website: http://www.stopthethyroidmadness.com

- Patient centric website presenting the experience of thyroid patients in an honest and direct way.

Mary Shomon's Thyroid Disease Website

Website: http://thyroid.about.com

- Provides a broad range of information for patients on all aspects of thyroid disease.

Thyroid Disease Manager

Website: http://www.thyroidmanager.org

- The purpose of the site is to assist physicians in managing patients who have, or may have thyroid disease. Information is provided on thyroid diseases, diagnosis and therapy. Provides a range of relatively up-to-date, technical information on thyroid hormones and thyroid hormone metabolism.

The National Academy of Hypothyroidism

Website: http://nahypothyroidism.org

- This is a non-profit, multidisciplinary medical society dedicated to the dissemination of new information on the diagnosis and treatment of hypothyroidism.

PubMed

Website: http://www.ncbi.nlm.nih.gov/pubmed/

- Resource for finding medical research papers. Millions of studies from researchers all over the world are summarised and available on PubMed.

Appendix C

References By Chapter

Chapter 2

1. Starr, M.: *Hypothyroidism Type 2: The Epidemic*. Columbia, Mark Starr Trust, 2010. Chapter 9, Pages 170-182.
2. Durrant-Peatfield, B.: *Your Thyroid and how to keep it healthy*. Second edition. London, Hammersmith Press Ltd, 2006. Chapter Nine, Pages 125-140.
3. The Association for Clinical Biochemistry.: UK Guidelines for the Use of Thyroid Function Tests. July 2006. <http://www.british-thyroid-association.org/info-for-patients/Docs/TFT_guideline_final_version_July_2006.pdf>
4. Conti, A., Studer, H., Kneubuehl, F., Kohler, H.: Regulation of Thyroidal Deiodinase Activity. *Endocrinology*, Vol. 102 (1):321-329, 1978.
5. Ikeda, K., Takeuchi, T., Ito, Y., Murakami, I., Mokuda, O., Tominaga, M., Mashiba, H.: Effect of thyrotropin on conversion of T4 to T3 in perfused rat liver. *Life Sciences*, Volume 38, Issue 20:1801-1806, 1986.
6. Ikeda, T., Honda M., Murakami, I., Kuno, S., Mokuda, O., Tokumori, Y., Tominaga, M., Mashiba, H.: Effect of TSH on conversion of T4 to T3 in perfused rat kidney. *Metabolism*, Volume 34, Issue 11:1057-1060, 1985.
7. Nicoloff, J.T., Fisher, D.A., Appleman, M.D. Jr.: The role of glucocorticoids in the regulation of thyroid function in man. *J. Clin. Invest.*, 49(10):1922–1929, 1970.
8. Brabant, A., Brabant, G., Shuermeyer, T., et al.: The role of glucocorticoids in the regulation of thyrotropin. *Acta Endocrinol.*, (Copen), 121:95-100, 1989.
9. Alford, F.P., Baker, H.W.G., Burger, H.G., de Kretser, D.M., Hudson, B., Johns, M.W., Masterton, J.P., Patel, Y.C., Rennie, G.C.: Temporal Patterns of Integrated Plasma Hormone Levels During Sleep and Wakefulness. I. Thyroid-Stimulating Hormone, Growth Hormone and Cortisol. *J. Clin. Endocrinol. Metab.*, Vol. 37 (6):841-847, 1973.
10. Lowe, J.C., Eichelberger, J., Manso, G., Peterson, K.: Improvement in euthyroid fibromyalgia patients treated with T3. *J. Myofascial Ther.*, 1(2):16-29, 1994.

Chapter 3

1. Wilson, J.L.: *Adrenal Fatigue The 21st Century Stress Syndrome*. USA, Smart Publications, 2001. Chapter 16, Pages 212-213.
2. Wilson, J.L.: *Adrenal Fatigue The 21st Century Stress Syndrome*. USA, Smart Publications, 2001. Chapter 17, Page 218.
3. Honeyman-Lowe, G., Lowe, J.C.: *Your Guide to Metabolic Health*. Boulder, McDowell Health-Science Books, 2003. Chapter 8, Pages 169-189.
4. Lowe, J.C.: *The Metabolic Treatment of Fibromyalgia*. Boulder, McDowell Publishing Company, 2000. Section 5.2, Pages 955-957.
5. Starr, M.: *Hypothyroidism Type 2: The Epidemic*. Columbia, Mark Starr Trust, 2010. Chapter 10, Pages 183-190.

Chapter 4

1. Dillman E, Gale C, Green W., et al.: Hypothermia in iron deficiency due to altered triiodothyronine metabolism. *Am J Physiol*. 239(5):R377-81. Nov.1980.

2. Beard J., Tobin B., Green W. Evidence for thyroid hormone deficiency in iron-deficient anemic rats. *J. Nutr.* 119(5):772-778. May 1989.
3. Stangl, G.I., Schwarz, F.J., Kirchgessner, M.: Cobalt deficiency effects on trace elements, hormones and enzymes involved in energy metabolism of cattle. *Int. J. Vitam. Nutr. Res.*, 69(2):120-126, 1999.
4. Holick, M.F.: Sunlight and vitamin D for bone health and prevention of autoimmune diseases, cancers, and cardiovascular disease. *Am. J. Clin. Nutr.*, Vol. 80, No. 6:1678S-1688S, 2004.
5. Friedman, T.C.: Vitamin D deficiency and thyroid disease. <http://www.goodhormonehealth.com/VitaminD.pdf>
6. Kharrazian, D.: *Why Do I Still Have Thyroid Symptoms? When My Lab Tests Are Normal.* New York, Morgan James Publishing, 2010. Chapter Two, Page 35.
7. Kharrazian, D.: *Why Do I Still Have Thyroid Symptoms? When My Lab Tests Are Normal.* New York, Morgan James Publishing, 2010. Chapter Three, Page 52-53.
8. Ross, A.C., Manson, J.E., Abrams, S.A., Aloia, J.F., Brannon, P.M., Clinton. S.K., Durazo-Arvizu, R.A., Gallagher, J.C., Gallo, R.L., Jones, G., Kovacs, C.S., Mayne, S.T., Rosen, C.J., Shapses, S.A.: The 2011 report on dietary reference intakes for calcium and vitamin D from the Institute of Medicine: what clinicians need to know. J. Clin. Endocrinol. Metab., 96 (1):53–58, 2011.
9. Lowe, J.C.: *The Metabolic Treatment of Fibromyalgia.* Boulder, McDowell Publishing Company, 2000. Section 5.5, Page 1033.
10. Van Dam, F. and van Gool, W.A.: Hyperhomocysteinemia and Alzheimer's disease: A systematic review. *Archives of Gerentology and Geratrics*, 48: 425-430 (2009).
11. Smith, A.D.: The worldwide challenge of the dementias: a role for B vitamins and homocysteine?. *Food Nutr Bull*, 29(2 Suppl): S143–72 (2008).
12. Hickey, S., Saul, A.W.: *Vitamin C: The Real Story.* Basic Health Publications Inc., 2008.
13. Hickey, S., Roberts, H.: *Ascorbate The Science of Vitamin C.* 2004.
14. Seelig, M.S.: *Magnesium Deficiency in The Pathogenesis of Disease.* Springer. 1980. Part II, Chapter 7.
15. Seelig, M.S., Rosanoff, A.: *The Magnesium Factor.* Avery. 2003. Chapter 1, Pages 14-17.
16. Beckett, G.J., MacDougall, D.A., Nicol, F., Arthur, J.R.: Inhibition of type I and type II iodothyronine deiodinase activity in rat liver, kidney, and brain produced by selenium deficiency. *Biochem. J.*, 259(3):887-892, 1st May 1989.
17. Arthur, J.R., Nicol, F., Beckett, J.G.: Selenium deficiency, thyroid hormone metabolism, and thyroid hormone deiodinases. *Am. J. Clin. Nutr.*, Vol. 57:236S-239S, 1993.
18. Gärtner, R., Gasnier, B.C., Dietrich, J.W., Krebs, B., Angstwurm, M.W.: Selenium supplementation in patients with autoimmune thyroiditis decreases thyroid peroxidase antibodies concentrations. *J. Clin. Endocrinol. Metab.*, Vol. 87, No. 4:1687-1691, 2002.
19. Al-Juboori, I.A., R. Al-Rawi, H. K. A-Hakeim.: Estimation of Serum Copper, Manganese, Selenium, and Zinc in Hypothyroidism Patients. *IUFS J Biol.* 68(2):121-126. 2009.
20. Brandão-Neto, J., de Mendonça, B.B., Shuhama, T., Marchini, J.S., Pimenta, W.P., and Tornero, M.T.T.: Zinc acutely and temporarily inhibits adrenal cortisol secretion in humans a preliminary report. *Biol Trace Elem Res.* Vol 24, No. 1, 83-89, Doi: 10.1007/BF02789143.
21. Kim, B.G., Adams, J.M., Jackson, B.A., Lindemann, MD: Effects of chromium(III) picolinate on cortisol and DHEAs secretion in H295R human adrenocortical cells. *Biol Trace Elem Res.* 2010 Feb;133(2):171-80.
22. Holford, P.: *The Optimum Nutrition Bible.* Judy Piatkus (Publishers) Ltd., 1998. Part 8, Pages 301-319.

Chapter 5

1. Starr, M.: *Hypothyroidism Type 2: The Epidemic.* Columbia, Mark Starr Trust, 2010. Pages 197-236.
2. Honeyman-Lowe, G., Lowe, J.C.: *Your Guide to Metabolic Health.* Boulder, McDowell Health-Science Books, 2003. Chapter 12, Pages 264-265.
3. Durrant-Peatfield, B.: *Your Thyroid and how to keep it healthy.* Second edition. London, Hammersmith Press Ltd. 2006. Chapter Four, Page 43.
4. Durrant-Peatfield, B.: *Your Thyroid and how to keep it healthy.* Second edition. London, Hammersmith Press Ltd., 2006. Chapter Four, Page 45.

5. Honeyman-Lowe, G., Lowe, J.C.: *Your Guide to Metabolic Health.* Boulder, McDowell Health-Science Books, 2003. Chapter 9, Pages 191-201.
6. Durrant-Peatfield, B.: *Your Thyroid and how to keep it healthy.* Second edition. London, Hammersmith Press Ltd., 2006. Chapter Seven, Pages 88-92.
7. Wood, J.D.: Histamine, mast cells, and the enteric nervous system in the irritable bowel syndrome, enteritis, and food Allergies. *Gut,* Vol. 55:445-447, 2006.
8. Lowe, J.C.: *The Metabolic Treatment of Fibromyalgia.* Boulder, McDowell Publishing Company, 2000. Section 5.2, Pages 662-663.
9. Kharrazian, D.: *Why Do I Still Have Thyroid Symptoms? When My Lab Tests Are Normal.* New York, Morgan James Publishing, 2010.

Chapter 7

1. Lowe, J.C.: *The Metabolic Treatment of Fibromyalgia.* Boulder, McDowell Publishing Company, 2000. Section 5.5, Page 1033.

Chapter 8

1. Beard, J., Tobin, B., Green, W.: Evidence for thyroid hormone deficiency in iron-deficient anemic rats. *Am. Inst. Of Nutr. Minerals and Trace Elements* 022-3166/89. Page 772.
   <http://jn.nutrition.org/content/119/5/772.full.pdf>

Chapter 10

1. Lowe, J.C.: DrLowe.com. Questions and answers about T3. July 2010.
   <http://www.drlowe.com/QandA/askdrlowe/t3.htm>

Chapter 11

1. Werner, C., Ingbar, H.: *The Thyroid a fundamental and clinical text.* Fourth Edition. Maryland, Harper and Row, Publishers, Inc., 1978. Chapter 49, Page 967.
2. Becker, K.L.: *Principles and Practice of Endocrinology and Metabolism,* Philadelphia, J.B. Lippincott Company. 1990. Chapter 235, Part XVI, Page 1720.
3. Lowe, J.C.: *The Metabolic Treatment of Fibromyalgia.* Boulder, McDowell Publishing Company, 2000. Section 5.4, Pages 1017-1019.
4. Kaplan, M.M., Swartz, S.L., Larsen, P.R.: Partial peripheral resistance to thyroid hormone. *Am. J. Med.,* 70 (5):1115-1121, May 1981.
5. Lowe, J.C.: *The Metabolic Treatment of Fibromyalgia.* Boulder, McDowell Publishing Company, 2000. Section 5.4, Page 1017.
6. Negi, C.S.: *Introduction to Endocrinology.* Prentice-Hall of India Pvt. Ltd., 2010. Page 124.
7. Werner, C., Ingbar, H.: *The Thyroid a fundamental and clinical text.* Fourth Edition. Maryland, Harper and Row, Publishers, Inc., 1978. Chapter 16, Page 329.
8. Melmed, S.: *The Pituitary.* Second Edition. Blackwell Publishing, June 2002. Chapter 5, Page 187.

Chapter 12

1. Starr, M.: *Hypothyroidism Type 2: The Epidemic.* Columbia, Mark Starr Trust, 2010. Chapter 8, Page 168.
2. Rowsemitt C.N., Najarian, T.: TSH is Not the Answer: Rationale for a New Paradigm to Evaluate and Treat Hypothyroidism, Particularly Associated with Weight Loss. *Thyroid Science* 6(4):H1-16, 2011 <www.ThyroidScience.com>
3. Najarian, T, Rowsemitt, C.N.: Hypothyroidism, Particularly Associated with Weight Loss: Evaluation and Treatment based on Symptoms and Thyroid Hormone Levels. *Thyroid Science* 6(6):CR1-7, 2011 <www.ThyroidScience.com>
4. Uzzan, B., Campos, J., Cucherat, M., Nony, P., Boissel, J.P., Perret, G.Y.: Effects on bone mass of long-term treatment with thyroid hormones: a meta-analysis. *J. Clin. Endocrinol. Metab.,* Vol. 81:4278-4289, 1996.
5. Starr, M.: *Hypothyroidism Type 2: The Epidemic.* Columbia, Mark Starr Trust, 2010. Chapter 7, Page 76.

6. Lowe, J.C.: *The Metabolic Treatment of Fibromyalgia*. Boulder, McDowell Publishing Company, 2000. Section 4.4, Pages 865-875.

7. Kaplan, M.M., Sarne, D.H., Schneider, A.B.: Editorial: In search of the impossible dream? Thyroid hormone replacement therapy that treats all symptoms in all hypothyroid patients. *J. Clin. Endocrinol. Metab.*, Vol. 88, No. (10):4540-4542, 2003.

8. Dullaart, R.P., vanDoormaal, J.J., Hoogenberg, K., Sluiter, W.J.: Triiodothyronine rapidly lowers plasma lipoprotein (a) in hypothyroid subjects. *Neth. J. Med.*, 46:179-184, 1995.

9. LeMar, H.J. Jr., West, S.G., Garrett, C.R., Hofeldt, F.D.: Covert hypothyroidism presenting as a cardiovascular event. *Am. J. Med.*, (5):549-552, 1991.

10. Mourouzis, I., Forini, F., Pantos, C., Iervasi, G.: Thyroid Hormone and Cardiac Disease: From Basic Concepts to Clinical Application. *J Thyroid Res.* 2011;2011:958626. Epub 2011 Jun 19.

Chapter 15

1. Werner, C., Ingbar, H.: *The Thyroid a fundamental and clinical text*. Fourth Edition. Maryland, Harper and Row, Publishers, Inc., 1978. Chapter 49, Page 967.

2. Werner, C., Ingbar, H.: *The Thyroid a fundamental and clinical text*. Fourth Edition. Maryland, Harper and Row, Publishers, Inc., 1978. Page Chapter 16, 329

3. Melmed, S.: *The Pituitary*. Second Edition. Blackwell Publishing, June 2002. Chapter 5, Page 187.

4. Silva, J.E., Larsen, P.R.: Pituitary nuclear 3,5,3'-triiodothyronine and thyrotropin secretion: an explanation for the effect of thyroxine. *Science*, Vol. 198, No. 4317:617–20, 1977.

5. Larsen, P.R., Frumess, R.D.: Comparison of the biological effects of thyroxine and triiodothyronine in the rat. *Endocrinology*, Vol. 100, No. 4:980–988, 1977.

6. Oppenheimer, J.H., Schwartz, H.L., Surks, M.I.: Propylthiouracil inhibits the conversion of L-thyroxine to L-triiodothyronine: an explanation of the antithyroxine effect of propylthiouracil and evidence supporting the concept that triiodothyronine is the active thyroid hormone. *J Clin Invest.*, 51(9):2493–2497, 1972.

7. Werner, C., Ingbar, H.: *The Thyroid a fundamental and clinical text*. Fourth Edition. Maryland, Harper and Row, Publishers, Inc., 1978. Chapter 18, Page 347.

Chapter 16

1. Becker, K.L.: *Principles and Practice of Endocrinology and Metabolism*. Philadelphia, J.B. Lippincott Company, 1990. Chapter 6, Pages 45-51.

2. Wilson, J.L.: *Adrenal Fatigue The 21st Century Stress Syndrome*. USA, Smart Publications, 2001. Chapter 22, Pages 265-267.

3. Russell, W., Harrison, R.F., Smith, N., Darzy, K., Shalet, S., Weetman, A.P., Ross, R.J.: Free triiodothyronine has a distinct circadian rhythm that is delayed but parallels thyrotropin levels. *J Clin Endocrinol Metab.* 93(6):2300-6. June 2008.

Chapter 25

1. Starr, M.: *Hypothyroidism Type 2: The Epidemic*. Columbia, Mark Starr Trust, 2010. Appendix A, Page 250.

Chapter 28

1. Lowe, J.C.: *The Metabolic Treatment of Fibromyalgia*. Boulder, McDowell Publishing Company. 2000, Section 2.6, Page 301.

2. Starr, M.: *Hypothyroidism Type 2: The Epidemic*. Columbia, Mark Starr Trust, 2010. Appendix A, Page 250. Chapter 6, Page 61.

3. Lowe, J.C. et al.: Fibromyalgia &Thyroid Disease. DrLowe.com, May 2000. <http://www.drlowe.com/france.htm>

4. Privalsky, M.L., Yoh, S.M.: Resistance to Thyroid Hormone (RTH) Syndrome Reveals Novel Determinants Regulating Interaction of T3 receptor with Corepressor. *Mol. Cell. Endocrinol.*, 159(1-2):109-124, 2000.

5. Durrant-Peatfield, B.: *Your Thyroid and how to keep it healthy*. Second edition. London, Hammersmith Press Ltd., 2006. Chapter Four, Pages 48-49.

6. Prescott, R.W., Yeo P.P., Watson M.J., Johnston I.D., Ratcliffe J.D., Evered D.C.: Total and Free Thyroid Hormone Concentrations after Elective Surgery. *J. Clin. Pathol.*, 32(4):321–324, 1979.

7. Merimee, T.J., Fineberg, E.S.: Starvation-Induced Alterations of Circulating Thyroid Hormone Concentrations in Man. *Metabolism*, 25, Issue 1:79-83, 1976.

Chapter 29

1. Van den Beld, A.W., Visser, T.J., Feedlers, R.A., Grobbee, D.E., Lamberts, S.W.J.: Thyroid Hormone Concentrations, Disease, Physical Function and Mortality in Elderly Men. *J. Clin. Endocrinol. Metab.*, Vol. 90, No. 12:6403–6409, 2005.

2. Escobar-Morreale, H.F., Obregon, M.J., Escobar del Rey, F., and Morealle de Escobar, G.: Replacement therapy for hypothyroidism with thyroxine alone does not ensure euthyroidism in all tissues, as studied in thyroidectomized rats. *J. Clin. Invest.*, 96(6):2828–2838, 1995.

3. Escobar-Morreale, H.F., Obregon, M.J., del Rey, F.E., de Escobar, G.M.: Only the Combined Treatment with Thyroxine and Triiodothyronine Ensures Euthyroidism in All Tissues. *Endocrinology*, 137(6):2490-2502, 1996.

4. Visser, WE, Friesema, EC, Jansen, J, Visser, TJ.: Thyroid hormone transport in and out of cells. *Trends Endocrinol Metab.*, 19(2):50-56, 2008.

5. Panicker, V., Saravanan, P., Vaidya, B., Evans, J., Hattersley, A.T., Frayling, T.M., Dayan, C.M.: Common Variation in the DIO2 Gene Predicts Baseline Psychological Well-Being and Response to Combination Thyroxine Plus Triiodothyronine Therapy in Hypothyroid Patients. *J. of Clin. Endocrinol. and Metab.*, Vol. 94, No. 5:1623-1629, 2009.

6. Rottem, M.: Chronic Urticaria and Autoimmune Thyroid Disease: Is there a Link? *Autoimmunity Reviews*, 2(2):69-72, 2003.

7. Lowe, J.C.: *The Metabolic Treatment of Fibromyalgia*. Boulder, McDowell Publishing Company. 2000. Section 3.13, Pages 662-663.

8. Hickey, S. and Saul, A.W.: *Vitamin C: The Real Story*. Basic Health Publications Inc. 2008. Page xi.

9. Faith, R.E, Murgo, A.J., Good, R.A., Plotnikoff, N.P.: *Cytokines Stress and Immunity*. CRC Press Inc, 2006. Pages 69-72.

10. Schatzberg, A.F. and Nemeroff, C.B.: *The American Psychiatric Publishing Textbook of Psychopharmacology*, 3rd ed. American Psychiatric Publishing, Inc. 2009. Page 211.

11. Pfaff, D.W.: *Hormones, Brain and Behaviour*. Vol. 5. Academic Press, 2002. Page 225.

12. Jingcheng, Yu, Koenig, R.J.: Regulation of Hepatocyte Thyroxine 5-'Deiodinase by T3 and Nuclear Receptor Coactivators as a Model of the Sick Euthyroid Syndrome. *J. Biol. Chem.*, 275(49):38296-38301, September 2000.

13. Kharrazian, D.: *Why Do I Still Have Thyroid Symptoms? When My Lab Tests Are Normal*. New York, Morgan James Publishing, 2010. Chapter Three, Page 48.

14. Lu, B., Moser, A.H., Shigenga, J.K., Feingold, K.R., Grunfeld, C.: Type II nuclear hormone receptors, coactivator, and target gene repression in adipose tissue in acute-phase response. *J Lipid Res.*, 47(10):2179-90, 2006.

15. Kimura, H., Caturegli, P.: Chemokine orchestration of autoimmune thyroiditis. *Thyroid*, 17(10):1005-1011, 2007.

16. Yamazaki, K., Suzuki, K., Yamada, E.,Yamada, T, Takeshita, F., Matsumoto, M., Mitsuhashi, T., Obara, T, Takano, K., Sato, K.: Suppression of iodide uptake and thyroid hormone synthesis with stimulation of type I interferon system by double-stranded ribonucleic acid in cultured human thyroid follicles. *Endocrinology*, 148(7):3226-3235, 2007.

17. Kwakkel, J., Wiersinga, W.M., Boelen, A.: Interleukin-1 beta modulates endogenous thyroid hormone receptors alpha gene transcription in liver cells. *J Endocrinol*, 194(2):257-265, 2007.

18. Boelen, A., Platvoetter-Schiphorst, M.C., Wiersinga, W.M.: Association between serum interleukin-6 and serum 3,5,3'-triiodo-thyronine in nonthyroidal illness. *J Clin Endocrinol Metab.*, 77:1695-1699, 1993.

19. Bartelena, L., Brogioni, S., Grasso, L.,Velluzzi, F., Martino, E.: Relationship of the increased serum interleukin-6 concentration to changes of thyroidal function in nonthyroidal illness. *J Endocrinol Invest.*, 17(4):269-274, 1994.

20. Scanlan, T.S.: 3-Iodothyronamine (T1AM): A New Player on the Thyroid Endocrine Team? *Endocrinology*, Vol. 150, No. 3:1108-1111, 2009

21. Refetoff, S., Dewind, L.T., DeGroot, L.J.: Familial syndrome combining deaf-mutism, stippled epiphyses, goiter and abnormally high PBI: possible target organ refractoriness to thyroid hormone. *J. Clin. Endocrinol. Metab.,* Vol. 27 (2):279-294, 1966.

22. Sakurai, A., Takeda, K., Ain, K., Ceccarelli, P., Nakai, A., Seino, S., Bell, G.I., Refetoff, S., DeGroot, L.J.: Generalized resistance to thyroid hormone associated with a mutation in the ligand-binding domain of the human thyroid hormone receptor b. *Proc. Natl. Acad. Sci. USA,* 86(22):8977-8981, 1989.

23. Usala, S.J., Tennyson, G.E., Bale, A.E. et al.: A base mutation of the c-erbAb thyroid hormone receptor in a kindred with generalized thyroid hormone resistance. Molecular heterogeneity in two other kindreds. *J. Clin. Invest.,* 85:93-100, 1990.

24. Refetoff, S., Weiss, R.E. & Usala, S.J.: The syndromes of resistance to thyroid hormone. *Endocr Rev.,* Vol. 14(3):348-399, 1993.

25. Harkonen, M.: Resistance to thyroid hormone. *Duodecim,* 110(21):2009-2011, 1994.

26. Ashizawa, K., Nagataki, S.: Pituitary resistance to thyroid hormone. *Japan J Clin. Med.,* 51(10):2726-2730, 1993.

27. Refetoff, S.: Thyroid Hormone resistance syndromes. Werner's *The Thyroid: A Fundamental and Clinical Text.* Edited by S.H. Ingbar and L.E. Braverman. J. B. Lippincott Co., 1986. Pages 1292-1307.

28. Mechain, C., Leger, A., Feldman, A., Kutten, F., Mauvais-Jarvis, P.: Syndrome pf resistance to thyroid hormones. *Presse Med.,* 22(37):1870-1875, 1993.

29. Refetoff, S.: Resistance to thyroid hormone: an historical overview. *Thyroid,* 1994; 4(3):345-349.

30. Myhill, S., Norman, E., Booth, N.E., McLaren-Howard, J.: Chronic fatigue syndrome and mitochondrial dysfunction. *Int. J. Clin. Exp. Med.,* 2,1-16, 2009.

31. Liewendahl, K.: Triiodothyronine binding to lymphocytes from euthyroid subjects and a patient with peripheral resistance to thyroid hormone. *Acta Endocrinol. (Copenh.),* 83(1):64-70, 1976.

32. Liewendahl, K., Rosengard, S., Lamberg, B.A.: Nuclear binding of triiodothyronine and thyroxine in lymphocytes from subjects with hyperthyroidism, hypothyroidism and resistance to thyroid hormones. *Clin. Chim. Acta.,* 83(1-2):41-48, 1978.

33. Ikekubo, K., Konishi, J., Endo, K., Nakajima, K., Mori, T., Nagata, I., Torizuka, K.,: Anti-thyroxine and anti-triiodothyronine antibodies in three cases of Hashimoto's thyroiditis. *Acta Endocrinol. (Copenh.),* 89(3):557-566, 1978.

34. Sakata, S., Nakamura, S., Miura, K.: Autoantibodies against thyroid hormones or iodothyronine. Implications in diagnosis, thyroid function, treatment, and pathogenesis. *Ann. Intern. Med.,* 103(4):579-589, 1985.

35. Staeheli, V., Vallotton, M.B., Burger, A.: Detection of human anti-thyroxine and anti-triiodothyronine antibodies in different thyroid conditions. *J Clin Endocrinol Metab.,* 41(4):669-675, 1975.

36. Ginsberg, J., Segal, D., Erlich, R.M., Walfish, P.G.: Inappropriate triiodothyronine (T3) and thyroxine (T4) radioimmunoassay levels secondary to circulating thyroid hormone autoantibodies. *Clin. Endocrinol. (Oxf.),* 8(2):133-139, 1978.

37. Vyas, S.K., Wilkin, T.J.: Thyroid hormone autoantibodies and their implications for free thyroid hormone measurement. *J. Endocrinol. Invest.,* 17(1):15-21, 1994.

38. Lans, M.C., Spiertz, C., Brouwer, A., Koeman, J.H.: Different competition of thyroxine binding to transthyretin and thyroxine-binding globulin by hydroxy-PCBs, PCDDs and PCDFs. *Eur. J. Pharmacol.,* 270(2-3):129-136, 1994.

39. Visser, T.J., Kaptein, E., van Toor, H., van Raaij, J.A., van der Berg, K.J., Joe, C.T., van Engelen, J.G., Brouwer, A.: Glucuronidation of thyroid hormone in rat liver: effects of in vivo treatment with microsomal enzyme inducers and in vitro assay conditions. *Endocrinology,* 133(5):2177-2186, 1993.

CPSIA information can be obtained at www.ICGtesting.com
Printed in the USA
BVOW080036250512

291051BV00003B/34/P

9 780957 099302